Lymphoreticular Disease

An introduction for the pathologist and oncologist

Edited by I. Carr and B.W. Hancock

Second edition

Blackwell Scientific Publications
Oxford London Edinburgh
Boston Palo Alto Melbourne

Lymphoreticular
Disease

© 1977, 1984 by
Blackwell Scientific Publications
Editorial offices:
Osney Mead, Oxford OX2 0EL
8 John Street, London WC1N 2ES
9 Forrest Road, Edinburgh EH1 2QH
52 Beacon Street, Boston
  Massachusetts 02108, USA
706 Cowper Street, Palo Alto
  California 94301, USA
99 Barry Street, Carlton
  Victoria 3053, Australia

First published 1977
Second edition 1984

Printed in Great Britain
at the Alden Press, Oxford
and bound by
R. J. Acford, Chichester

DISTRIBUTORS

USA
  Blackwell Mosby Book Distributors
  11830 Westline Industrial Drive
  St Louis, Missouri 63141

Canada
  Blackwell Mosby Book Distributors
  120 Melford Drive, Scarborough
  Ontario, M1B 2X4

Australia
  Blackwell Scientific Book Distributors
  31 Advantage Road, Highett
  Victoria 3190

British Library
Cataloguing in Publication Data

Lymphoreticular disease.—2nd ed.
  1. Reticulo-endothelial system—Diseases
  I. Carr, Ian, 19 -   II. Hancock, Barry W.
  616.4′2   RC645.5

  ISBN 0-632-00779-6

In memory of
Professor W.A.J. Crane
of the University of Sheffield
in appreciation

Contributors

Ian Carr MD, PhD, FRCPath, FRCPC
Professor of Pathology, University of Manitoba
and St Boniface Hospital, Winnipeg
Formerly Senior Lecturer in Pathology, University of Sheffield
and Honorary Consultant Pathologist
Weston Park Hospital, Sheffield

Barry W. Hancock MD, DCH, MRCP
Senior Lecturer in Medicine, University of Sheffield
Honorary Consultant Physician, Royal Hallamshire and
Weston Park Hospitals, Sheffield

Laurence Henry MD, FRCP, FRCPath
Professor of Pathology, University of Sheffield
Honorary Consultant Pathologist
Royal Hallamshire Hospital, Sheffield

A. Milford Ward MA, MB, FRCPath
Senior Lecturer in Immunology, University of Sheffield
Honorary Consultant Immunologist
Sheffield Area Health Authority (Teaching)
Director, Supraregional Protein Reference Unit

L.F. Skinnider MB, FRCPC
Professor of Pathology, University of Saskatchewan, Saskatoon

W.R. Timperley MA, DM, FRCPath
Consultant Neuropathologist, Royal Hallamshire Hospital
Honorary Clinical Lecturer, University of Sheffield

Illustrator

A. Sylvester FIMLS
Senior Chief Technician, Department of Pathology
Weston Park Hospital, Sheffield

Contents

Preface to the First Edition

This book gives a brief account of diseases of the lymphoreticular system as seen mainly in a cancer hospital in a British provincial city by two histopathologists, a physician and an immunologist. It is intended for the histopathologist, the physician and the oncologist in training—as an introduction. This is a field where it is of particular importance that the clinician be aware of the variations in histological structure in the lesions he deals with; I hope that the histopathological chapters are intelligible to the clinician. Conversely the histopathologist must be aware of the potentially dangerous therapy to which a histopathological diagnosis admits (or condemns) a patient.

The manner of presentation of the material in many of the chapters relates to the manner of presentation of the primary problem—what is the histological structure of this adenopathy? While an account of immunological correlations is clearly necessary it is not intended to give a description of clinical immunology. Diseases which are properly the province of the haematologist, and tropical disorders, have not been considered so that the field is essentially that which is diagnosed by biopsy of the lymphoreticular system in a temperate climate.

I have attempted to edit individually written chapters to form a cohesive whole.

We are grateful to many colleagues for their criticisms, and in particular to Professor J. Richmond and Dr G.M. King for help with the clinical section, and Dr T. Powell for X-rays, to Dr A.J. Coup, Dr A. Kennedy, Professor C.W. Potter, Mr P. Price, Dr W. Timperley, Dr A. Tait Smith, Dr J.C.E. Underwood and Professor D.H. Wright for material, to Drs K. Henry, M. Bennett and G. Farrer-Brown for a substantial illustrated contribution to chapter 5, to Mr P. Norris and Mrs J. Rhodes for electron microscopic and photographic help, to the technical staff of the Department of Pathology, Weston Park Hospital and the secretarial staff of the Departments of Pathology and Medicine, University and Weston Park Hospital. The errors are our own.

Ian Carr

Preface to the Second Edition

The second edition has been updated where necessary. It is intended as an introduction and not a reference book. Two new authors have contributed chapters suggested by reviewers of the first edition; the resultant text, for geographic reasons, has not been edited into a whole but is a group of separate chapters.

Ian Carr
Barry Hancock

Lymphoreticular Disease

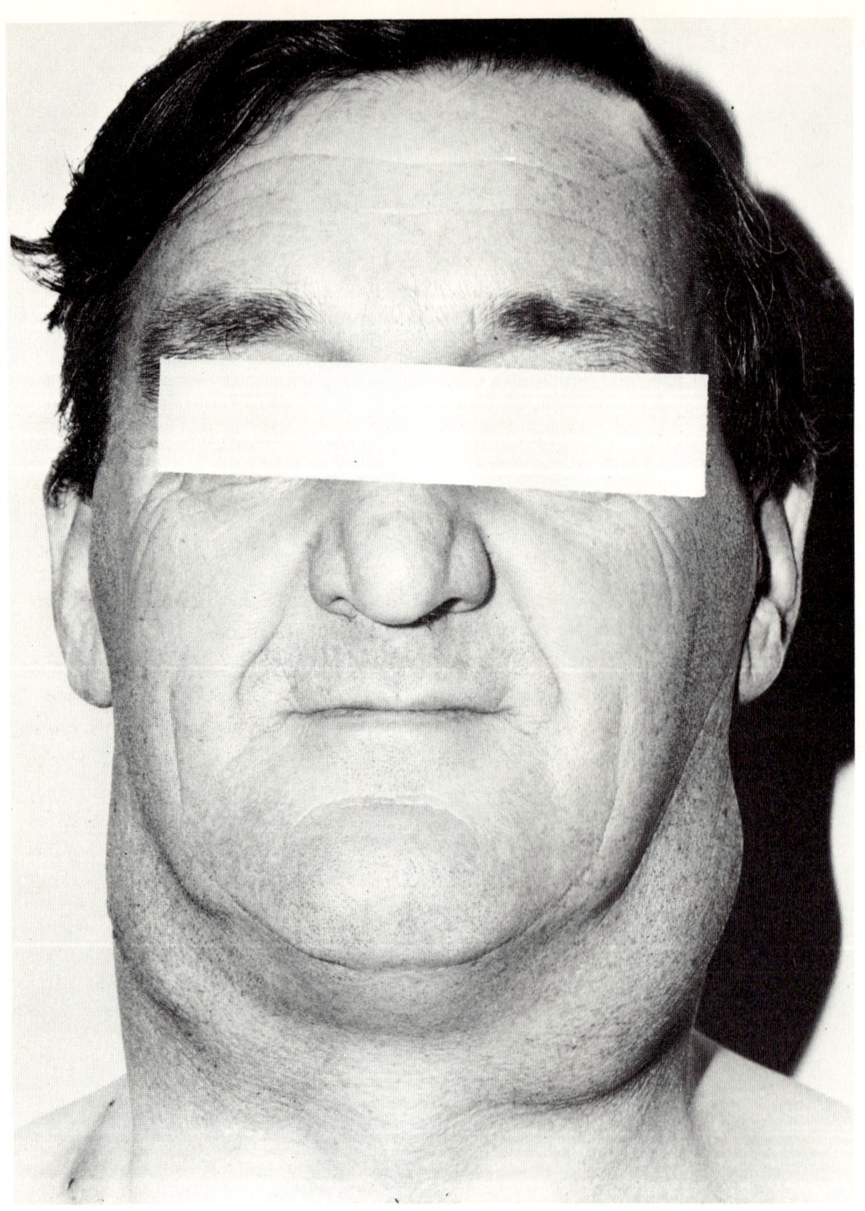

Frontispiece. A patient with Hodgkin's disease involving cervical lymph nodes.

Chapter 1

Introduction: The lymphoreticular tissues and their diseases

The lymphoreticular tissues comprise the lymph nodes, the spleen, the thymus, the gut-associated lymphoid tissues, the bone marrow in its non-haemopoietic function, and scattered macrophages and lymphocytes elsewhere. Two main families of cells are involved, the macrophages (the mononuclear phagocyte system) and the lymphocytes and their derivatives (the lymphoid system). These cells lie in a complex fibro-vascular stroma containing some other cell types not all fully identified. Together these two systems, macrophage and lymphocyte make up the lymphoreticular system. The term reticuloendothelial system is so imprecise as to be of little scientific value, and has been formally abolished at two major gatherings of experts in the field. (Other experts, however, still hold congresses in its name and honour.) A rose by any other name will smell as sweet. In this introductory chapter a brief account of the component cells of this tissue will be given, followed by an account of the manner in which they migrate and react.

THE CELLS OF LYMPHORETICULAR TISSUES

Lymphoreticular organs consist, like others, of a connective tissue framework, in which some cells reside and through which others migrate, some in an ordered pattern of actual circulation. There is a blood vascular and lymph vascular system running through them, through which these fluids circulate. Unlike other organs it is not always possible to be certain whether individual cells or cell groups are moving or static. The following cells are found in lymphoreticular organs—lymphocytes, plasma cells, macrophages, endo-thelial cells, fibroblasts, other vascular cells and nerves, and dendritic cells.

THE LYMPHOCYTE

Lymphocytes range in size from 6 μm to 12 μm and can conveniently be described as small and large (Figs 1.1 and 1.2). The term large lymphocyte is in the main synonymous with lymphoblast. The small lymphocyte has a nucleus which stains heavily in standard light and electron microscopic preparations due to the density of the chromatin. The scanty cytoplasm contains a few small mitochondria, a centriole, and some ribosomes; there are few cytomembranes. There may be a few small cytoplasmic processes, but the outline of the cell is usually relatively smooth. When moving on a flat surface, such as a glass slide, the lymphocyte characteristically shows a projecting handle-like process trailing behind it. The lymphocyte is freely motile in tissue culture.

The large lymphocyte or lymphoblast has a nucleus with less dense chromatin in an open meshwork. There is much more cytoplasm than in the small lymphocyte; this has a basophilic staining reaction at the light microscopic level. At the ultrastructural level this is accounted for by the presence of numerous polyribosomes. When cell division is stimulated in lymphoid tissue as in an immune reaction, both thymidine uptake and mitosis are seen in large lymphocytes. In descriptions of the changes occurring in tissues during immune responses a separate cell type is described by several authors as the 'immunocyte' or 'immunoblast'. This term refers to the functional properties of differentiating forms of one type of lymphocyte.

Thymic (T) lymphocytes derive originally from the bone marrow but immediately from the thymus. Their life span may be fairly long (months or years). Many lymphocytes recirculate round the body, leaving the blood stream through the postcapillary venules to enter peripheral lymphoid organs and draining with the lymph back into the venous circulation. The major part of the recirculating pool is composed of T-lymphocytes. T-lymphocytes are found in the deep cortical and interfollicular areas in lymph nodes, in the periarteriolar regions of the spleen and in the perifollicular areas in Peyer's patches. T-lymphocytes enlarge and divide *in vitro* when treated with phyto-haemagglutinin (PHA). T-lymphocytes are responsible for cell mediated immunity and co-operate with B-lymphocytes in the humoral immune response to some

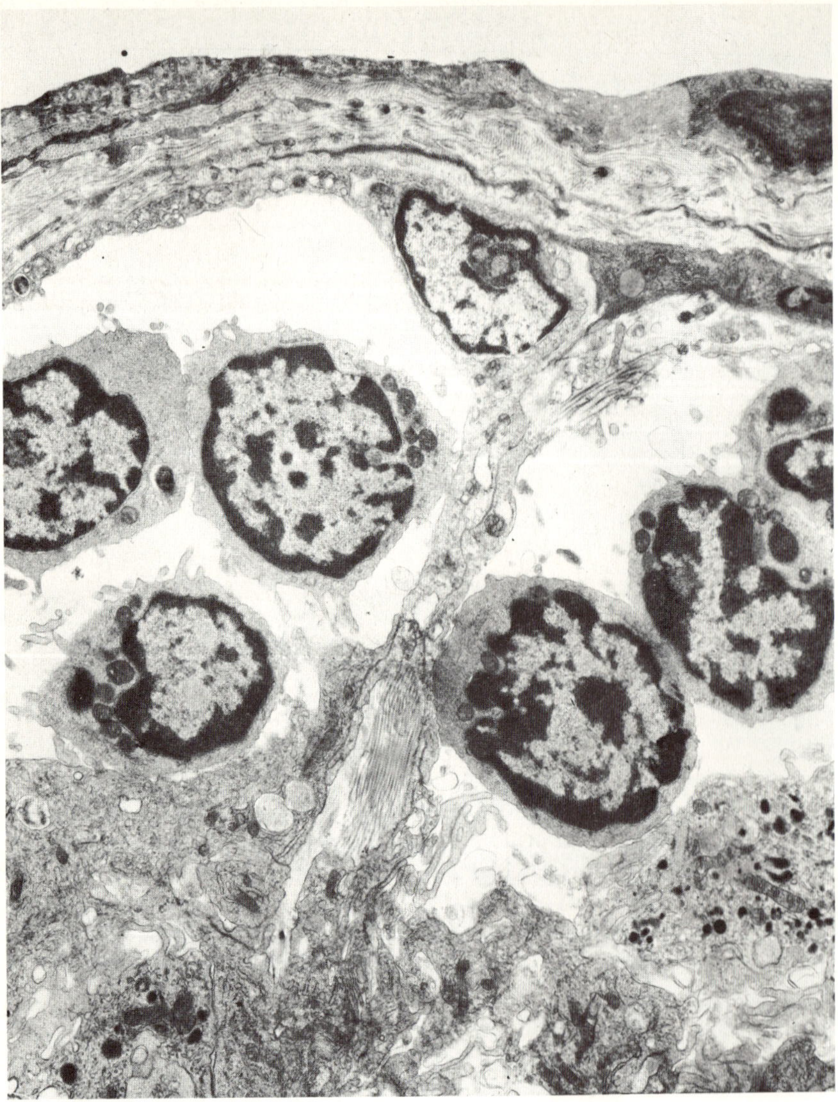

antibodies, though they are not responsible for the actual synthesis of antibody. T-lymphocytes are involved in the phenomenon of immunological memory. T-lymphocytes carry less surface immunoglobulin than B cells, but form rosettes when incubated *in vitro* with sheep red blood cells (Fig. 1.3).

Subclasses of T-lymphocytes have different functions. Thus helper T cells improve the efficiency with which B-lymphocytes produce antibodies. Cytotoxic T cells recognize and destroy host cells displaying foreign antigens. Suppressor T cells limit the extent to which the host mounts either a cell-mediated or a humoral response.

Bursa-dependent or B-lymphocytes derive ultimately from the marrow. In birds they derive immediately from the Bursa of Fabricius, a hind gut diverticulum. In mammals, including man, their origin is less clear; although intestinal lymphoreticular tissue may be the site of development of some B-lymphocytes, the majority develop and mature within the bone marrow. B cells have a shorter life—days or weeks—rather than months and are a less important component of the

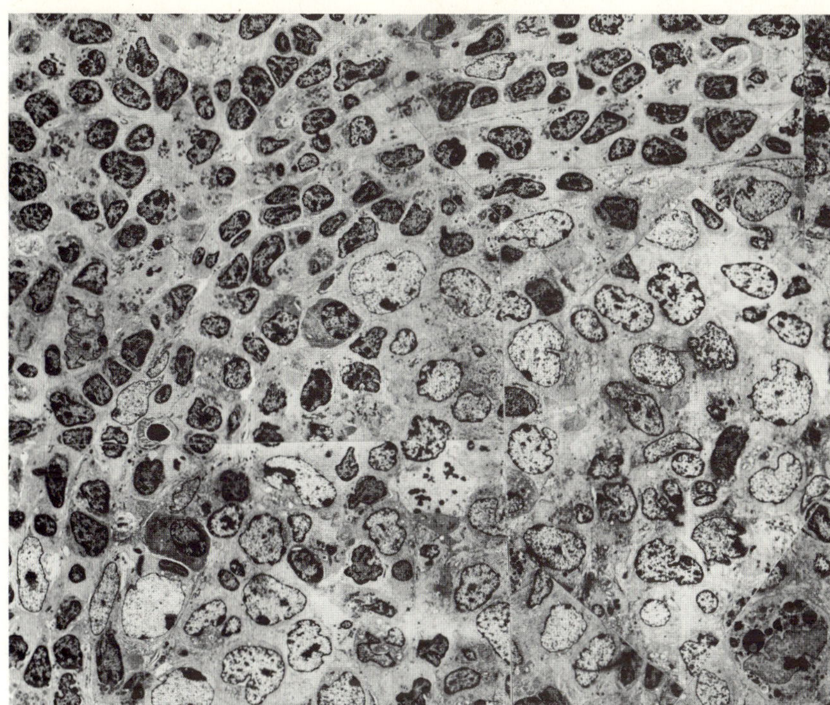

Fig. 1.2. Montage of germinal centre from normal human lymph node. Around the edge of the centre is a rim of small lymphocytes. In the centre are small and large lymphocytes of various sizes. One cell is in mitosis. A large macrophage ('tingible body macrophage') contains fragments of degenerating lymphocytes. Between all of these cells and around the edge of the follicles run the fine processes of the dendritic cells. × 1,200.

recirculating pool. B-lymphocytes are found in the subcapsular and medullary areas of lymph nodes and in the germinal centres, in the peripheral white pulp and red pulp of the spleen, and in the central follicles of Peyer's patches. B-lymphocytes do not respond to PHA, and are not an important component of cell-mediated immunity; they inter-

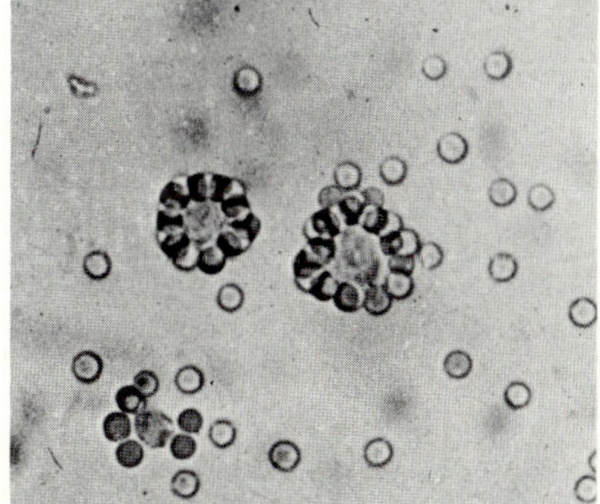

Fig. 1.3. T cell rosetting. Phase contrast micrograph of sheep red blood cells forming a rosette around two T-lymphocytes.

act with T-lymphocytes in the induction of many humoral immune responses—though other responses are T cell independent. B-lymphocytes carry a prominent and easily recognizable surface immunoglobulin component (of the order of 10^5 molecules per cell), and mature into plasma cells, producing immunoglobulin at various stages during maturation. B-lymphocytes also carry surface receptors for complement enabling them to bind antigen–antibody complexes. Some of the characteristics of T- and B-lymphocytes are indicated in Table 1.1. It is difficult to identify a characteristic morphologic difference between T- and B-lymphocytes. By transmission EM both T- and B-lymphocytes show a wide range of appearances depending on their stage of maturation. Some lymphocytes bear no evidence of T or B cell markers—so-called null cells.*

Lymphocytes produce a wide range of biologically active soluble factors during the cellular immune response. These materials are produced as a response to the presence of transplantation antigens on the surface of cells, neoantigens on tumour cells, viral antigens and microbial or soluble antigens presented on the surface of macrophages. These

* See Henry and Goldman (1975); Ford (1978); Owen (1978); Weissman *et al.* (1978) for reviews of aspects of lymphocyte biology.

	T	B
Origin (ultimate)	Marrow	Marrow?
(proximate)	Thymus	
Recirculation	Important	Less important
Longevity	More are long-lived	Fewer are long-lived
Site		
Lymph node	Interfollicular	Subcapsular
		Medullary
		Germinal centres
Spleen	Periarteriolar	Peripheral white pulp
		Red pulp
Peyer's patch	Perifollicular	Follicular
Response to mitogens		
PHA	Marked	Less marked
Pokeweed	Less marked	Marked
Function		
Cell mediated immunity	Important	Trivial involvement
Humoral immunity		
Induction	Important	Important
Antibody synthesis	Uninvolved	Important
Memory	Important	Important
Surface characteristics	Less prominent surface Ig	Prominent surface Ig

substances in general are known as lymphokines or mediators of delayed hypersensitivity; by altering the function of other cells they provide a mechanism of amplifying the effects of the reaction of antigen with a very few sensitized lymphocytes into a well marked mononuclear cell response.

The cells involved in production of soluble mediators are T-lymphocytes and the substances are small molecular weight (MW 20–50,000) proteins or glycoproteins. The factors include migration inhibition factor which inhibits macrophage movement; factors which activate macrophages and cause chemotaxis; non-specific factors toxic to cells; interferon which inhibits viral growth; a factor which stimulates osteoclasts, and transfer factor which transfers cell-mediated immunity.

THE PLASMA CELL AND IMMUNOGLOBULIN PRODUCTION

The mature plasma cell is characterized by a nucleus with prominent peripheral speckles of chromatin, and cytoplasm with a marked affinity for basic dyes due to the presence of very well developed granular endoplasmic reticulum (Fig. 1.4). Immunoglobulin is demonstrable within the cisterns of the endoplasmic reticulum, using as a specific stain antibody labelled with fluorescein on peroxidase. Antibody production occurs in lymphoblasts and is most active in young plasma cells (plasmablasts). The older larger plasma cells often contain crystalline aggregates of immunoglobulin within the endoplasmic reticulum. These may be stainable and visible with light microscopy as eosinophilic masses (Russell bodies).

Immunoglobulins

The biological product of the plasma cell is the immunoglobulin molecule or antibody protein. In man five main structural types or classes are recognized—IgG, IgA, IgM, IgD and IgE. Further division into subclasses is also recognized. Each class and subclass has distinct physico-chemical and functional characteristics. Each immunoglobulin molecule consists of a basic four polypeptide chain structure interlinked by disulphide bonds. The basic unit consisting of a pair of 'heavy chains' antigenically distinct for each class and subclass, and a pair of 'light chains'. The light chains are of two antigenic types which are common to all immunoglobulin classes. This structure holds for all immunoglobulin classes except for IgM which appears as a pentameric molecule made up of five basic units linked by an additional polypeptide chain, and for IgA in external secretions (SIgA) which is present as a dimeric molecule composed of two basic units linked by an additional polypeptide chain and associated with a secretory component which is synthesized by epithelial cells.

Experimental studies on the IgG molecule show that it can be cleaved by the action of papain into three fragments. Two of these are identical and will combine with antigen to form soluble complexes. These univalent antibody fragments are termed Fab. The third fragment does not react with antigen and is termed the Fc fragment. Further analysis of the Fab fragment shows that it consists of a single light chain and a portion of the heavy chain termed the Fd fragment. Pepsin cleaves the IgG molecule into a larger divalent antigen binding fraction, $F(ab')_2$, and subunits of the Fc fragment.

Electron microscopy of purified IgG molecules visualized

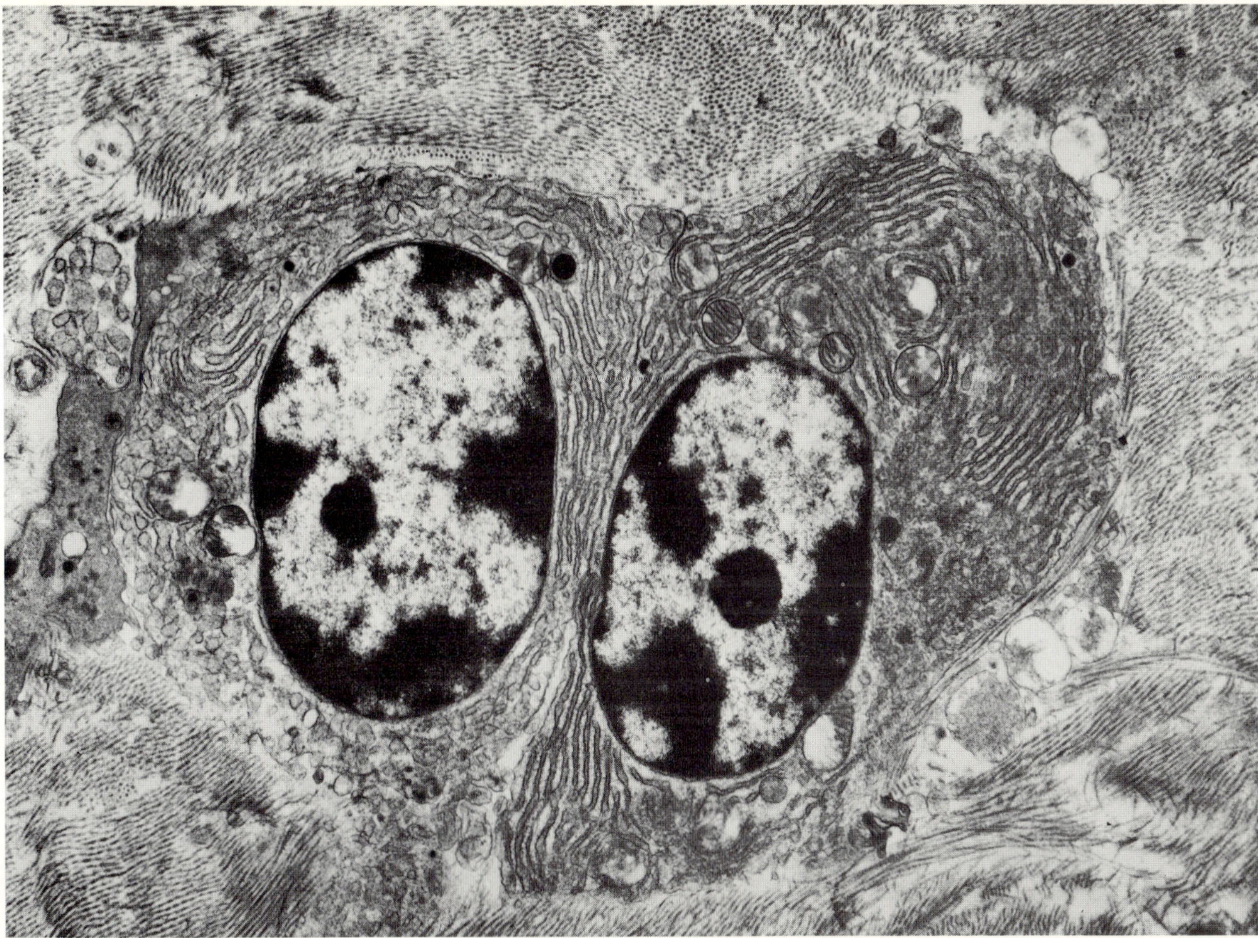

Fig. 1.4. Two human plasma cells lying in dense collagenous connective tissue. × 3,800.

by negative staining techniques show the molecule to have a Y-shape, the limbs of the Y being able to swing outwards on combining with antigen around a 'hinge' region.

Immunoglobulin class characteristics

The physicochemical characteristics and functional aspects of the immunoglobulin classes are shown in Tables 1.2 and 1.3. The immunoglobulins and their functional properties have been extensively reviewed by Hong (1972).

THE MACROPHAGE

Macrophages are medium to large sized cells (12–30 μm) in diameter characterized by avid phagocytic ability and usually high content of lysosomal enzymes (see Carr and Daems 1980 for reviews). They have irregular surfaces due to the presence of cytoplasmic processes, usually flap-like, a moderate content of mitochondria and prominent granular endoplasmic reticulum (Figs 1.5 and 1.6). Mature macrophages often carry on their surfaces a receptor which specifically recognizes certain classes of immunoglobulin, the Fc receptor. They contain numerous lysosomal dense bodies, some small and homogeneous in structure, probably primary lysosomes composed of newly formed lysosomal enzymes, and others larger and more heterogeneous containing ingested foreign material, red cell debris, lipid etc. The lysosomes contain a wide variety of hydrolytic enzymes capable of breaking down proteins to the level of small peptides or aminoacids. Characteristically the

Table 1.2 Physicochemical characteristics of the immunoglobulin classes

WHO nomenclature	IgG	IgA	IgM	IgD	IgE
Subclasses	1–4	1, 2	1, 2	—	—
Sedimentation coefficient	7S	7–11S	19S	7S	8S
Molecular weight	150,000	160,000 +polymers	900,000	185,000	200,000
Heavy chain antigen	γ	α	μ		E
Light chain antigen	κ and λ	κ and λ	κ and λ	κ and λ	κ and λ
Antigen valency	2	2 +polymers	5(10)	2	2
Serum half-life	24 days	6 days	5 days	3 days	2 days
Concentration in normal adult serum	6–16 g/l; 70–150 U/ml	1.2–4.2 g/l; 70–150 U/ml	0.5–1.7 g/l; 65–200 U/ml	3–300 mg/l	*; 0–400 U/ml

* The international Unit of IgE is *approximately* equal to 2.4 ng, but by convention mass concentration terms are not used for this immunoglobulin class.

Table 1.3 Biological characteristics of the immunoglobulin classes

	Placental transfer	Complement fixation	Fix to lymphocytes	Fix to macrophages	Fix to mast cells
IgG					
1	++	+++	−	+++	−
2	±	+	−	+	−
3	++	+++	−	+++	−
4	++	±	++	±	−
IgA					
1	−	polymer only	−	−	−
2	−		−	−	−
IgM					
1	−	+++	−	+++	−
2	−	−	+++	−	−
IgD	−	?	?	?	−
IgE	−	−	−	−	+

surface of the macrophage to interact there with the lymphocyte. Under circumstances where an excessive pool of antigen is present in the body, it may be mopped up by macrophages preventing the development of immunological tolerance. Macrophages have a role in lipid metabolism, phagocytosing particulate lipid and being able to esterify and solubilize such lipids as cholesterol. They are responsible for phagocytosis of effete erythrocytes and for storing the iron derived therefrom. Lastly they have considerable secretory properties being able to produce notably pyrogen, interferon, lysozyme, and the third component of complement. Macrophages in inflammatory lesions and in many other sites derive from blood monocytes and ultimately from a rapidly dividing marrow precursor justifying the use of the term mononuclear phagocyte system. Local division in many sites takes place and macrophages long resident in peripheral sites acquire distinctive cytochemical characteristics. The word 'histiocyte' means, in a strict sense, a tissue macrophage. It is loosely used to mean a large cell in lymphoreticular tissue, often of B-lymphocyte origin.

A granuloma is a focal aggregate of macrophages and lymphocytes often with areas of central necrosis. The macrophages derive in the main from circulating monocytes which are immobilized in the site by factors produced by the interaction of sensitized lymphocytes with antigen. The mature macrophages divide and also coalesce with recently emigrated monocytes to form giant cells or macrophage polykaryons of variable, usually low, phagocytic activity. Some macrophages enlarge, come to contain numerous large moderately electron-lucent vacuoles and are then known as epithelioid cells. These cells are probably not highly phagocytic and may well be secretory in nature. It is likely that they as well as other macrophages secrete lysosomal enzymes and other biologically active substances into the surrounding tissue.

DENDRITIC CELLS

It has been evident for many years that cells are present in lymphoreticular tissues which do not fit the above categories. These have often been called 'reticular' or 'reticulum' cells, terms no longer useful. Recent studies (reviewed by Tew *et al.* 1982) have established that many of these cells are poorly phagocytic, or not phagocytic, have long processes extending in several directions and have irregular nuclei. They have been grouped as 'dendritic' cells, and fall into several subclasses, not yet perfectly defined. Follicular dendritic cells

cytoplasm contains numerous 6 nm microfilaments probably representing actin.

Macrophages are responsible for the phagocytosis of bacteria and viruses, and are involved in chronic granulomata. They take up antigen but their precise role in the immune response is not clear. They are necessary in the immune response to some large particulate antigens to break up the antigenic material to a form which can be dealt with by the lymphocyte. Alternatively, antigen may be retained on the

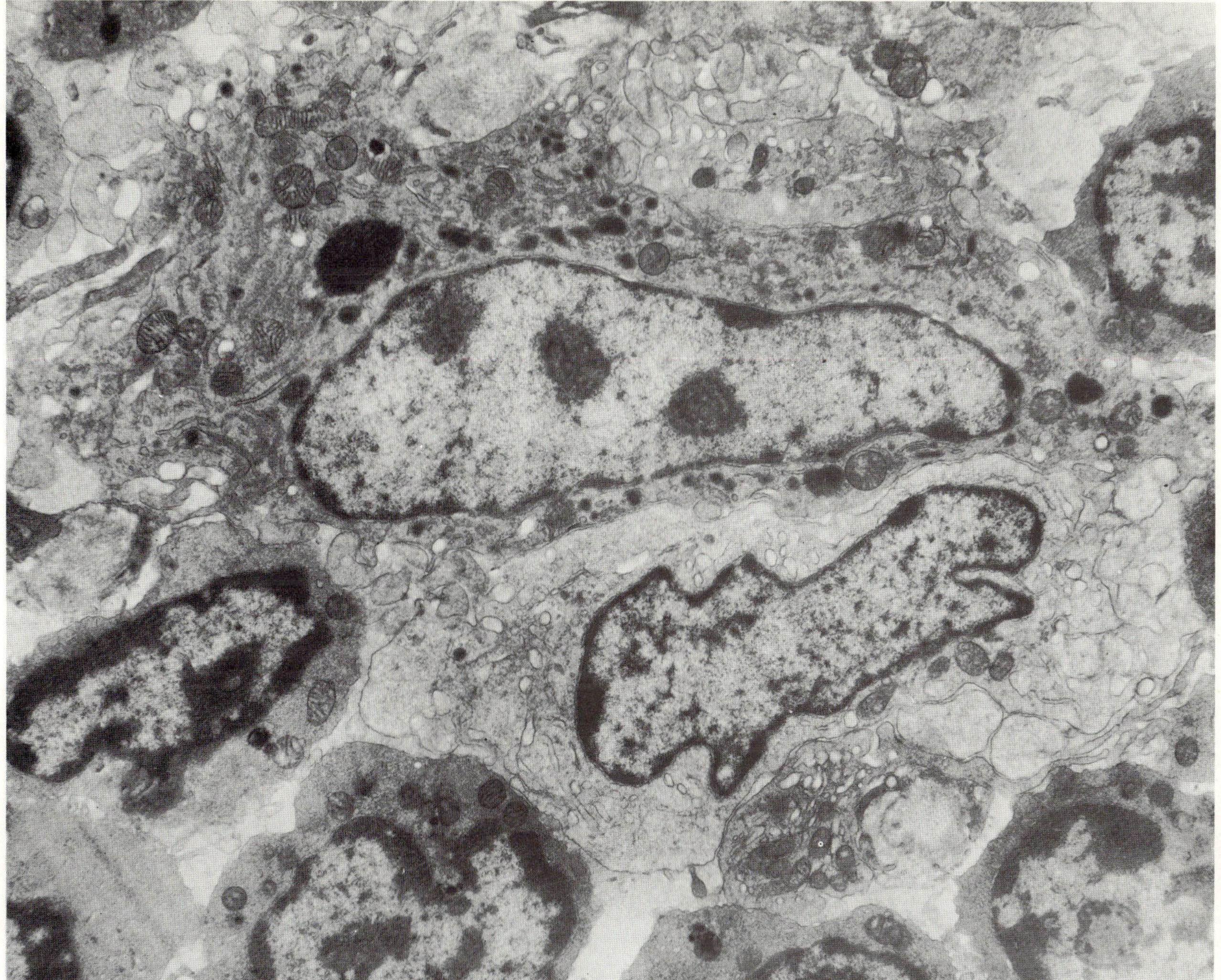

Fig. 1.5. Electron micrograph of human lymph node showing a macrophage with many primary and secondary lysosomes and numerous cytoplasmic membranous profiles and an adjacent histio-cytic cell—a large cell with voluminous cytoplasm and few or no lysosomes. × 8,200.

are identified by EM in sections of lymphoid follicles and are able to trap and retain antigen–antibody complexes on their surfaces. Lymphoid dendritic cells were identified in cell suspensions of lymphoid tissues, are rich in Ia antigen but lack Fc and C_3 receptors and are potent stimulators of certain immunologically related cellular reactions, e.g. the mixed leucocyte reaction. Interdigitating dendritic cells are found by electron microscopy in T-dependent areas of lymphoid tissues, interlock with adjacent lymphocytes, and may be important in their maturation. Langerhans cells may be very similar to interdigitating dendritic cells; they are identified in skin by general morphology rather similar to that of a macrophage. Their characteristic feature is the presence of a granule, the Birbeck granule about 42 nm in external diameter with a core 11 nm in diameter with a repeating density.

THE HISTOLOGICAL STRUCTURE OF LYMPHORETICULAR ORGANS

The structure of normal lymphoreticular organs is well described by Weiss (1977). The present section is a summary

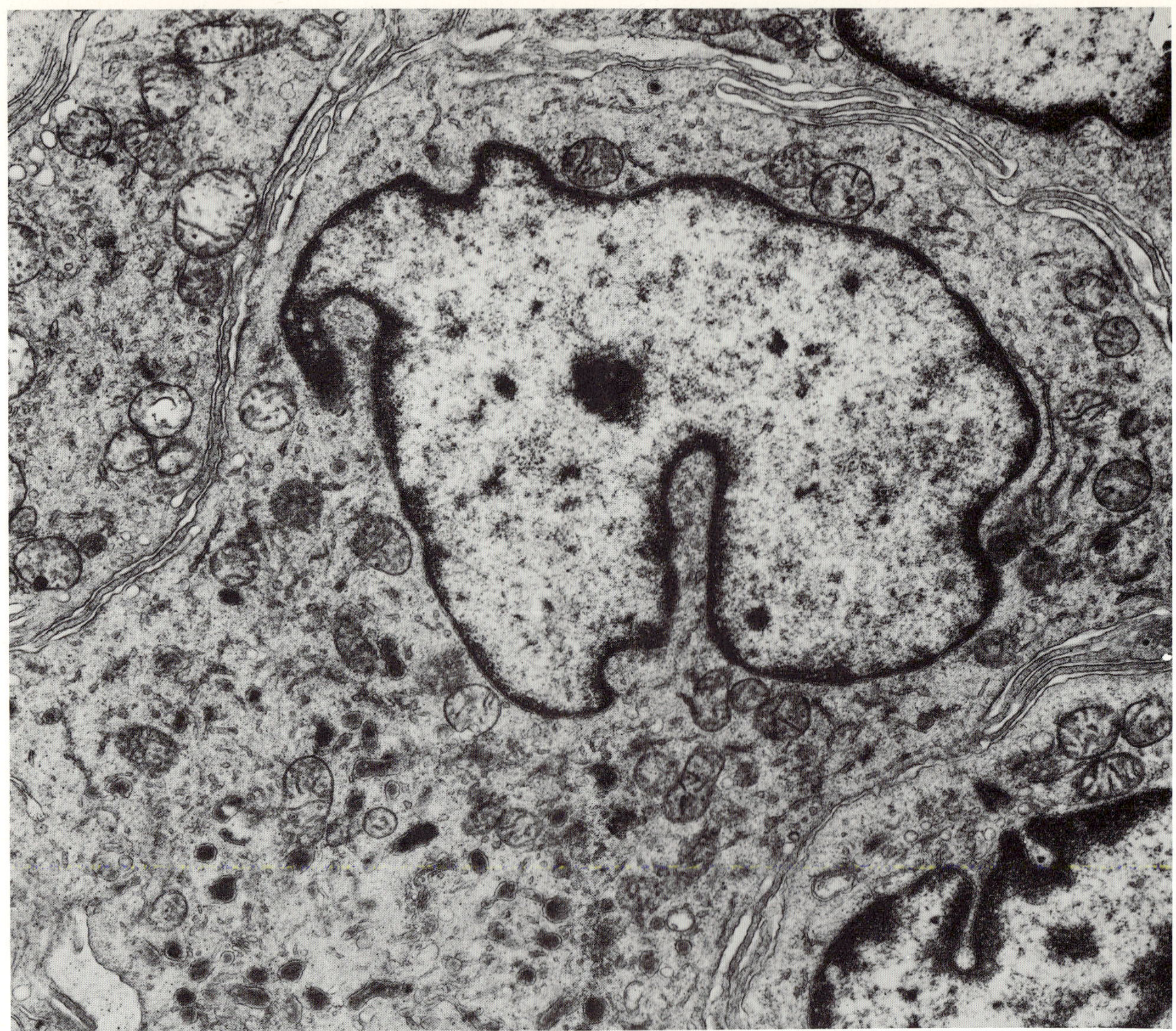

Fig. 1.6. Electron micrograph of macrophage from sarcoid granuloma showing numerous lysosomes, interdigitating cytoplasmic processes and areas of adhesion. × 14,000.

of the facets of normal structure necessary for the appreciation of the histopathology of these organs.

LYMPH NODES

The structure of normal lymph nodes varies with site and age. A normal cervical lymph node from a young adult is bean shaped and measures 1–2 cm in maximum diameter. The capsule is composed of two or three layers of fibroblasts and the collagen which they lay down. Below the capsule lies a subcapsular sinus lined peripherally by endothelial cells, and elsewhere by macrophages with gaps between them (see Fig. 1.1). Across the sinusoid run strands of collagen, covered by the cytoplasm of endothelial cells. The macrophages lining the inner layer of the sinusoid lie on a layer of collagen in which are a few fibroblasts. The subcapsular sinus is continuous with radial sinusoids and these with anastomosing medullary sinusoids which in their turn join to form the efferent ducts of the node. The structure of the wall of all of the sinusoids is similar. Macrophages form a particularly prominent part of the wall of the medullary sinusoids.

The parenchyma of the lymph node outside the sinusoids is built on a framework of elongated fibroblasts with numerous long spidery processes each lying upon and surrounding a trabecula of collagen. This is often described as the reticulin framework of the node. In between there are packed lymphocytes and other lymphoreticular cells in varying proportions; the areas of the parenchyma are conveniently divided as follows (Cottier *et al.* 1973):

1 *The outer cortex*
2 *The germinal centres and lymphocytic follicles*
3 *The inner cortex or paracortex*
4 *The medullary cords*

1 *The outer cortex* is composed of undifferentiated areas which contain predominantly small lymphocytes with a few plasma cells.

2 *The germinal centres and lymphocytic follicles:* The germinal centre is spherical and surrounded by small lymphocytes. It is composed of large lymphocytes and blast cells. Sometimes a lighter staining superficial zone is less densely packed and may show a few plasma cells while in a darker staining deep zone, mitosis is very evident. The background framework contains dendritic cells and conventional macrophages often with prominent ingested dead cells (the tingible body macrophages of Flemming; see Fig. 1.2). Germinal centres vary in structure showing cyclical activity. After stimulation of the node mitosis may be very prominent. Later mitosis is less prominent but there may be numerous macrophages containing cell debris. Sometimes the centre may be largely replaced by epithelioid macrophages. Lastly a centre may have a very dense thick peripheral cuff of lymphocytes but show little central activity. Dense aggregates of small lymphocytes, so-called primary lymphoid follicles, may represent an extremely inactive form of germinal centre. Germinal centres have a 'light' and a 'dark' zone classified on the staining qualities of the cells and the light zone has a peripheral 'cap' of darkly staining lymphocytes. This 'cap' points to the direction from which the lymph flows, and thus by implication, the antigenic stimulus, is coming. The pattern is reversed in the pig lymph node where the lymph flows from the hilum outwards, and the 'medulla' is at the periphery of the node. It is thought though by no means proved that B-lymphocytes migrate into the follicle, enlarge and develop irregularly shaped nuclei, divide and ultimately leave the follicle as immature plasma cells.

3 *The inner cortex or paracortex.* The deeper part of the cortex is composed of rather more loosely arranged lymphoid tissue; most of the lymphocytes in this area are thymus derived at least in experimental animals and there is a moderate number of macrophages. When scanty these produce a 'starry sky' effect and when plentiful nodular aggregates. These nodular aggregates do not contain plasma cells and are found in reactive lesions and notably in dermatopathic lymphadenitis. They are commoner in superficial glands. High-walled postcapillary venules are found in this area; the apparent thickness of the wall is due to emigrating T-lymphocytes. During a cell-mediated immune response this area becomes oedematous due to blockage of the sinusoids; numerous lymphocytes migrate through the wall of the postcapillary venules into the paracortex and there proliferate.

4 *The medullary cords* are the areas of lymphoid tissue which lie between the medullary sinusoids. They are packed with plasma cells during an immune response.

The variations in structure of lymph nodes which occur during lymph node reactions will be treated in detail in Chapter 3. Basically the following things may happen:

1 A stimulation of germinal centre activity
2 Plasma cell proliferation and maturation
3 Maturation and enlargement and division of sinus and interstitial macrophages
4 Increased cell traffic through the node:
   (*a*) as increased passage of monocytes and lymphocytes in the afferent lymph
   (*b*) as increased migration and maturation of T-lymphocytes
   (*c*) as a banal acute inflammatory reaction
   (*d*) as increased monocyte immigration, macrophage maturation and formation of granulomata, often with epithelioid cells.

Variations occur in normal lymph node structure under physiological circumstances: nodes vary with site, age and with antigenic stimulation.

Substantial variations occur in lymph node structure with site in the body. As compared to cervical nodes, nodes derived from sites draining the alimentary tract tend to have prominent sinusoids and active germinal centres. Nodes from the groin often show a considerable amount of fibrous tissue often arranged in trabeculae intersecting the node; germinal centres in this site may be few. DNA synthesis varies considerably with site. There is a considerable traffic of cells through even a normal lymph node in resting conditions.

Substantial variations also occur with age. The lymph node of the child, like all juvenile tissues contains little fibrous tissue. Immunological reactions occurring in juvenile lymphoid tissue are particularly vigorous and the degree of cellular pleomorphism present may be marked. With age there is a generalized atrophy of lymphoid tissues; the lymph nodes shrink in size; few germinal centres are present, or they may be quite absent. Nodes become infiltrated with adipose tissue and a variable degree of fine fibrosis occurs. This atrophy occurs more markedly in the cervical, axillary and inguinal nodes. In extreme old age lymph nodes may be very hard to find.

The tissue changes in lymph nodes in the immune response have been studied in pure form by injecting antigens into the feet of rodents and sheep and subsequently serially examining uptake of antigen in the popliteal node, cell proliferation in the node, output of cells from the node by cannulating the efferent lymphatic and production of immunoglobulins both in the node as detected by immunofluorescence and in the serum (reviewed by Mulligan 1974). The process may be summarized as follows. Antigen drains to the lymph node in the lymph, or possibly is carried there by macrophages. It is presumably retained in minute amounts on the surface of dendritic cells in the germinal centre. Adjacent B-lymphocytes are stimulated in a manner which is not clear, to mature, to proliferate and to make antibody. About a week after the primary stimulus, there will therefore be visible mitosis in germinal centres and proliferation of lymphocytes in and around the centres: pyroninophilic large lymphocytes become visible in and around the germinal centres and then in the medullary cords of lymphoid tissue. Similar cells are exported in the efferent lymph of the node and go off to colonize other parts of the lymphoreticular system; and about ten days after the primary stimulus detectable immunoglobulin appears in the blood. When the stimulus is repeated a similar but accelerated and exaggerated pattern of events occurs. Antigen retention in the germinal centres is well-marked, cell proliferation is very prominent and cell output by the node much greater. Many more mature plasma cells appear in the node, notably in the medullary cords and immunoglobulin produc-

tion is rapid and sustained, both in the popliteal node and in the other lymphoreticular organs which were colonized during the primary response and where, therefore, a similar pattern of events is occurring.

When the antigen used to stimulate the node is of the type which elicits a delayed hypersensitivity type of response—there is a massive migration of lymphoid cells through the postcapillary venules and the paracortical areas become stuffed with dividing large lymphoid cells which are then passed out in the efferent lymphatics in large numbers. In addition there is an increase in cellular traffic in the efferent lymphatics and sometimes, e.g. after BCG, but not always, many macrophages may appear in the node. The degree of congestion of the node may apparently be so intense as to close the postcapillary venules.

The histological differences between a lymph node undergoing a humoral immune reaction and a lymph node undergoing a cellular immune reaction may be summarized as follows: in the former germinal centres are prominent and contain many dividing immunoblasts; the medullary cords contain many plasma cells. In the latter the paracortical areas fill with newly arrived immunoblasts which proliferate and block the sinusoids but do not mature into plasma cells. Most natural immune responses contain both components and most lymph nodes are engaged most of the time in responding to one or several antigens.

Some, such as the popliteal node, will show little activity until an antigen enters its drainage area, others, for example, the mesenteric nodes, normally being exposed to a number of bacterial antigens from the gut show greater evidence of immunological activity even in the 'resting' state. Again, antigens encountered in the daily course of life are not purified and their portal of entry may vary. Even the same antigen given under different conditions may produce humoral or cellular immunity and therefore in the human, a rather mixed histological picture occurs. Many antigens affecting the human are bacterial or viral in nature and these will be self-replicating in the body. If they are not therefore, eliminated rapidly, the primary and secondary responses will merge as the organism continues to produce antigen over a period of time, with a consequent blurring of the morphologic changes. If the antigen is organismal in nature its presence in the node may elicit an inflammatory as well as an immunological reaction rendering the distinction between 'reactive hyperplasia' and 'lymphadenitis' less exact. It is worth noting that in practice a 'normal resting' human lymph node is rarely encountered.

The structure of the spleen (normal weight up to 250 g) may be best understood by reference to the pathway of blood through it. The branches of the splenic artery run in fibrous trabeculae which are continuous with the splenic capsule. Branches emerge from the trabeculae into masses of lympho-reticular tissue, the white pulp. Each mass of white pulp has an eccentric artery; some of its blood is distributed by capillary branches in the white pulp, or into the marginal sinusoids at the edge of the white pulp. Other small arteries run direct from the white pulp into the red pulp, and branch into small straight (penicilliary) arterioles with little smooth muscle in their walls, sometimes ending in capillaries with a sheath of macrophages. These open into venous sinusoids either directly or via the interstitial tissue of the red pulp and thence into trabecular veins.

The structure of these components of the spleen which are relevant to human histopathology will now be summarized;

The proportion of white pulp to red pulp is normally

Fig. 1.7. Sinusoid of spleen showing lymphocyte and red blood cells migrating between the lining endothelial cells of the splenic sinus. ×2,375.

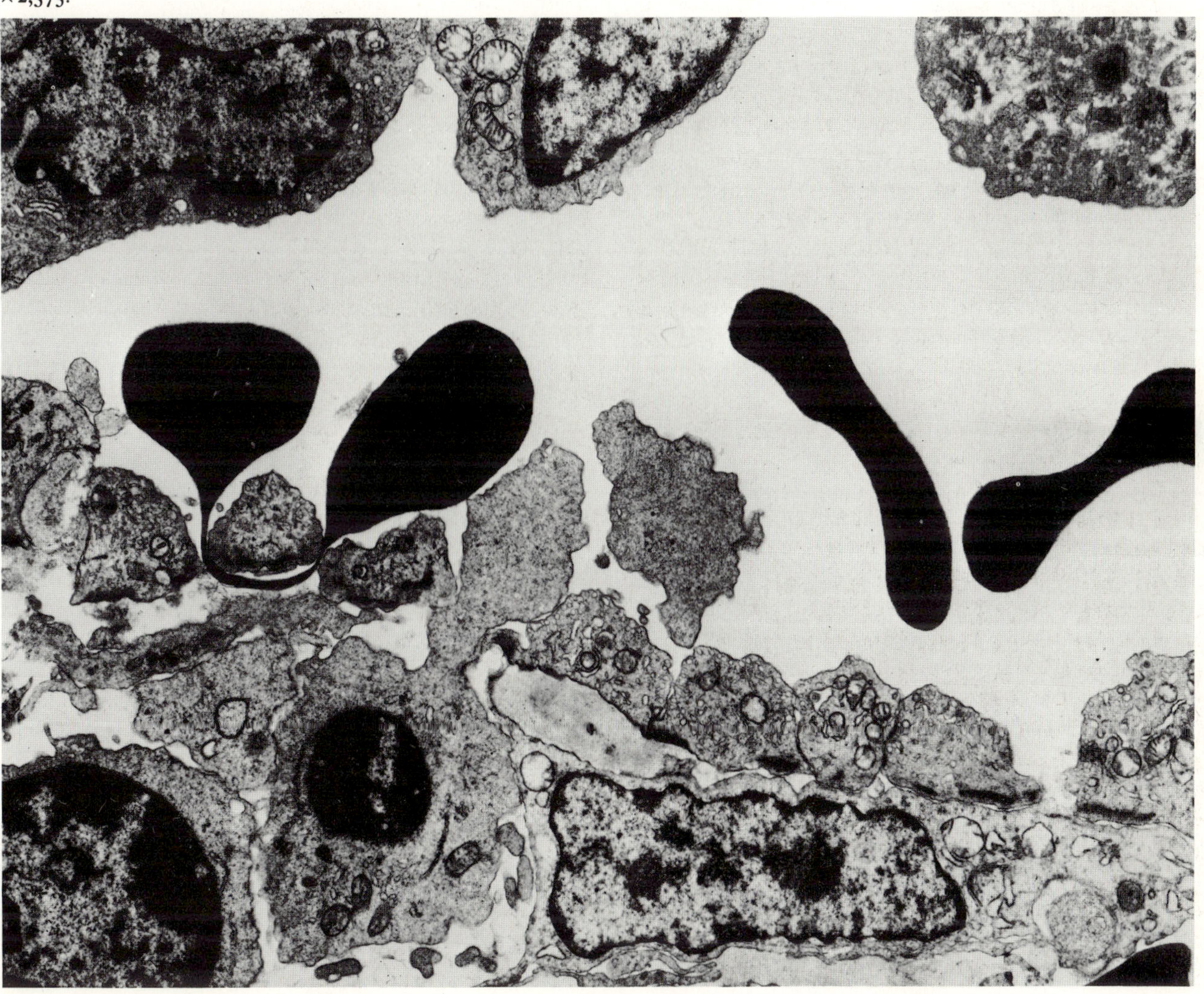

within the range 1:3 to 1:6. The white pulp is composed of lymphoreticular tissue densely packed with small lymphocytes. The area around the small arteries (the periarteriolar lymphocytic sheath) contains interdigitating cells; macrophages on which T cells home and within which they are thought to mature. Elsewhere in the white pulp lie germinal centres similar to those seen in lymph nodes and similarly containing antigen-retaining dendritic cells. Germinal centres in spleen often contain trabeculae of hyaline eosinophil largely collagenous material and may show similar changes to those described as occurring in lymph nodes.

The red pulp is composed of sinusoids lined by poorly phagocytic endothelial cells containing clusters of prominent microfilaments which suggest their (known) contractility. Red cells leak readily between these endothelial cells (Fig. 1.7). The interstitial area of the red pulp is composed of cords of irregularly arranged macrophages showing good evidence of phagocytosis of red and other cells. Lying among these are erythrocytes and leucocytes in transit. Normally scattered polymorphs in small clusters of not more than two or three are seen; eosinophils are present in the spleens of those who have died suddenly, though often absent when death is protracted. The normal spleen contains some iron as shown by the Prussian blue reaction.

After intravenous administration of antigens, the spleen shows morphological changes similar to those occurring in lymph nodes after local administration (reviewed by Mulligan 1974). Antigen is retained on dendritic cells in germinal centres, there is a proliferation of lymphoid cells which mature into plasma cells and migrate firstly to the edge of the red pulp and then into it. The spleen of an animal or human subject undergoing an active humoral immune response will therefore show much white pulp with many germinal centres and numerous plasma cells. Similarly if an active systemic delayed hypersensitivity response is going on, the spleen will show prominent white pulp with cellular proliferation outside germinal centres.

The major morphological change occurring with age is inactivity and then atrophy of white pulp. Germinal centres are infrequent over the age of 30 and white pulp often almost absent in old age.

OTHER ELEMENTS OF THE LYMPHORETICULAR SYSTEM

Other scattered lymphoreticular elements exist. A major fraction (perhaps 10%) of the population of macrophages exist in the liver as Kupffer cells. The hepatic sinusoid is formed of two types of cells, poorly phagocytic endothelial cells lying on a basement membrane and bound to one another by desmosomes, and flattened macrophages with long processes floating freely in the sinusoid and variably attached to the wall. The macrophages are highly phagocytic.

The bone marrow is a significant lymphoreticular organ. Blood percolates through a system of sinusoids lined by endothelial cells which though not true macrophages are moderately phagocytic, probably more so than those of spleen. When colloids are injected intravenously some is taken up immediately by the endothelial cells and more at a later period by the interstitial macrophages.

Localized aggregates of lymphoreticular cells are found scattered throughout the body; these generally are not sufficiently organized to possess specialized postcapillary venules. One site in which the macrophages require some comment because of their history rather than their peculiarities is the brain. Microglia are small cells with elongated deeply basophilic nuclei and scanty cytoplasm, found in both grey and white matter. Their cytoplasm has the characteristic ultrastructural appearance of a rather immature macrophage. They derive embryologically from circulating mononuclear cells and recruitment largely stops at or around birth. Similar cells are found around vascular sheaths and in the connective tissue membranes of the brain and are clearly identified as macrophages. In an inflammatory lesion or infarct, local microglia mature into large phagocytically active macrophages ('compound granular corpuscles') and there is also renewed active immigration of monocytes into the area.

THE THYMUS

Embryologically, the thymus develops from the third pharyngeal pouch in company with parathyroid tissue; during development it descends until it occupies its final position in the upper part of the anterior mediastinum. As a result an ectopic thymus may occur in the neck or anterior mediastinum. Thymomas have been found in the pleura and lung and therefore thymic tissue can become displaced laterally beyond the bounds of its normal embryological descent. Because of the association of the thymus with parathyroid, the latter tissue may be found embedded in a normally situated thymus and in rare cases may give rise to a parathyroid adenoma in the anterior mediastinum. Conversely, thymic tissue has been demonstrated in the wall of a parathyroid cyst; the cystic element is derived presumably from a remnant of the third pharyngeal pouch.

The structure of the thymus is best seen in the newborn child when it is a prominent and highly cellular organ. It is divided into lobules by fine connective tissues and each lobule is clearly demarcated into a cortex with many densely packed lymphocytes and a less highly cellular medulla. Since in the earliest stages of development the rudimentary organ contains only epithelial cells derived from the pharyngeal pouch, the basic framework of the thymus depends on a cell of epithelial origin, the epithelial reticular cell.

The epithelial reticular cell of the thymus is large—12 μm or more in diameter with a leptochromatic nucleus and cytoplasm which stains pale pink with eosin and has a number of characteristics which denote its epithelial origin. Many of the cells have a prominent granular endoplasmic reticulum and contain PAS positive electron dense secretory granules; many contain intracellular microcysts into which cytoplasmic processes protrude. Others contain aggregated cytoplasmic

Fig. 1.8. Epithelial reticular cell of thymus showing aggregates of microfilaments resembling keratin and vacuoles containing microvilli. × 22,150.

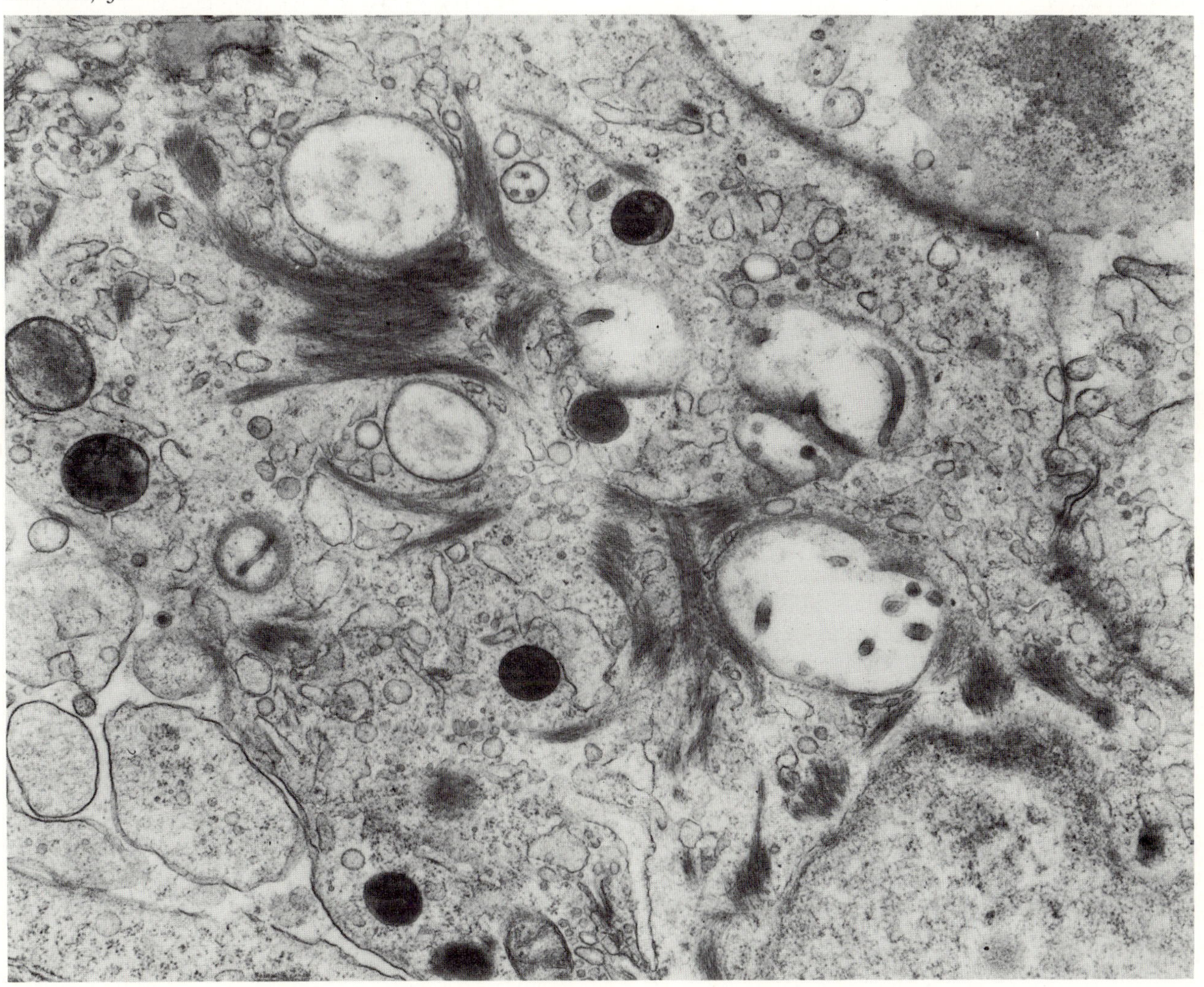

microfilaments resembling keratin. Epithelial cells are attached to one another by means of desmosomes forming a cellular framework throughout the organ (Fig. 1.8). Epithelial cells and their processes form a variably complete sheath around the thymic blood vessels. In the medulla aggregates of dead and dying keratinizing epithelial cells form the well-known Hassall's corpuscles.

The thymic parenchyma is composed of a framework of these epithelial reticular cells. In the cortex these are relatively few and closely packed with lymphocytes, mainly small lymphocytes and some macrophages. In the medulla lymphocytes are fewer and the epithelial reticular cells much more obvious. To be distinguished from epithelial reticular cells are normal connective tissue macrophages, present in both cortex and medulla. In situations where there is considerable necrosis of lymphocytes these ingest lymphocytes and become large and prominent. Also seen in small numbers in the thymus are myoid cells—mesenchymal cells which contain actin and myosin filaments identifiable ultrastructurally and immunohistologically. Eosinophils are also present, especially at the corticomedullary junction and some Hassall's corpuscles may contain large numbers of these cells. Plasma cells are seen in the fibrous septa and in the paraseptal areas within the organ, but within the deeper thymic parenchyma, appear only as scattered cells. However, larger pyroninophilic cells may be seen in the cortex. Whether these latter are immature plasma cells or not is difficult to ascertain, but they undoubtedly have an immunological function. Mast cells are only seen in the fibrous septa between the lobules or in perivascular areas within the thymic parenchyma. Lymphoid follicles and germinal centres do not appear in the normal thymus, but do occur in association with some diseases. They have been found in some control series of normal persons undergoing accidental death. Whether these represent a 'normal' constituent of the thymus or a latent pathological process is uncertain. The blood vessels are arranged in a capillary system which enters the cortical surface and drains from the medulla. Lymphatic vessels drain out to the tracheobronchial lymph nodes. There is a continual circulation of lymphocytes through the thymus and also a considerable local production of these cells. Many of the lymphocytes produced in the thymus, however, never leave the organ, and these may be ingested by macrophages which are present in the thymic cortex.

The lymphocyte content of the organ can be profoundly altered by the administration of cortisone, which induces a rapid decay of lymphocytes in the thymic cortex with phagocytosis of cell fragments; some lymphocytes are resistant to the effect of cortisone. The majority of the cells disappearing during the first two days after cortisone administration are immunologically inert, the total immunological potential of the organ remaining unaffected. The immunocompetent cells left, largely in the medulla, are rather larger than the other thymic lymphocytes and are relatively radioresistant. After stopping cortisone, regeneration is rapid and the organ is normal again in fourteen days.

The immunological function of the thymus

In experimentally thymectomized animals cell-mediated immunity is deficient and the paracortical areas of lymph nodes and periarteriolar sheath of the white pulp of the spleen fail to develop. An analogous situation is present in the rare human thymic aplasia. It is probably true that two thymic products are of importance in this process, a thymic hormone and thymic lymphocytes; the interaction between these is not yet totally clear. Thymic grafts in millipore chambers restore immunological function in thymectomized animals as do extracts of thymus—the hormone, not yet fully characterized, is described as thymosin, is a sulphated mucosubstance and may be produced by epithelial reticular cells. Thymic lymphocytes probably derive ultimately from the marrow but massive proliferation occurs in the thymus, from which they emerge probably by migrating into venules at the corticomedullary junction, to home on to the peripheral thymic dependent areas where they mature, probably within the so-called 'interdigitating' macrophages.

INTESTINAL LYMPHORETICULAR TISSUE

Nodules of lymphoreticular tissue are found in large numbers in the mucosa of the small intestine, some are small, under 1 mm in size while others, found notably in the ileum, are macroscopically visible masses up to 2 cm in diameter. The structure of these nodules resembles that of the parenchyma of lymph nodes, but without sinusoids. They are covered by columnar epithelium and have both germinal centres and postcapillary venules similar to those seen in lymph nodes.

Similar nodules of lymphoreticular tissue are found in the tongue, oropharynx and nasopharynx, the largest of these being the tonsils. The covering epithelium here (stratified squamous) often deeply invaginates the lymphoreticular tissue.

AGEING CHANGES IN LYMPHORETICULAR TISSUE

These have been fully reviewed by Marshall (1961). There are certain species variations but the following account is broadly true for man. The anatomical mass of lymph nodes and spleen reaches a maximum at a period variously estimated between 12 and 25 years, followed by a prolonged steady state though relative mass of lymphoreticular tissue to body weight is maximal in childhood. Lymphoreticular mass in general falls after 50 years.

In lymph nodes germinal centres become prominent in the first year of life in response to antigenic stimulation. After puberty there is a relative decrease in cortical tissue and increase in hyaline connective tissue, notably in the hilar area, and with the years an increasing amount of fat. In old age germinal centres tend to disappear and the node, apart from adipose infiltration looks a solid mass of small lymphocytes. A reduction in germinal centres also occurs in people dying of chronic diseases. A similar involution of the white pulp of the spleen and reduction in the number of prominent germinal centres starts about the age of thirty years and progresses slowly thereafter. The changes of old age in lymphoreticular tissue are reflected in a diminution in immunological responsiveness.

The most spectacular age changes however are those occurring in the thymus, which weighs some 10 g at birth, increases to a maximum of 30–40 g at puberty and there after involutes so that by the age of 30 years it is not usually obvious and in old age may be difficult to demonstrate even histologically, when only a few clusters of lymphocytes and epithelial reticular cells may be left lying in adipose and fibrous tissue. There is a progressive loss of cortical lymphocytes and increase in fibrous tissue notably around blood vessels so that the organ appears excessively lobulated. There is an increase in mast cells and an initial increase followed by disappearance of plasma cells; later epithelial reticular cells reduce in numbers and adipose replacement occurs progressively. These ageing changes should be distinguished from those of 'accidental involution', occurring in severe stress and presumably due to glucocorticoids; here there is an acute loss of lymphocytes; the dead cells and debris are ingested by macrophages which come to contain much birefringent lipid—giving a 'starry sky' appearance.

THE IDENTIFICATION OF CELL TYPES IN LYMPHORETICULAR TISSUE

The precision of identification of cell types in lymphoreticular tissue increases with the sophistication of the techniques used. As has been described it is possible to identify many cells in H & E sections when cut thinly and carefully stained. The small lymphocyte has a round dense nucleus and very little cytoplasm. The small (B) lymphocyte of follicular origin has a nucleus which departs from the spherical in shape and is sometimes, particularly in smear preparations, visibly indented or cleaved. The large lymphocyte is more difficult to identify precisely but has a leptochromatic nucleus and rather more cytoplasm which is often basophilic and pyroninophilic; the nucleus is often cleaved. The macrophage or histiocyte (non-neoplastic) has a reniform nucleus, bulky cytoplasm whose edges may appear irregular or frilly and which contains visible inclusions, often basophilic. The plasma cell often has a nucleus with a characteristic 'cartwheel' arrangement of chromatin and bulky cytoplasm staining purplish in H & E sections and positively with pyronin. With the electron microscope more precise identification is possible. Macrophages can be positively identified by their numerous pseudopodia, numerous lysosomes, and prominent cytoplasmic membranous components. With the use of immunological cell marker techniques further refinements are possible. B cells can be identified by making a cell suspension and staining cell surface immunoglobulin using fluorescein-conjugated goat antihuman antisera. B cells, T cells and cells of the monocyte-macrophage series can be identified by rosette techniques. In its simplest form this technique is applied to T cells; these form rosettes *in vitro* with sheep red blood cells by a poorly understood and probably non-immunological mechanism—the E rosette (see Fig. 1.3). B-lymphocytes carry a receptor for the third component of complement (C_3) and therefore form rosettes with red cells treated with IgM antibody and complement (the EAC rosette). Monocytes and macrophages carry a C_3 receptor and also form EAC rosettes; in addition they carry a receptor for IgG and therefore form rosettes with red cells treated with IgG (the EA rosette).

The E, EAC and EA rosetting techniques can also be used, with appropriate modifications, on fresh frozen tissue sections. In addition B cells can be identified by their affinity for radiolabelled soluble antigen–antibody complexes. Immunoperoxidase techniques may be used to define the membrane and intracellular immunoglobulin of B cells. The availability of monoclonal antibodies to surface determinants of T cells, T cell subsets, and macrophages further increases the immunological discriminant within the tissue section. The cellular response to mitogens and lectins can only be tested in cell suspensions. Cytochemical examination of cell suspensions or of frozen or appropriately prepared paraffin sections can give useful information. Acid phosphatase and α naphthyl acetate esterase are demonstrable in small amounts, as a 'dot-like' reaction in T-lymphocytes; and in large amounts in histiocytes. Adenosine triphosphate is found in many B cell lymphomas. Tartrate-resistant acid phosphatase is found only in the hairy cells of hairy-cell leukaemia. Peroxidase and naphthol-AS-D chloroacetate esterase are found in myeloid cells (Chilosi *et al.* 1981).

These reactions are summarized in Table 1.4. Some of these techniques are tricky and not universally available.

Table 1.4 Distinguishing lymphoreticular cells

	LZM	ACP	ANAE	CAE	TRAP	Ig	Rosettes
Macrophage	++	+	+	(±)	−	−	EAC, EA
T-lymphocyte	−	(+)	(+)	−	−	−	E
B-lymphocyte	−	−	−	−	−	+	−
Myeloid cell	+	(±)	−	+	−	−	−
Hairy-cell	−	−	−	−	+	−	−

Some enzyme markers on lymphoid cells may be of diagnostic interest, for example adenosine deaminase, 5′ nucleotidase and terminal deoxynucleotidyl transferase (TdT). The latter, measured either by a quantitative enzyme assay or immunofluorescence, is an enzyme that catalyses addition of deoxyribonucleotide triphosphates to ribonucleotides, without a template. It is present in significant amounts in immature and proliferating T cells or null cells, but not significantly in B cells. It is therefore found in normal thymocytes, many thymomas, acute lymphocytic leukaemia and lymphoblastic lymphoma and sometimes in the blast crisis of chronic myeloid leukaemia or diffuse histiocytic lymphoma, but is not found in most B-derived lymphomas, hairy-cell leukaemia, Hodgkin's disease or in the mature T cells of Sezary's syndrome (Blatt *et al.* 1980).

THE CLASSIFICATION OF LYMPHORETICULAR DISEASE

Lymphoreticular disease excluding leukaemia is in general classified in relation to histological appearances in a biopsy, usually of a lymph node. Such a biopsy may show one of four basic changes:

1 Hypoplasia; this is rare and is found in the immune deficiency states. This is considered in Chapter 2.

2 Reactive hyperplasia with a variable even dominant inflammatory component. This is considered in Chapter 3.

3 Neoplasia, secondary and primary; the former is not essentially lymphoreticular disease and will be considered only briefly in this text. Some primary lymphoreticular neoplasms may be associated with an excess of neoplastic leucocytes in the peripheral blood. Where this is the initial or major manifestation the condition is a leukaemia; the tissue manifestations of leukaemia are considered in Chapter 9. Primary neoplasia of the lymphoreticular system can best be classified according to whether the neoplastic process is localized, forming a lump or mass, or diffusely infiltrative. It is convenient to refer to one of the former disorders as a **lymphoma**—the major lymphomas are considered in Chapters 4 and 5, and to the latter as **histiocytosis**—and discussed in Chapter 8. An alternative to the latter term was reticulosis; this term unfortunately was sometimes used to include the lymphomas and sometimes merely to mean a lymphoreticular reaction; being therefore ambiguous it will not be used here. The term **reticuloendotheliosis** implying a neoplastic proliferation of undefined cells of lymphoreticular origin has been used in several contexts; it will here be used to relate only to a specific condition—leukaemic reticuloendotheliosis (hairy-cell leukaemia). Neoplasms of plasma cell origin are considered in Chapter 10.

4 Storage disorders or thesauroses—where there is abnormal storage of normal or abnormal materials in macrophages. These conditions are rare and at present seem to shade imperceptibly into the histiocytoses, with which they will be considered.

Inevitably in this systematic consideration of lymphoreticular disease major attention will be given to lymph node pathology. A brief recapitulation of the histopathology of the spleen and thymus is given in Chapters 11 and 12. Finally the diagnosis and management of the most important lymphoreticular diseases will be considered in Chapter 13. This includes a discussion of the value of marrow biopsy in lymphoreticular disease. A brief schema of lymphoreticular disease follows

(Table 1.5); this will be amplified in the section on neoplasia.

Most of this book is concerned with malignant neoplasia of the human lymphoreticular system of unknown aetiology.

Table 1.5 The pathological classification of lymphoreticular disease excluding leukaemia

1 **Hypoplasia**—the immune deficiency states.
2 **Hyperplasia**—including inflammatory changes.
3 **Neoplasia**
  A Hodgkin's disease (HD)
    Lymphocyte predominant   (LP)
    Nodular sclerosing   (NS)
    Mixed or classical   (M)
    Lymphocyte depleted   (LD)
  B Non-Hodgkin's lymphoma   (NHL)
    Pattern   Cell type
    Nodular (Follicular)   *Lymphocytic small*
    Diffuse   Lymphocytic large ⎫
                         Histiocytic ⎭ Large cell
    State whether with fibrosis and whether primarily extranodal.
  C Histiocytosis and reticuloendotheliosis
    Malignant histiocytosis (MH) (histiocytic medullary reticulosis)
    Malignant histiocytosis of childhood (e.g. Letterer Siwe)
    Differentiated histiocytosis
    Leukaemic reticuloendotheliosis   (LRE)
  D Multiple myeloma
    The indicated abbreviations are used often enough to be commonly intelligible and will be used in the text. Italicized lesions are of fairly good prognosis.

REFERENCES

Blatt J., Reaman G. & Poplack D.G. (1980) Current concepts: Biochemical markers in lymphoid malignancy. *New Engl. J. Med.* **303**, 918–22.

Carr I. & Daems W.Th. (1980) *The Reticuloendothelial System. A Comprehensive Treatise. Vol. 1. Morphology.* Plenum Press, New York.

Chilosi M., Pizzolo G., Menestrina F., Iannucci A.M., Bonetti F. & Fiore-Donati L. (1981) Enzyme histochemistry on normal and pathologic paraffin-embedded lymphoid tissues. *Amer. J. Clin. Path.* **76**, 729–36.

Cottier H., Turk J. & Sobin C. (1973) A proposal for a standardized system of reporting human lymph node morphology in relation to immunological function. *J. Clin. Path.* **26**, 317–31.

Ford W.L. (1978) Lymphocytes. 3 Distribution. Distribution of lymphocytes in health. *J. Clin. Path.* **32**, (Suppl. 13), 63–9.

Henry K. & Goldman J.M. (1975) In *Recent advances in Pathology*, vol. 9, pp. 30–72 (Eds. Harrison C.V. & Weinbren K.). Churchill Livingstone, Edinburgh.

Hong (1972) In *The Immunoglobulins in Clinical Immunobiology*, vol. 1, pp. 29–46 (Eds Bach F.M. & Good R.A.). Academic Press, London.

Marshall A.H.E. (1961) In *Structural Aspects of Ageing*, pp. 5–7 (Ed. Bourne G.H.). Pitman Press, London.

Mulligan R.M. (1974) Morphology and metabolism of lymphoid cells. *Pathology Annual* **9**, 385–420.

Owen J.J.T. (1978) Immunodeficiency. Maturation of the immune system and immunodeficiency. *J. Clin. Path.* **32** (Suppl. 13), 1–4.

Tew J.G., Thorbecke G.J. & Steinman R.M. (1982) Dendritic cells in the immune response: Characteristics and recommended nomenclature (a report from the Reticuloendothelial Society Committee on Nomenclature). *J. Reticuloendothelial Soc.* **31**, 371–80.

Weiss L. (1977) *The Blood Cells and Hematopoietic Tissues.* McGraw Hill, New York.

Weissman I.L., Warnke R., Butcher E.C., Rouse R. & Levy R. (1978) The lymphoid system. *Human Pathology* **9**, 25–45.

Immunodeficiency syndromes

Chapter 2

IMMUNODEFICIENCY DISORDERS:
CLASSIFICATION:
GENERAL CONSIDERATIONS

Immunodeficiency disorders represent a diverse group of disorders which share one common feature—an increased susceptibility to infection. Many of the disorders are congenital or inherited so that patients are, for the most part, infants or children. The initial nomenclature of the various disorders was confusing and terminology depended on the whim of the original author. The classification and terminology was rationalized by the WHO report of 1971, and it is this nomenclature that is used throughout this chapter (Table 2.1).

In the same manner in which the defence mechanisms may be considered under separate headings—antibody, cellular mechanisms and phagocytosis—so Immune Deficiency Syndromes can be considered as anomalies affecting these three systems either alone or in combination. All primary immunodeficiencies are rare, but over 1,000 cases have been reported in the literature with many others undiagnosed or unreported. The MRC Working Party on Hypogammaglobulinaemia in the United Kingdom (1969 and 1971) estimated the overall incidence of antibody deficiency syndromes as 1 per 100,000. The true incidence may be somewhat higher than this estimate due to the very strict criteria involved in the study, only those cases with a serum IgG level of less than 2 g/l or other *convincing* evidence of immune disturbance being included in the calculations. For children under 6 months of age the IgG limit was further reduced to 1 g/l. These figures did not include the other groups of immune deficiency and did not include those infants who died before a diagnosis could be made, so that the true overall incidence may be nearer to 2 per 100,000 live births. Table 2.2 shows the relative incidence of the various broad categories of primary immune deficiency.

Hobbs (1966) showed that the hypogammaglobulinaemia of immaturity was at least as common as primary immuno-

Table 2.1 Classification of primary immunodeficiencies (modified from *Bull. Wld. Hlth. Org.* (1971), **45**, 125–42)

Type	Suggested cellular defect		
	B cells	T cells	Stem cells
Infantile X-linked agamma-globulinaemia	+		
Selective immunoglobulin deficiency (IgA)	+ (some)		
Transient hypogammaglobulinaemia of infancy	+		
X-linked immunodeficiency with hyper IgM	+		
Thymic hypoplasia (pharyngeal pouch syndrome, Di George's syndrome)		+	
Episodic lymphopenia with lymphocytotoxin		+	
Immunodeficiency with or without hypoimmunoglobulinaemia	+	+ (some-times)	
Immunodeficiency with ataxia telangiectasia	+	+	
Immunodeficiency with thrombocytopenia and eczema (Wiskott–Aldrich syndrome)	+	+	
Immunodeficiency with thymoma	+	+	
Immunodeficiency with short-limbed dwarfism	+	+	
Immunodeficiency with generalized haematopoietic hypoplasia	+	+	+
Severe combined immunodeficiency			
autosomal recessive	+	+	+
X-linked	+	+	+
sporadic	+	+	+
Variable immunodeficiency (common, largely unclassified)	+	+ (some-times)	

Table 2.2 Classification of immunodeficiency disorders (WHO)

	Percentage of total cases
Humoral immunodeficiency	50–75
Combined immunodeficiency	10–25
Cellular immunodeficiency	5–10
Phagocytosis defects	1–2
Dyscomplementaemia	<1

deficiency and that secondary immunodeficiency accounted for 70% of all cases of immunodeficiency amongst hospitalized patients, with an overall incidence of 2.3%.

The age at diagnosis of humoral immunodeficiency is described in the MRC report as follows: 17% of cases occur in infants younger than one year, 26% in children between one and five years of age, 15% in children between six and 15 years of age, and 42% in adults. Humoral immunodeficiency is more common in males than in females although there are some age-related differences in the male : female ratio. Below 15 years of age over 80% of cases are male while above 15 years about 60% of cases occur in females.

Several of the disorders are associated with recessive genes having either X-linked or autosomal recessive modes of inheritance (Table 2.3). Other disorders have a less obvious inheritance pattern and adult humoral immunodeficiency tends to be a sporadic illness which occurs more commonly in females than in males. Genetic factors may, however, be operative in that cases have been described in cousins and

Table 2.3 Mode of inheritance in primary immunodeficiency

X-linked
    Infantile agammaglobulinaemia
    Severe combined immunodeficiency
    Immunodeficiency with hyper IgM
    Immunodeficiency with thrombocytopenia and eczema
    Chronic granulomatous disease

Autosomal recessive
    Severe combined immunodeficiency
    Immunodeficiency with lymphopenia and normal immuno-
        globulins
    Immunodeficiency with ataxia telangiectasia
    Immunodeficiency with short limbed dwarfism

Inheritance uncertain
    Adult humoral immunodeficiency
    Selective IgA deficiency

siblings. Families with humoral immunodeficiency tend to show an increased frequency of collagen disorders (Fudenberg *et al.* 1962). The subject has been reviewed by Denman (1980).

CLINICAL FEATURES

The major presenting feature is an increased susceptibility to infection. The patients have infections more frequently and more severely, their infections last longer and end more often in severe complications. The offending organisms are often of low pathogenicity. The main presenting systems involved are shown in Tables 2.4 and 2.5. The majority of patients present

Table 2.4 Main presenting symptoms in children with primary immunodeficiency

	%
Respiratory infections	88
Failure to thrive	2.5
Diarrhoea	2
Skin infections	1
Urinary tract infections	0.5
Generalized vaccinia	0.5

Table 2.5 Systems involved in presenting illness in children with primary immunodeficiency

	%
Lower respiratory tract	63
Upper respiratory tract	41
Skin and eyes	23
Gastrointestinal tract	16
Central nervous system—meninges	13

with single system involvement—usually the respiratory tract—despite classical descriptions of multisystem involvement. Of the upper respiratory tract infections, chronic middle ear disease is the most severe, leading to chronic osteomyelitis and deafness. The organisms most commonly reported are the pneumococci, staphylococci and *Haemophilus influenzae*, whilst *Pneumocystis carinii* pneumonia shows a marked increase in frequency in the children with combined immune deficiency syndromes.

MALIGNANCY AND IMMUNODEFICIENCY

Malignant disease is a not infrequent finding in patients with primary immunodeficiency syndromes. 10% of patients with ataxia telangiectasia and the Wiskott–Aldrich syndrome die of malignant disease, and it appears even more frequent in patients with the variable immunodeficiencies. Lymphoid-malignancy is common although the incidence of epithelial malignancy is unexpectedly high. Acute leukaemia has been reported in a number of cases of X-linked infantile agamma-globulinaemia; since the latter is a rare disease, this may represent a genuinely increased incidence of leukaemia.

AUTOIMMUNE DISEASE

Auto-antibodies with or without overt autoimmune disease are common. The reason for this association is not clear but may be due to the basic genetic anomaly or to the effects of immunodeficiency on latent viral infection.

ANTIBODY DEFICIENCY SYNDROMES

X-LINKED INFANTILE HYPOGAMMAGLOBULINAEMIA

Both the X-linked infantile hypogammaglobulinaemia (Bruton 1952) and the non-sex-linked form of the disorder are characterized by the lack of serum and secretory immunoglo-bulins (see Table 2.1), recurrent bacterial infections and a relatively normal cellular immune function. Lymphocytes are present in the peripheral blood in normal numbers and are apparently normal functionally although there is often some mild depression of transformation with PHA at low dose (Hosking *et al.* 1971).

The thymus is usually atrophic. Hassall's corpuscles are present but show degenerative changes and calcification. The appearances are those of accelerated involution associated with severe infection.

The lymph nodes may be slightly enlarged, but there is a complete absence of cortical development with a lack of follicles and germinal centres. Lymphocytes are plentiful but there is no evidence of plasma cell maturation. Cortico-medullary differentiation is poor.

The spleen shows poorly developed small Malpighian corpuscles without reaction centres. There is no alteration in the periarteriolar lymphoid sheath. Plasma cells are absent from the splenic pulp.

The normal lymphoreticular aggregates are largely absent from both the small and large intestinal wall. Plasma cells are absent. Where lymphoid aggregates are seen, germinal centres are absent.

COMBINED DEFICIENCY SYNDROMES

SEVERE COMBINED IMMUNODEFICIENCY

First described by Glanzmann and Riniker (1950) this has become known as the Swiss type agammaglobulinaemia. The syndrome is characterized by the early onset of severe infections with lymphopenia, thymic aplasia, and a deficiency of both humoral and cellular immune function. The clinical findings in 70 cases are reviewed by Hitzig *et al.* (1968). In this series the mean age of onset of symptoms was 2.7 months and mean age at death was 6.8 months. 89% of cases had evidence of pneumonia, 86% diarrhoea, 79% thrush, 67% some form of skin involvement and 57% generalized sepsis. The most characteristic feature is the general lack of lymphoid elements both centrally and peripherally.

The thymus is aplastic or markedly dysplastic. In the series reported by Hitzig *et al.* (1968) 82% had a thymus weight of less than 5 g; it was apparently absent in 10%. Where thymic elements are present there is extreme lymphoid depletion. There is no differentiation between cortex and medulla and Hassall's corpuscles are absent. The overall architecture is disturbed to the extent that normal lobulation is lost with an increase in fibrous tissue. The most prominent cell is the thymic epithelial cell. When lymph nodes can be identified, lymphocytes are scanty and there is no evidence of cortical or follicular development. The capsule of the node is thickened and fibrotic, with obliteration of the peripheral sinus. Plasma cells are absent. There is an apparent increase in hystiocytic cells and fibroblasts. The spleen is usually small and may be almost unrecognizable as such. There is a complete absence of Malpighian corpuscles, the trabeculae being separated by congested sinusoids.

The gastrointestinal lymphoid aggregates are completely absent; Peyer's patches are largely replaced by necrotic fibrous tissue; the appendix is devoid of lymphocytes, follicles and plasma cells. There is usually an associated intestinal villous anomaly with a loss of villous architecture and a general thinning of the mucosa.

IMMUNODEFICIENCY WITH ATAXIA TELANGIECTASIA

This autosomal recessive disorder is characterized by telangiectasia, an abnormal gait leading to progressive ataxia, and a variable immunodeficiency involving both cellular and humoral immune systems. Although most patients with ataxia telangiectasia have some form of immune defect, there is no consistent pattern. Ammann *et al.* (1969) showed that 60% of patients had defects in cell-mediated immunity or humoral immunity or both, and that the humoral immune defect was usually a lack of IgA and IgE. There has been considerable difficulty in explaining the multisystem involvement in this disease on the basis of a single pathogenetic mechanism. Ammann and Hong (1971) suggest that the basic anomaly is one of thymic abnormality and that the multisystem manifestations are resultant upon autoimmunity or recurrent infection or both.

Thymic abnormalities ranging from aplasia and hypoplasia to extreme atrophy are described. Hassall's corpuscles are absent or only poorly developed and corticomedullary demarcation is absent. The overall cellularity is only marginally reduced. Where lymphocytes are reduced in numbers the epithelial reticular cells are prominent. Lymph nodes show variable morphology but generally there is poor follicular development with an absence of germinal centres. Antigenic stimulation will invoke follicular development. There is commonly severe depletion of the paracortical regions with poor corticomedullary demarcation. The lymphoid depletion is age-related, and progressive.

The lymphoid aggregates of the gastrointestinal tract are poorly developed with absence of follicular development. The spleen shows poorly developed Malpighian corpuscles with scanty reaction centres. There is severe depletion of lymphocytes in the region of the splenic arterioles.

IMMUNODEFICIENCY WITH ECZEMA AND THROMBOCYTOPENIA

The Wiskott–Aldrich syndrome is an X-linked recessive immune deficiency syndrome characterized by thrombocytopenia, eczema, recurrent infections and an inability to produce antibody to polysaccharide antigens. Cooper *et al.* (1968) have shown that thymus and lymph node morphology is normal in the initial instance and that plasma cell development is established normally. They proposed that the immunologic defect was an apparent defect involving an inability to handle polysaccharide antigen. The presence of normal numbers of plasma cells and normal levels of immunoglobulin in the early stages of the disease indicate integrity of the efferent limb of the immune system. The inability to handle polysaccharide antigen leads to a progressive disorganization of the lymphoid system so that by the age of 4 most patients show morphological abnormalities with lymphocytic depletion from both thymic and bursa dependent zones. This theory of the development of the immunological defect is supported by experimental studies in mice (Ekstedt and Hayes 1967).

The thymus is normal in structure early in life, but shows accelerated involution and lymphocyte depletion though with normal Hassall's corpuscles. The changes are very variable.

In young children lymph nodes show only slight lymphoid depletion of thymic dependent paracortical regions. Lymphoid follicles are usually normally formed and plasma cell development well established. In older patients, however, both cortex and paracortical regions are severely depleted of cells. Germinal centres are absent.

The spleen is usually somewhat enlarged but severely depleted of lymphocytes in both the periarteriolar lymphoid sheath and the rest of the white pulp.

There is no marked depletion of gastrointestinal lymphoreticular tissue and most patients show normal lymphoid aggregates with adequate follicular development.

CELLULAR DEFICIENCY SYNDROMES

THYMIC HYPOPLASIA (PHARYNGEAL POUCH SYNDROME)

This disorder is characterized by congenital tetany, an unusual facies and an increased susceptibility to infection. There is absence or hypoplasia of thymus and parathyroid glands following failure of development of the IIIrd and IVth pharyngeal pouches. The syndrome was characterized by Di George (1965) and further described by Taitz *et al.* (1966).

Since the thymus has failed to develop properly either no thymus can be found or only a shrunken residue with a scanty epithelial component, no Hassall's corpuscles and few lymphocytes.

The lymph nodes show complete failure of development of

the paracortical areas with normal cortex, follicles and germinal centres. Plasma cell development is normal.

In the spleen the periarteriolar lymphoid sheath is absent but the rest of the white pulp develops normally. The gastrointestinal lymphoreticular tissue develops normally.

DYSPHAGOCYTOSIS SYNDROMES

These are not strictly lymphoreticular disease but will be briefly mentioned for convenience. The association of adequate numbers of circulating phagocytes with normal host defence has been appreciated for many years. Leucopenia, either congenital or acquired due to malignancy or chemotherapy, results in an increased susceptibility to infection particularly from bacterial pathogens. Functional anomalies of the phagocyte system have only been recognized relatively recently. Chronic granulomatous disease of childhood and the Chediak–Higashi syndrome are associated with defective bactericidal capacity and severe bacterial disease; Job's syndrome, although not definitely proven as a phagocyte dysfunctional state, with recurrent staphylococcal abscesses, has many similar characteristics and can conveniently be considered in the same context.

CHRONIC GRANULOMATOUS DISEASE OF CHILDHOOD

This is an inherited defect of leucocyte bactericidal capacity characterized by granulomatous lesions in the skin, lungs, and lymph nodes, together with hypergammaglobulinaemia, anaemia, and leucocytosis. All the children in the early reports died in the first decade and the condition became known as 'a fatal granulomatous disease of childhood'. The relentless progression and poor prognosis is not wholly warranted, and the 'fatal' has now been deleted. Tests of bacterial phagocytosis show that the actual process of engulfment is normal, but that intact, viable, bacteria persist within the phagocytes. In the leucocytes of chronic granulomatous disease 80–100% of ingested bacteria will remain viable after 120 minutes incubation, whereas with normal leucocytes less than 1% of ingested bacteria will be viable after much shorter incubation periods (Quie *et al.* 1971). The inability to kill bacteria is accompanied by an inability to kill fungi, and *Candida albicans* has become a widely used test organism. The abnormality is not restricted to polymorphonuclear phagocytes and also

affects eosinophils and macrophages. The reduction of Nitro Blue Tetrazolium (NBT) is used as a histochemical means of identifying oxidase activity during phagocytosis. Whereas 80–90% of normal leucocytes will reduce NBT to a blue formazan on phagocytosis, only 10% of leucocytes in chronic granulomatous disease will produce the blue colouration. This test must, however, be confirmed by the demonstration of defective intracellular bacterial killing.

The clinical features of this condition were reviewed by Johnston and McMurray (1967). The areas primarily affected are those which receive constant bacterial challenge such as the skin, lungs and perianal tissues. Recurrent infection leads to lymphadenopathy and splenomegaly with suppuration and granuloma formation. The precise metabolic defect is the subject of considerable debate. The normal polymorph in the resting state metabolizes only 1% of its glucose-6-phosphate via the hexose monophosphate shunt. This is increased 10-fold during phagocytosis and is accompanied by an increased oxygen uptake with accumulation of hydrogen peroxide, NADH and NADPH. Polymorphs in chronic granulomatous disease are incapable of increasing their utilization of the hexose monophosphate shunt and fail to accumulate peroxide. The fact that the polymorphs of patients with chronic granulomatous disease can kill organisms which produce peroxidase such as pneumococci and streptococci suggests that the basic defect lies in the early part of the leucocyte metabolism pathways.

The lymph nodes show reactive hyperplasia with numerous granulomata consisting of mononuclear cells, many of which contain prominent deposits of lipochrome pigment, in juxtaposition with suppurative lesions consisting of effete polymorphs and numerous bacteria. The spleen shows reactive hyperplasia with granulomata and numerous abscesses.

JOB'S SYNDROME

This condition was originally described as affecting fair, red-headed girls (Davis *et al.* 1966) and is associated with 'cold' staphylococcal abscesses in the skin, subcutaneous tissues and lymph nodes. Despite the claim by Bannatyne *et al.* (1969) that this is chronic granulomatous disease occurring in the female, reports on polymorph bactericidal capacity have been variable. Episodic lymphadenopathy with reactive lymphadenitis and suppuration without granuloma formation are usual.

TREATMENT OF PRIMARY IMMUNODEFICIENCY

Treatment involves the prompt antimicrobial treatment of intercurrent infections and the attempt to correct the underlying defect. Humoral defects involving lack of IgG may be partially corrected by gammaglobulin replacement therapy, though hypersensitivity reactions are fairly common and desensitization may be required. Transfusion of fresh frozen plasma may also be employed. Deficiency of IgA and IgM rarely benefits from replacement therapy. The treatment of cellular immunity defects is difficult. Transfer factor or whole leucocyte transfusion may be tried. Reconstitution of immunity with thymus or bone marrow grafts is still only in the semi-experimental stage of development although some spectacular successes have been achieved. Dysphagocytosis syndromes may require fresh leucocyte transfusion in the event of severe infection.

SECONDARY IMMUNODEFICIENCY

Impairment of lymphocyte function has been demonstrated in a number of diseases but in only a few instances does this become clinically relevant (Table 2.6).

Depression of cellular immunity is a feature of generalized Hodgkin's disease and humoral immunity of lymphocytic and plasma cell tumours. Depression of neutrophil phagocytic function may be a feature of myeloid leukaemia. The commonest cause of immunodeficiency at the present time is probably the use of immunosuppressive drugs (particularly corticosteroids).

In the acquired immunodeficiency syndrome characteristically found in young homosexual males, generalized lymph node enlargement is common. The nodes show reactive follicular and sinusoidal hyperplasia. The medullary sinuses are packed with monomorphic round cells containing muramidase, and with polymorphs. Granulomata with small foci of necrosis, and generalized lymphocytic depletion of the node are found less commonly (Guarda *et al.* 1983).

The most important consequence of immunodepression is the increased likelihood of infection, particularly with opportunistic organisms of fungal, protozoal and viral type. Humoral immunodepression may be associated with severe recurrent and even fatal bacterial infections.

The increased incidence of malignancy and autoimmune disease with immunodepression is recognized (Crowther 1974) but further long-term experience is necessary before drawing valid conclusions on causative relationships.

Treatment of secondary immunodeficiency is only needed in patients suffering from recurrent infections (Webster 1974). Humoral immune defects can sometimes be improved by regular administration of immunoglobulin. In cellular defects various forms of immunotherapy are undergoing extensive trial. Transfer factor, a low molecular weight substance isolated from sensitized lymphocytes is capable of transferring cell-mediated immune responses to previously unreactive recipients (Lawrence 1969) and may have therapeutic potential in certain primary and secondary immunodeficiency syndromes (Levin *et al.* 1973; Kirkpatrick 1980). The immunomodulating compound levamisole (Willoughby and

Table 2.6 Secondary immunodeficiency

Disease	System affected		
	Cellular immunity	Humoral immunity	Phago-cytosis
Malignancy			
Hodgkin's disease	+ +	+	−
Non-Hodgkin's lymphoma	+	+ +	−
Chronic lymphatic leukaemia	±	+ +	±
Acute leukaemia	+	+	+ +
Myelomatosis	±	+ +	−
Macroglobulinaemia	±	+ +	−
Carcinomatosis	+	+	+
Infection			
Measles	±	−	−
Leprosy	+	−	−
Tuberculosis	+	−	−
Sarcoidosis	+	−	−
Autoimmune disorders	+ +	−	±
Metabolic disorders			
Malnutrition	+	±	±
Renal failure	+	±	±
Protein losing diatheses	−	+	−
Surgery			
Major surgery/severe trauma	+	+	−
Splenectomy	+	+ +	±
Thymectomy	+ +	+	−
Drugs			
Corticosteroids	+ +	+	±
Cytotoxic drugs	+ +	+	±
(Radiotherapy)	+	±	±

Wood 1977) influences cellular immunity in various experimental and clinical models; its therapeutic role has yet to be established however. Interferons are highly active glycoproteins released from cells infected by virus; they probably act by inhibiting the translation of viral messenger-RNA and are undergoing clinical trials in various situations, including prophylaxis against acquired viral infections in immunosuppressed hosts (Scott and Tyrrell 1980). The most important concept however, as in any secondary state, is treatment of the underlying disease.

REFERENCES

AMMANN A.J., CAIN W.A., ISHIZAKA K., HONG R. & GOOD R.A. (1969) Immunoglobulin E deficiency in Ataxia telangiectasia. *New Eng. J. Med.* **281**, 469–72.

AMMANN A.J. & HONG R. (1971) Autoimmune phenomena in Ataxia telangiectasia. *J. Pediat.* **78**, 821–6.

BANNATYNE R.M., SKOWRON P.N. & WEBER J.L. (1969) Job's syndrome—a variant of chronic granulomatous disease. Report of a case. *J. Pediat.* **75**, 236–42.

BRUTON O.C. (1952) Agammaglobulinaemia. *Pediatrics* **9**, 722–8.

COOPER M.D., CHASE H.P., LOMAN J.T., KRIVIT W. & GOOD R.A. (1968) Wiskott–Aldrich syndrome: an immunologic deficiency disease involving the afferent limb of immunity. *Amer. J. Med.* **44**, 499–513.

CROWTHER D. (1974) Immunosuppression. *Medicine (London)*, **29**, 1729–1733.

DAVIS S.D., SCHALLER J. & WEDGWOOD R.J. (1966) Job's syndrome—Recurrent 'cold' staphylococcal abscesses. *Lancet* **i**, 1013–15.

DENMAN A.M. (1980) Immunodeficiency and general medicine. *Brit. Med. J.* **281**, 1376–8.

DI GEORGE A.M. (1965) *in discussion. J. Pediat.* **67**, 907–8.

EKSTEDT R.D. & HAYES L.L. (1967) Runt diseases induced by non-living bacterial antigens. *J. Immunol.* **98**, 110–18.

FUDENBERG H.H., GERMAN J.L. & KUNKEL H.G. (1962) The occurrence of rheumatoid factor and other abnormalities in families of patients with agammaglobulinaemia. *Arthritis Rheum.* **5**, 565–88.

FUDENBERG H.H., GOOD R.A., GOODMAN H.C., HITZIG W., KUNKEL W., ROITT I.M., ROSEN F.S., ROWE D.S., SELIGMANN M. & SOOTHILL J.R. (1971) *Bull. W.H.O.* **45**, 125–42.

GLANZMANN E. & RINIKER P. (1950) Essentielle Lymphocytophise. Ein neues Krankheitsbild aus der Säuglinspathologie. *Ann. Paediat. (Basel)* **175**, 1–32.

GUARDA L.A., BUTLER J.J., MANSELL P., HERSH E.M., REUBEN J. & NEWELL G.R. (1983) Lymphadenopathy in homosexual men. Morbid anatomy with clinical and immunologic correlations. *Am. J. Clin. Pathol.* 559–68.

HITZIG W.H., BARANDUN S. & COTTIER H. (1968) Die Schweizerische Form der Agammaglobulinämie. *Ergebn. Inn. Med. Kinderheilk.* **27**, 79–154.

HOBBS J.R. (1966) Disturbances of the immunoglobulins. *Sci. Basis Med. Ann. Rev.* 106–27.

HOSKING C.S., FITZGERALD M.G. & SIMONS M.J. (1971) Quantified deficiency of lymphocyte response to phytohaemagglutinin in immune deficiency diseases. *Clin. Exp. Immunol.* **9**, 467–76.

JOHNSTON R.B. & McMURRAY J.S. (1967) Chronic familial granulomatosis: Report of five cases and review of the literature. *Amer. J. Dis. Child.* **114**, 370–87.

KIRKPATRICK C.H. (1980) Therapeutic potential of transfer factor. *New Eng. J. Med.* **303**, 390–1.

LAWRENCE H.S. (1969) Transfer factor. *Adv. Immunol.* **11**, 195–266.

LEVIN A.S., SPITLER L.E. & FUDENBERG H.H. (1973) Transfer factor therapy in immune deficiency states. *Ann. Rev. Med.* **24**, 175–208.

MEDICAL RESEARCH COUNCIL (1969) Hypogammaglobulinaemia in the United Kingdom. *Lancet* **i**, 163–8.

MEDICAL RESEARCH COUNCIL (1971) Hypogammaglobulinaemia in the United Kingdom. *Special Report Series No. 310.* HMSO.

QUIE P.G., KAPLAN E.L., LAXDAL T. & DOSSETT J. (1971) In *Immunologic Incompetence* (Eds Kagan B.M. & Stiehm E.R.). Yearbook Medical Publishers, Chicago.

SCOTT G.M. & TYRRELL D.A.J. (1980) Interferon: therapeutic fact or fiction for the eighties? *Brit. Med. J.* **1**, 1558–62.

TAITZ L.S., ZORATE SALVADOR C. & SCHWARTZ E. (1966) Congenital absence of the parathyroid and thymus glands in an infant (III and IV Pharyngeal Pouch Syndrome). *Pediatrics* **38**, 412–18.

WEBSTER A.D.B. (1974) Immunodeficiency. *Medicine (London)* **29**, 1707–14.

WILLOUGHBY D.A. & WOOD C. (1977) The history and development of levamisole, in "Forum on immunotherapy," vol. 1, pp. 3–11. Royal Society of Medicine, London.

The patient with enlarged lymph nodes can present a difficult, sometimes impossible clinical and pathological problem. Lymphadenopathy can be an incident in a systematic disease whose other manifestations make the diagnosis obvious. The purpose of this chapter is to discuss secondary lymphadenopathy presenting as a histopathologic diagnostic problem—that is the conditions to be discussed are those other than primary neoplasms of the lymphoreticular system. This problem should *always* be considered in the light of a knowledge of the patient's clinical condition and it is often necessary to defer definitive histological diagnosis until the results of full clinical, radiological, haematological and immunological investigations are available. Histopathological reports on lymph nodes should carry comments where possible on possible immunological inferences to be drawn from histology. It should also be remembered that lymph node morphology changes with age and site, the number of germinal centres becoming less as age progresses (Luscieti *et al.* 1980).

Two allied but distinguishable occurrences can happen in a lymph node. Firstly the node may react to a stimulus; the changes seen are known as reactive hyperplasia. Secondly the organisms or other causative substances may elicit an actively inflammatory reaction in the lymph node with migration into the node of all the components of an inflammatory reaction, notably polymorphs and macrophages. These two occurrences, reaction and inflammation, often co-exist but an attempt will be made to separate them. Interpretation of many of the older descriptions of reactive lymph node changes is rendered difficult by their being couched in out of date terminology.

The problems of diagnosis of reactive lymph nodes have been discussed by Butler (1968) and Dorfman and Warnke (1974). Three different things can happen: (a) sinus hyperplasia; (b) proliferation of reactive follicles; (c) proliferation of pulp elements. Often these things happen together. In sinus hyperplasia the sinus macrophages increase in size and number producing on occasions a solid packing of sinuses (Fig. 3.1). In addition there may be an increased traffic of monocytes and macrophages through the node. In follicular hyperplasia there are large numbers of large reactive follicles scattered throughout the node. The overall reticulin pattern of the node is retained. The follicles may vary widely in size and shape sometimes being dumb-bell shaped but usually have a rim of small lymphocytes clearly demarcating the periphery. Within the follicle are seen the usual cellular components. Mitosis is common and there may be many large 'tingible body macrophages' containing cellular debris. There may be well marked nuclear pleomorphism. The interfollicular pulp is compressed (Figs 3.2 and 3.3). Proliferation of pulp elements as the main reaction is best seen in immune reactions, when the interfollicular tissue becomes packed with immunoblasts and plasma cells (Fig. 3.4). Postcapillary venules in the paracortical areas may be prominent, crowded with emigrating lymphocytes and surrounded by maturing immunoblasts. This may be accompanied by infiltration with varying numbers of neutrophil and eosinophil polymorphs (Litt 1972). All combinations of these forms of hyperplasia may occur and may be compounded by inflammatory changes. The changes of inflammation as seen in a lymph node are similar to those seen elsewhere. In acute inflammation the sinusoids are packed with polymorphs and suppuration may occur; in chronic inflammation there is accumulation of macrophages, giant cell formation and granuloma formation. A rare reaction in lymph nodes is vascular transformation and fibrosis of the subcapsular sinus attributed to venous obstruction (Haferkamp *et al.* 1971).

It may be very difficult to distinguish reactive conditions from neoplasia. Occasionally a lymph node will show such profound hyperplasia that the cellular morphology becomes atypical and the architecture of the node appears to be obliterated, even as demonstrated by reticulin stains. In the study of Saltzstein (1965) a lymph node biopsy was diagnostic in only 72/177 patients. In the remaining non-diagnostic category 35 patients were under investigation for lymphadenopathy and of these 6 subsequently developed a malignant lymphoma. Firat *et al.* (1965) in a study of 60 cases of giant follicular lymphoid disease found that difficulty in

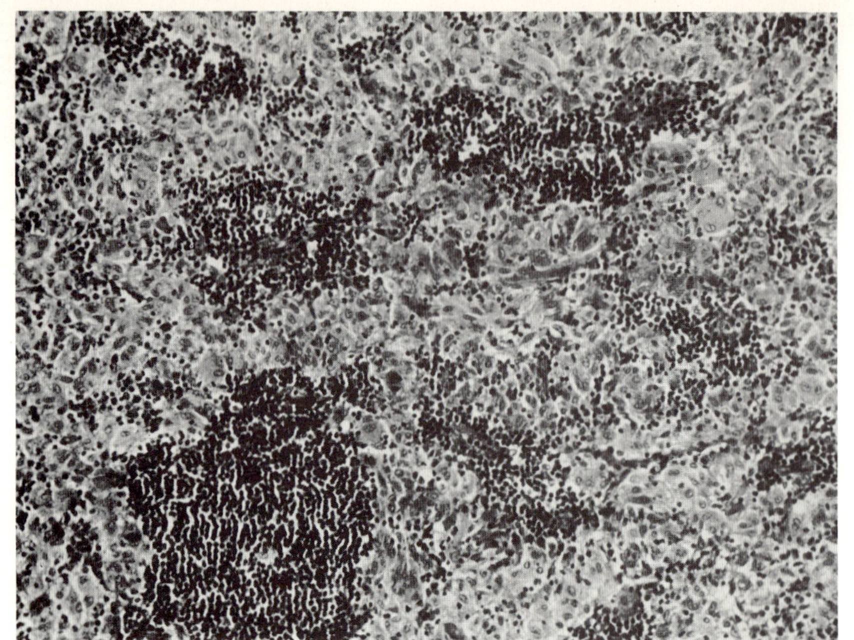

Fig. 3.1. Lymph node draining a chronic inflammatory focus. The proportion of lymph node occupied by sinusoid is increased; the sinusoids themselves show large prominent eosinophilic macrophages and also have an increased number of monocytes in transit. ×150.

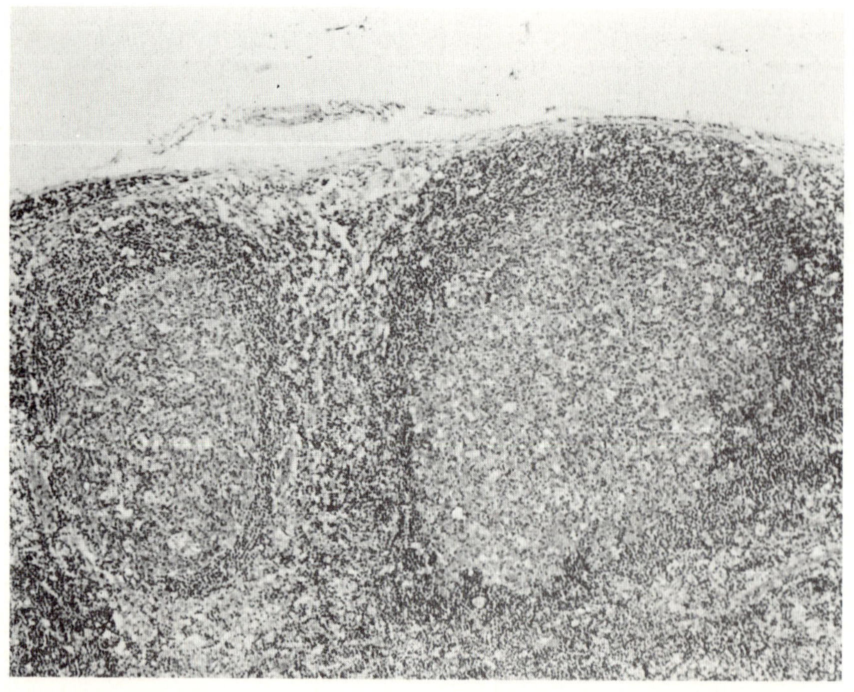

Fig. 3.2. A lymph node showing prominent reactive germinal centres—non-specific follicular hyperplasia. Note that the structure of the follicle is quite normal. ×45.

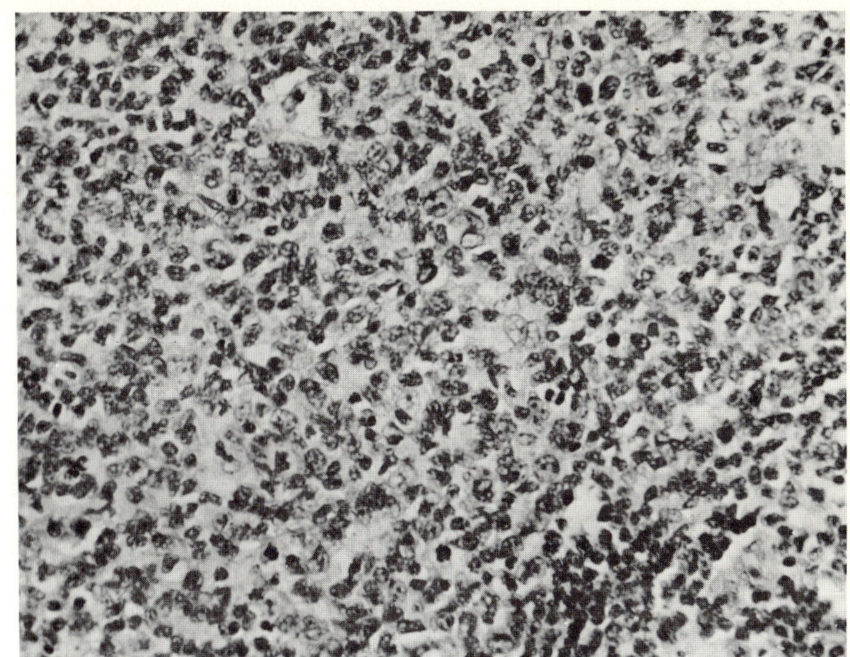

Fig. 3.3. Detail of the large lymphocytes seen in the centre of a reactive germinal centre. Mitotic figures are moderately frequent. ×215. Considering that this is not neoplastic tissue, there is a considerable degree of nuclear pleomorphism.

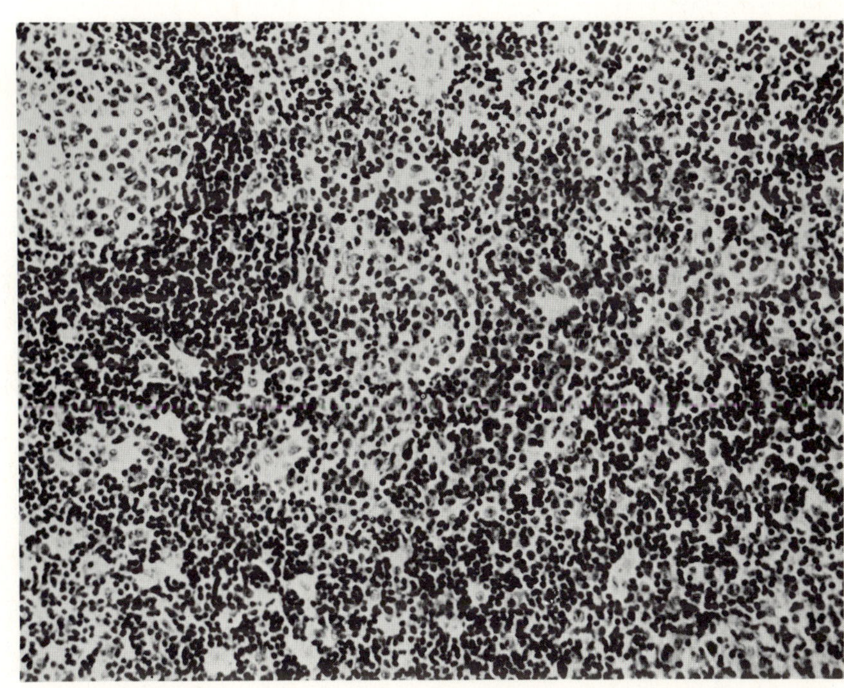

Fig. 3.4. A lymph node showing pulp or para follicular proliferation. Outside the small germinal centre there are numerous large lymphoblasts and histiocytic cells with a moderate number of mitotic figures. Plasma cells are not prominent. ×108.

pathological interpretation was experienced in nearly half of the cases. Perhaps the most difficult diagnostic distinction is between reactive follicular hyperplasia and follicular lymphoma. This has been discussed by Rappaport *et al.* (1956) and by Harrison (1966). In the malignant lymphomas the architecture tends to be obliterated whereas in follicular hyperplasia it is, if anything, accentuated, especially if there is a co-existent sinus reaction. In the reactive node the follicles vary widely in size and shape but rarely coalesce; they have a clearly demarcated mantle of small lymphocytes and contain numerous mitotic figures and tingible body macrophages; they do not spill out into or excessively compress the intervening interfollicular pulp. In the neoplastic node, the nodules tend to be of uniform size and distribution throughout the node, spill out into and compress the adjacent pulp, and contain abnormal cells. Gross pleomorphism may be evident but the mitotic rate is often low. Tingible body macrophages are not commonly seen, but their presence does not negate absolutely a diagnosis of neoplasia. The interfollicular areas usually contain a diffuse proliferation of neoplastic cells similar to those present in the nodules in contrast to the more mixed content of cells seen in reactive conditions. The distinction between reactive and neoplastic conditions may, however, be difficult if the cellular proliferation is diffuse rather than nodular. Schroer and Franssila (1979) found that in 70 such cases 37% developed a malignant lymphoma during the subsequent 10-year period, and commented that in equivocal cases further biopsies should be taken.

REACTIVE AND INFLAMMATORY LYMPHADENOPATHY

1 Non-specific lymphadenopathy (mixed reactive and inflammatory)

PREDOMINANTLY REACTIVE

2 Toxoplasmosis
3 Rheumatoid disease
4 Viruses
   (*a*) vaccinia
   (*b*) measles
   (*c*) infectious mononucleosis
5 Drugs—phenytoin

6 Lipid
   (*a*) exogenous
   (*b*) endogenous
7 Idiopathic
   (*a*) angiofollicular hyperplasia
   (*b*) immunoblastic lymphadenopathy
   (*c*) sinus histiocytosis with massive lymphadenopathy (SHML)
8 Acute febrile mucocutaneous lymph node syndrome
9 Neoplasm

PREDOMINANTLY INFLAMMATORY

10 Tuberculosis
11 Leprosy
12 Sarcoidosis and sarcoid-like reactions
13 Syphilis
14 Brucellosis
15 Chlamydial infections
16 Yersinial infections
17 *Pneumocystis carinii* infection
18 Fungal infections
19 Degenerative lesions
   (*a*) amyloid lymphadenopathy
   (*b*) lymph node infarction

1 Non-specific lymphadenopathy

It is not uncommon to examine lymph nodes removed either because of enlargement, or as part of a pathological specimen removed for other reasons, and to identify varying degrees of the reactions described above without finding an obvious cause. An inflammatory component may be present, indicated by the presence of a few polymorphs in the sinusoids, and this may lead to fibrosis. Search for obvious infective foci in the drainage area of the node should be carried out and serological tests, where appropriate for infectious mononucleosis, toxoplasmosis, rheumatoid disease etc., recommended. In not a few instances no good cause for the adenopathy will be identified. A few of these patients later develop lymphoma and it seems likely that the node initially examined is one peripheral to a lymphomatous focus. It is for this reason that a surgeon carrying out lymph node biopsy should always remove not the most accessible but the largest and most obviously abnormal node.

2 Toxoplasmic lymphadenopathy

Toxoplasmosis is a world-wide zoonosis caused by the protozoon parasite *Toxoplasma gondii*. This is a crescentic organism, probably a coccidian (Work and Hutchison 1969), which can exist extracellularly but usually multiplies within the cytoplasm of cells by a remarkable process known as endodyogeny whereby the daughter organisms develop at first within the parent, which subsequently degenerates, liberating the new trophozoites. The parasite may exist as a 'terminal colony' within the cytoplasm of a host cell, but may also continue to divide forming cysts containing many thousands of closely-packed organisms. The organism may be of varying degrees of virulence, occasionally rapidly fatal and may be transmitted via the placenta to produce congenital disease. Acquired disease in the human, however, is usually subclinical, involving a strain of low-virulence. When they do occur, clinical manifestations are numerous (review by Beverley 1969) but by far the commonest is the lymphadeno-pathic form. This may range from the enlargement of a solitary node to a generalized lymphadenopathy with pyrexia resembling glandular fever.

The main histological findings in an involved lymph node (Piringer-Kuchinka *et al.* 1958; Saxen and Saxen 1959; Stansfeld 1961) are preservation of the architecture and a follicular hyperplasia with germinal centres in which 'tingible body macrophages' are prominent. Small aggregations of large epithelioid macrophages are prominent in the interfollicular cortex; no giant cells are seen and there is no caseation. The sinusoids are densely packed with macrophages, some 'monocytoid macrophages' (Stansfeld 1961) and some mature sinus macrophages and epithelioid histiocytes. Many plasma cells are present throughout the node and in the capsule. In an experimental study in rabbits using a strain of low-virulence Henry *et al.* (1973) reproduced many of the above changes. Organisms are rarely seen, although toxoplasma cysts have occasionally been found (Stanton and Pinkerton 1953; Stansfeld 1961), and it is probable that the lymph node changes represent an immunological reaction to the organism rather than an actual inflammation of the node (Figs 3.5 and 3.6).

The intense follicular reaction in the cortex and production of plasma cells in the medulla would suggest a response of a humoral nature and a circulating antibody is readily demonstrable (Sabin and Feldman 1948). However, a toxoplasmin skin test is positive following infection, indicating delayed hypersensitivity, and Frenkel (1967) has suggested that lymphocytes are in fact more important than humoral antibody. It is nevertheless difficult to detect a paracortical

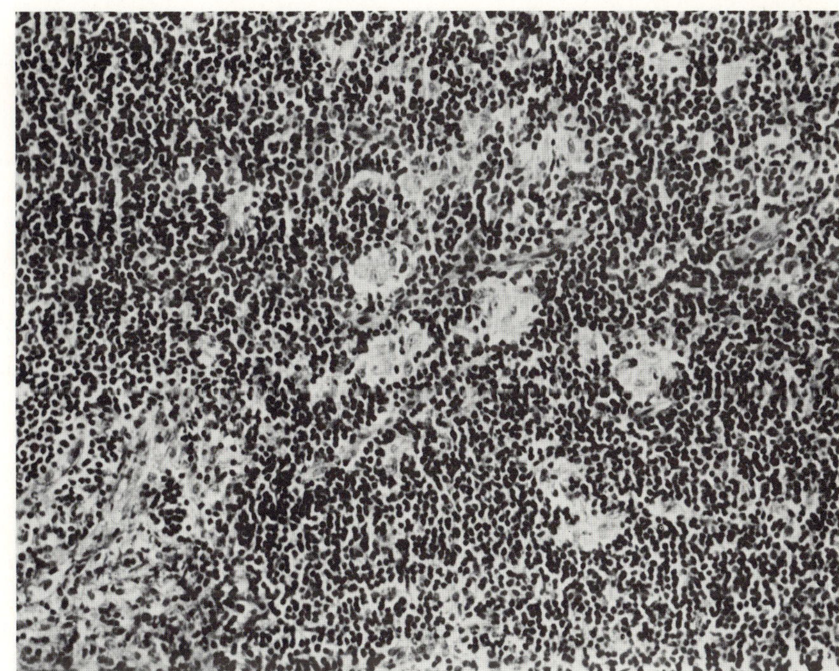

Fig. 3.5. Toxoplasmic lymphadenopathy. Clusters of large pale macrophages are scattered throughout the node—notably in the medulla. × 1,080.

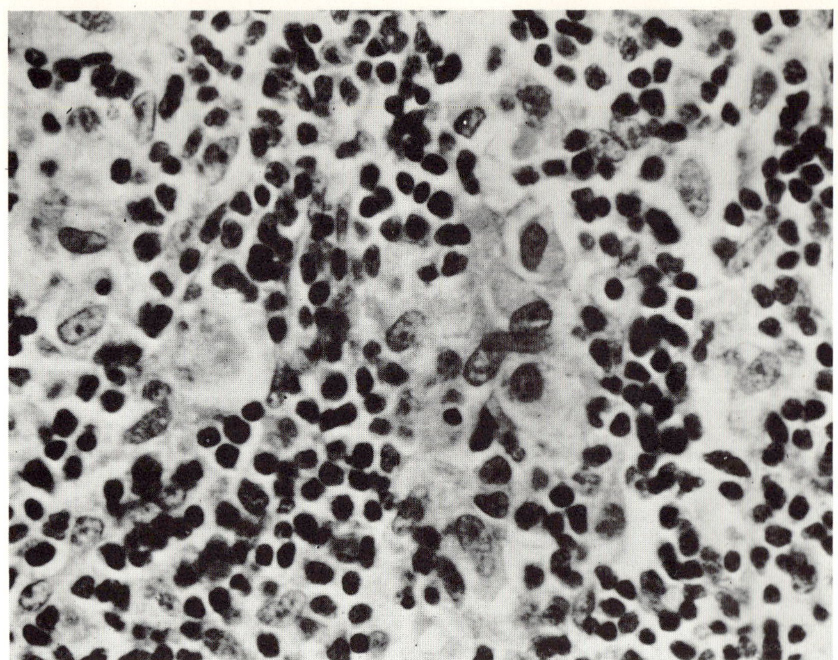

Fig. 3.6. Toxoplasmic lymphadenopathy. Detail of a cluster of macrophages. These often contain basophilic cellular debris. ×426.

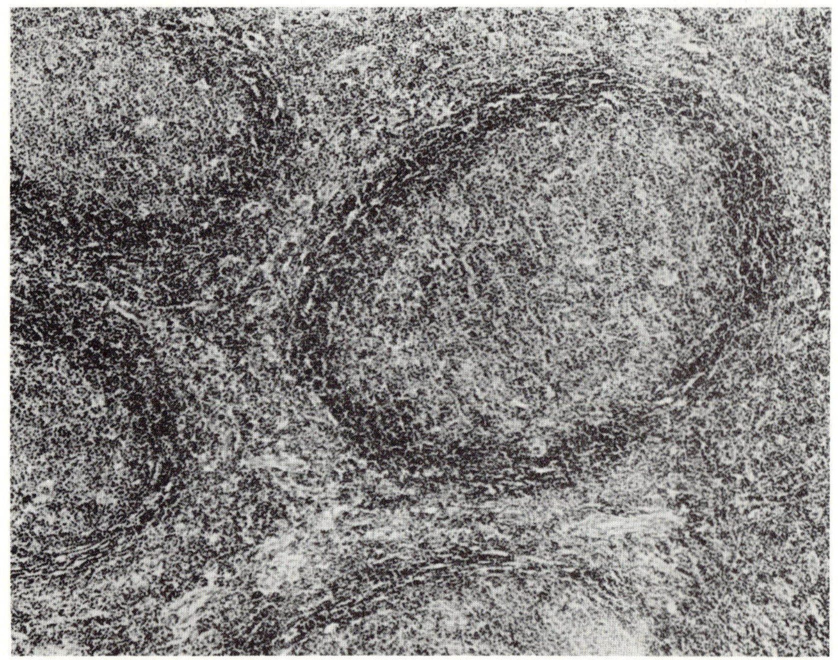

Fig. 3.7. Rheumatoid lymphadenopathy. A lymph node showing prominent follicular hyperplasia. ×45.

reaction, either in the human or experimental condition, although it is present to some extent when the high-virulence strain is used.

When the histological changes are matched with the dye-test findings, it would appear that the presence of well-marked germinal centres exhibiting cellular phago-cytosis coupled with the presence of epithelioid histiocytes is sufficient for a provisional diagnosis of toxoplasmosis, pending the result of the dye test. The only exception to this is a diagnosis of infectious mononucleosis (q.v.) which should be excluded by a Paul–Bunnell reaction.

3 Rheumatoid disease

Some 50–75% of patients with rheumatoid disease have enlargement of the lymph nodes, but since this aspect of the condition rarely creates a diagnostic problem, the nodes are rarely excised. In cases where this has been done the nodes show extreme follicular hyperplasia with follicles in both cortex and medulla. Germinal centres are well-marked and show tingible body macrophages. There is a prominent plasmacytosis in the interfollicular pulp with Russell body formation and occasional histiocytes, neutrophils and eosino-phils may be seen. The vascular endothelial cells are hypertrophied and there may be formation of new connective tissue in the node. Periadenitis may be seen and occasional nodes show a little sinus reaction. In a small number of cases amyloid deposition can be demonstrated. The differential diagnosis is mainly from the follicular forms of lymphoma (Motulsky *et al.* 1952; Cruickshank 1958; Nosanchuk and Schnitzer 1969), (Fig. 3.7), and from the rare plasmacytoma which may involve lymph nodes (Addis *et al.* 1980).

4 Virus infections

Little is known about the detailed fashion in which lymph nodes respond to virus infections. Many such infections may be associated with general or regional lymphadenopathy, but this forms part of a general febrile illness, and since the diagnosis can be made by other means, lymph node biopsy is rarely indicated. However, occasionally an enlarged node is removed to exclude a diagnosis of lymphoma in the absence of other symptoms and the histological changes may be sugges-tive of a virus aetiology although this may never be proven. The few studies that are available allow certain patterns of reaction to be defined.

a POSTVACCINIAL LYMPHADENOPATHY

Cases of this were described by Hartsock (1968) and in an experimental study by Mehrotra (1978). A variety of histolo-gical changes were present in the nodes (usually axillary). The basic nodal architecture was always preserved but there was considerable hyperplasia which may be diffuse or, later, follicular. An increased number of large cells, probably derived from transformed lymphocytes was seen with many mitotic figures, and the sinusoids contained a mixed popula-tion of lymphocytes, plasma cells and eosinophils. Focal collections of eosinophils were present in the nodal paren-chyma but no Reed–Sternberg cells were identifiable. Peri-capsular involvement was also seen. Sinus histiocytes occurred in two cases. Plasma cells were present in abundance in cases biopsied more than ten days following vaccination and follicular hyperplasia was not in evidence after 15 days. Similar changes are seen in herpes zoster (Butler 1968; Patterson *et al.* 1980).

The extreme cell proliferation and atypia, and the accumu-lation of eosinophils and plasma cells mimics the appearance of a malignant lymphoma, especially Hodgkin's disease, but the clinical history, the absence of Reed–Sternberg cells and the fact that the architecture, although distorted, is not obliterated will allow the diagnosis of lymphoma to be excluded. However a few cases of postvaccinal lymphadenitis subsequently developing Hodgkin's disease have been reported (Bichel 1976). This not only highlights the difficulty of making a diagnosis in some cases but is also of interest when considering the possible viral aetiology of Hodgkin's disease (q.v.).

b MEASLES

Warthin (1931) and Finkeldey (1931) described the cells which bear their name in the tonsils of children in the prodromal stage of measles. These are syncytial giant cells having up to 100 nuclei in a grape-like cluster in the centre of the cell, occurring both in the sub-epithelial area and in the germinal centres. Such cells are also seen in lymph nodes and in the lymphoid tissue of the gut, especially the appendix which may be removed following a clinical diagnosis of appendicitis. Allen *et al.* (1966) report a case of a lymph node removed from a child following administration of live measles vaccine. The node showed a distortion of the architecture with hyperplasia of histiocytic cells, some of which were atypical, and swelling of the capillary endothelial cells.

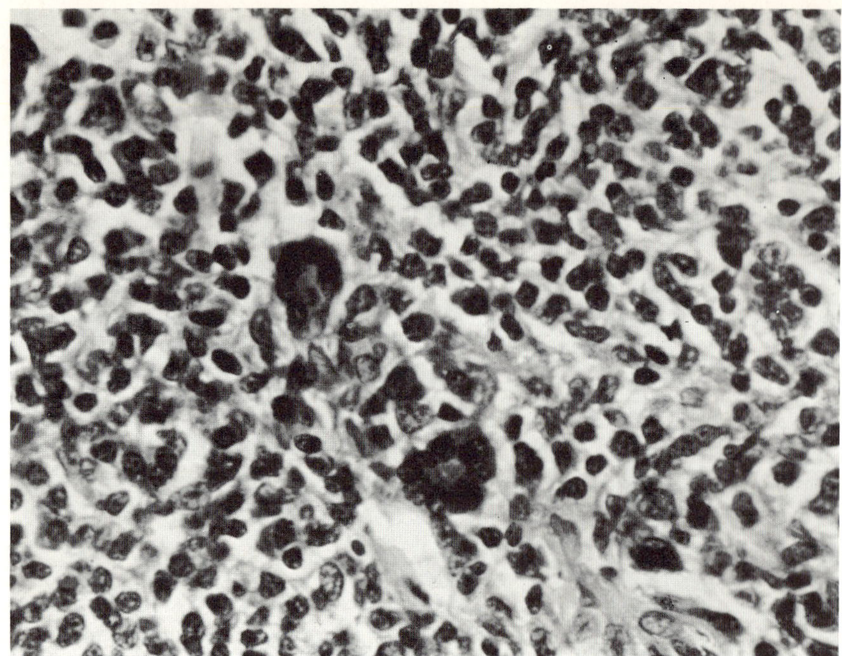

Fig. 3.8. Measles lymphadenopathy. Multinucleate, so-called Warthin–Finkeldey, giant cells are present. ×430.

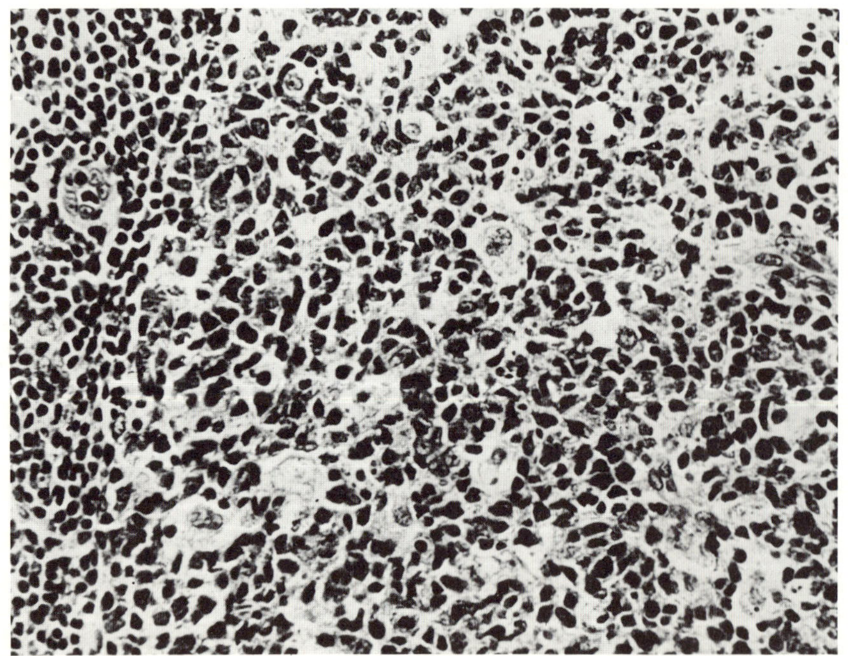

Fig. 3.9. Infectious mononucleosis. The edge of a large reactive germinal centre. There is gross nuclear pleomorphism; numerous large macrophages contain variable amounts of cell debris. The patient had grossly enlarged lymph nodes, a positive Paul–Bunnell reaction and was well four years later. ×216.

Warthin–Finkeldey giant cells were scattered throughout the substance of the node (Fig. 3.8).

c INFECTIOUS MONONUCLEOSIS

Since the diagnosis can be made by haematological means and the Paul–Bunnell reaction, lymph node biopsy is rarely undertaken. Biopsy is more likely to be performed in the atypical case and mistakes in diagnosis can occur. The histologic features have been described by several authors (Downey and Stasney 1936; Gall and Stout 1940; Custer and Smith 1948; Beswick 1955) and are related to wider aspects of the disease by Carter and Penman (1969). The appearance varies with the stage of the disease. At first the architecture of the node is preserved, with some degree of follicular hyperplasia. The germinal centres become prominent and contain tingible body macrophages and show mitotic activity. The interfollicular cortex shows histiocytic cell hyperplasia and collections of epithelioid histiocytes. The sinus pattern is maintained but some sinuses may contain lymphocytes and larger cells apparently identical with the circulating atypical mononuclear cells. The sinus-lining cells undergo hyperplasia and the medullary cords show a proliferation of lymphocytes and atypical mononuclear cells, although few plasma cells are seen. There may be infiltration of the capsule and pericapsular tissues by lymphocytes (Fig. 3.9).

At this stage the histologic appearance of the node is virtually identical with that seen in toxoplasmosis; the only point of difference is the plasma cell content of the medullary cords. The condition may now regress and the lymph node reverts to normal. However, some nodes may show a continuing hyperplasia. The germinal centres enlarge and fuse, distorting the architecture and producing solid areas of tissue where the follicular structure is indistinct or altogether absent. At the same time there is a hyperplasia of histiocytic cells with abundant mitotic activity. Although such areas may be focal, the resemblance of this stage to a malignant lymphoma may create serious diagnostic problems which are intensified by reports of cases of malignant lymphoma, particularly Hodgkin's disease following infectious mononucleosis. However, although the architecture of the node is distorted, it is not destroyed and although some histiocytic cells may be atypical, no abnormal mitoses are seen. The finding of cells resembling Reed–Sternberg cells in the disease constitutes an added diagnostic hazard in histologically difficult cases. A histological diagnosis of infectious mononucleosis always requires serological confirmation.

The investigation of a family with cancer in boys led Purtilo *et al.* (1977) to the discovery of an X-linked recessive lymphoproliferative syndrome. Manifestations of this included American Burkitt's lymphoma, mononucleosis or histiocytic lymphoma. An aproliferative phenotype was also described showing aplastic anaemia, agranulocytosis or hypogammaglobulinaemia. The proliferative forms are regarded as an abnormal response to infection with the Epstein–Barr virus (Purtilo *et al.* 1978).

LEUKAEMIA VIRUSES

It is possible though not yet proved that human leukaemia is caused by viruses. A pre-neoplastic stage obviously is not recognizable in man but studies in animals infected by leukaemogenic viruses show an early, non-specific hyperplasia of the sinus-lining cells in lymph nodes. Non-neoplastic histiocytic cells in the cortex then take up the virus. After 24 hours there is a hyperplasia of cells in the germinal centres which may proliferate to such an extent that the follicular pattern is lost. Subsequently, virus-containing cells are seen in the marrow and leukaemia supervenes (Hanna *et al.* 1970; Metcalf *et al.* 1959; Siegler *et al.* 1973). While such changes are not recognizable in the human, there may be a parallel in human patients who show only reactive hyperplasia in an early lymph node biopsy, developing lymphoma at a later stage.

5 Lymphadenopathy due to anticonvulsant drugs

Considering the vast usage of anticonvulsant drugs, lymphadenopathy is a rare complication. However, when it does occur, it presents a confusing histological picture which may simulate a lymphoma, or be diagnosed as such, especially if the drug history is not available to the pathologist. Many of the early cases reported were without histology but in 1959 Salzstein and Ackerman reviewed the literature on 75 cases and described the histology of seven of their own. Several drugs may be implicated but phenytoin is the commonest. The cervical lymph nodes are usually enlarged, other groups less frequently. This may be accompanied by fever, eosinophilia, hepatosplenomegaly, conjunctivitis and a variety of dermatological and haematological findings. Occasionally an arteritis similar to polyarteritis nodosa may occur.

Histologically the nodes show varying degrees of distortion of the architecture with a proliferation of atypical histiocytic cells showing a high mitotic rate. Plasma cells, eosinophils and immature lymphoid cells are seen. Focal areas of necrosis may be present in the cortex and some capsular infiltration may be seen (Krasznai and Gyory 1968). These authors also reported a variable follicular enlargement, but this is not recorded by others. The condition obviously mimics Hodgkin's disease and diagnosis may be extremely difficult especially if the architecture of the node appears to be obliterated (Rosenfeld *et al.* 1961). However, typical Reed–Sternberg cells are not seen, there is no invasion of blood vessel walls and on close inspection the architecture is distorted rather than destroyed (Hyman and Sommers 1966). Usually the lymphadenopathy regresses on cessation of the drug but occasionally it does not and may persist or resolve and then recur, even though the administration of the drug has not been resumed. In these cases, distinction from a lymphoma is difficult; matters are made more difficult by the rare development of true lymphoma in such patients. One of Saltzstein and Ackerman's patients subsequently died of a malignant lymphoma (Saltzstein 1962) and Hyman and Sommers (1966) reported six such cases, three with Hodgkin's disease and three with lymphosarcoma. Gams *et al.* (1968) report a case diagnosed histologically as a malignant lymphoma of a pleomorphic histiocytic type. On stopping the drug a complete regression of the disease ensued only to be followed by a recurrence 20 months

later and death from a malignant lymphoma of the type previously seen. It may be that such patients have had a malignant lymphoma unrelated to the drug administration but it is also possible that the anticonvulsant acts in such a way as to induce neoplasia in rare instances.

Reactions may occur with other drugs, among them para-amino salicylic acid and phenylbutazone and similar histological appearances may be seen in lymph nodes in serum sickness.

6 Reaction of lymph nodes to lipid

Injected lipid passes to the local lymph nodes and is taken up by macrophages, first in the capsular sinuses and then in the medulla. The fat may remain within macrophages, giving their cytoplasm a foamy appearance, to form small globules of lipid in the substance of the node which may incite an inflammatory reaction in the adjacent parenchyma. Fat derived endogenously may also be taken up by the lymph node. There are a number of common causes of this phenomenon which may be divided into exogenous and endogenous as follows:

a EXOGENOUS

Lymphangiography. Bronchography. Inhalation lipoid

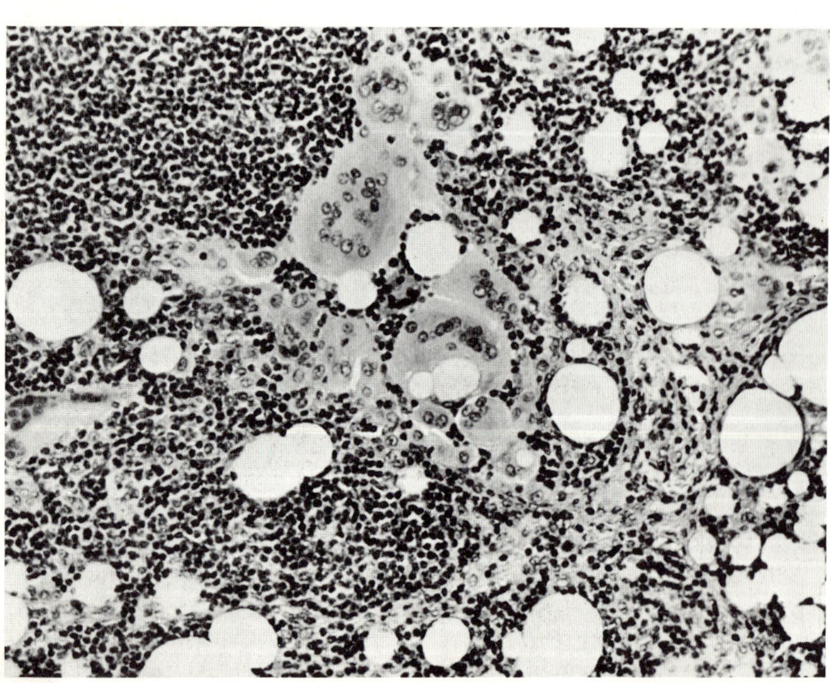

Fig. 3.10. Lymph node showing a granulomatous reaction to lipid. Numerous multinucleate giant cells are related to oil vacuoles. Postlymphangiography granuloma. × 108.

pneumonia. Injection of haemorrhoids with lipid-based material. Injection of Freund's adjuvant (in animals).

b ENDOGENOUS

Dermatopathic lymphadenopathy and lipogranulomatosis.

RESPONSE OF LYMPH NODES TO LYMPHANGIOGRAPHY

The response to iodine-containing contrast media in an oily base is described by Harrison (1966). The medium is injected directly into a lymphatic vessel and passes to the lymph node where it forms large droplets in the subcapsular and medullary sinuses, reaching a diameter of up to 100 μm; after 4 days a reaction is seen round the oil droplets with prominent giant-cell formation. The architecture of the node is not distorted and after 10 days or so resolution commences. The nodes may eventually return to normal, though only after a prolonged period (Fig. 3.10).

DERMATOPATHIC LYMPHADENOPATHY

This condition was first described by Pautrier and Woringer in 1937 and is reviewed by Harrison (1960). It is a lymphadenopathy associated with a variety of skin conditions and characterized by the accumulation of lipid material, melanin and occasionally haemosiderin in the node. It may be occasioned by the skin condition itself or by the associated scratching. It usually resolves as the primary skin condition heals.

The affected node shows some follicular reaction but the prominent feature is an accumulation of pale macrophages in the outer medulla or in the cortex, widely separating the follicles with some distortion of architecture. These cells contain lipid, usually cholesterol, and melanin, or occasionally both. Haemosiderin was present in three of the 13 cases reported by Nairn and Anderson (1955). There is some sinus hyperplasia and sometimes infiltration with plasma cells and eosinophils (see Fig. 3.22).

LIPOGRANULOMATOSIS

This term was used by Warner and Friedman in 1956 to refer to the reaction in lymph node or spleen to any lipid material often arising from such endogenous sources as haematomas, tumours, cholesterol deposits, xanthomatous lesions, fat embolism and fat necrosis. In practice the only condition presenting as a diagnostic problem is lipogranulomatosis of the nodes draining the biliary system, particularly the cystic lymph node. In 84 of a series of 125 cases of cholelithiasis described by Spain (1957), the disordered handling of lipid by the gall bladder caused lipid accumulation in the cystic node with the formation of a giant cell granuloma and ultimate fibrosis. Birefringent sudanophilic lipid was seen both intracellularly and extracellularly. The condition was twice as frequent in men, suggesting a sex difference in the handling of lipid. Similar lesions occur in the spleen, curiously more commonly in North America than in the UK (Cruickshank 1975 personal communication).

7 Idiopathic

This group includes three distinct lesions of differing histological structure and prognosis accompanied by differing and various systemic manifestations and degrees of immunological dysfunction.

a ANGIOFOLLICULAR LYMPH NODE HYPERPLASIA

This condition has been reported under various synonyms since 1921 (Symmers 1921) as a condition involving haemolymph nodes (Pemberton *et al.* 1950). It usually presents as a mediastinal mass to be distinguished from a thymoma (Thorburn *et al.* 1952; Iverson 1956). In 1954 Castleman and Towne reported a case of hyperplasia of the mediastinal lymph nodes and 13 such cases were subsequently recorded (Castleman *et al.* 1956). These showed follicular hyperplasia with or without germinal centre formation, but a blood vessel at the centre of the follicle showed endothelial hyperplasia. The perivascular region contained a proliferation of concentrically arranged pale cells with areas of hyalinization giving a superficial resemblance to Hassall's corpuscles, and simulating a thymoma. Varying numbers of plasma cells and eosinophils were present. Castleman considered these changes as a response to continued chronic inflammation.

Since 1954, over 100 of these cases have been reported and their diverse nomenclature indicates that the nature of the condition is far from settled. The literature to 1967 is reviewed by Tung and McCormack (1967) and from then by Anagnostou and Harrison (1972). The majority of cases occur in the mediastinum but similar changes may be seen in the cervical, retroperitoneal or mesenteric lymph nodes and a variety of other sites. The name 'angiofollicular lymph node hyperplasia' was given by Harrison and Bernatz (1963), but

Lattes and Pachter (1962), finding the disease in sites unrelated to lymph nodes, felt that a hamartomatous nature was more likely. Zettergren (1961), however, thought that the lesion was probably neoplastic and termed it as 'follicular lymphoreticulum'. However, the clinical outcome of these cases is universally good and thus the condition is unlikely to represent a malignant lymphoma, although a benign neoplasm cannot be excluded. Multicentric cases however, have been reported with a clinical presentation similar to angioimmunoblastic lymphadenopathy and a rapid decline (Bartoli *et al.* 1980).

Approximately 10% of cases have systemic symptoms which are cured by surgical removal of the lesion. These include fever with a raised ESR, sweating and fatigue, haematological abnormalities including thrombocytopenia and anaemia (Kahn *et al.* 1973) and immunological disorders including hyperglobulinaemia (Ballow *et al.* 1974). An isolated case has been reported as associated with myasthenia gravis (Emson 1973). In these patients, the follicles in the lesion contain germinal centres and Flendrig, quoted by Anagnostou and Harrison (1972) suggests that on this basis the condition falls into two groups termed by Keller *et al.* (1972) the 'hyaline-vascular' and 'plasma cell' types.

'Hyaline-vascular' type (systemic symptoms rare)

Follicular masses of lymphocytes are evenly distributed throughout the lesion but germinal centres are small. A capillary blood vessel at the centre of the follicles has plump endothelial cells, the surrounding cells being flattened and coming to resemble a Hassall's corpuscle. There is a considerable amount of hyaline fibrous tissue both around the central blood vessel and in the interfollicular tissue, with occasional areas of calcification. The lymphocytes in the centre of the follicles are arranged in a concentrically laminated fashion. Between the follicles there is an abundance of small capillaries and a mixed cell infiltrate of lymphocytes, plasma cells, immunoblasts, eosinophils and histiocytes. In 44 of the 74 cases in this group, areas of normal lymph node structure could be identified, although in the lesion itself no sinusoids were present. In 17 cases, sections of adjacent lymph nodes showed plasma cell accumulation or hyaline follicles.

Plasma cell type (systemic symptoms common)

Sheets of mature plasma cells are seen in the interfollicular tissue. Occasional sinusoids are present. Germinal centres are

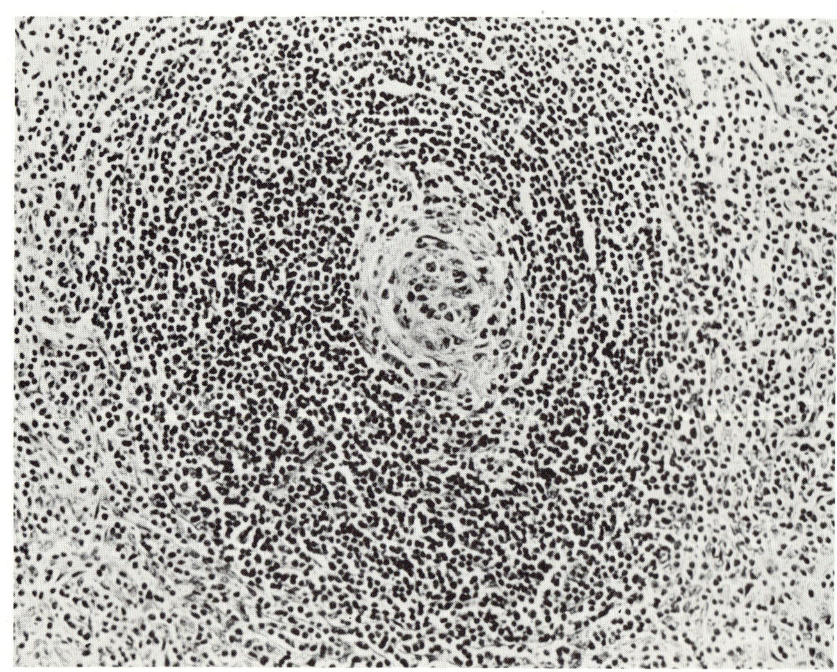

Fig. 3.11. Lymph node showing angiofollicular hyperplasia. In the core of a nodule of small lymphocytes lies a mass of hyaline connective tissue with a blood vessel. × 108.

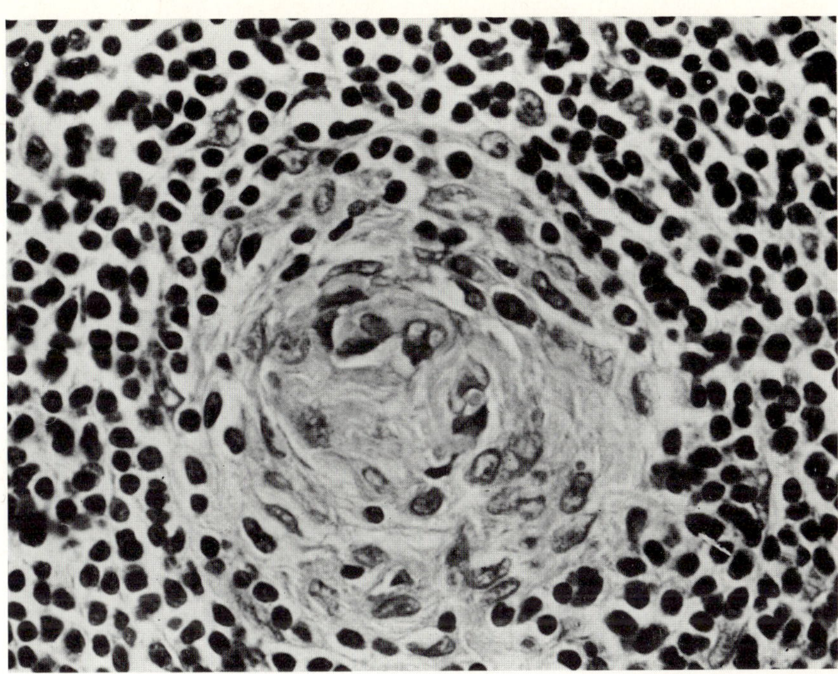

Fig. 3.12. Detail of nodule in angiofollicular hyperplasia showing a collagenous core with a small blood vessel. ×430.

present in the follicles and may attain a large size, containing mitotic figures, nuclear debris and histiocytes, but no central blood vessel is seen and no hyalinization. Remnants of lymph node architecture are present and some follicles are of the hyaline-vascular type. The clinical mass is usually a collection of discrete lymph nodes.

The connection between these two types is emphasized by cases showing areas of both hyaline-vascular and plasma cell configuration. Keller *et al.* (1972) conclude that the condition is reactive rather than hamartomatous, although the primary stimulus remains to be defined. They postulate that the two types represent phases of a single process, the plasma cell type being the early response later transposing to the hyaline-vascular (Figs. 3.11 and 3.12).

Differential diagnosis is from a follicular lymphoma, Hodgkin's disease, thymoma and reactive conditions with a large plasma cell content such as rheumatoid disease. A reticulin stain is often valuable to emphasize the vascularity of the lesion.

b ANGIOIMMUNOBLASTIC LYMPHADENOPATHY WITH DYSPROTEINAEMIA (AILD)

A disease syndrome in which there is a lymphoma-like clinical pattern and a non-neoplastic histological picture has been described by Frizzera *et al.* (1974) and by Lukes and Tindle (1975). It presents usually in people over 60 with severe constitutional symptoms—fever, sweats, chills and malaise, accompanied by leucocytosis, and anaemia. The lymph node architecture is diffusely, but only partially obliterated by immunoblasts of varying maturity (Fig. 3.13), and a proliferation of small blood vessels, often with a high endothelium similar to lymph node postcapillary venules. There may be an accumulation of PAS-positive intercellular material. None of these features is specific if taken individually (Brearley *et al.* 1979) but when considered as a whole, together with the clinical picture, a characteristic pattern emerges. There is usually polyclonal gammopathy, sometimes a cryoglobulinaemia, neutrophil or eosinophil leucocytosis and often anaemia, sometimes haemolytic with a positive Coombs' test; there may be nephropathy due to immunoglobulin deposition in the glomerulus (Wood and Hawkins 1979), and may be accompanied by a variety of autoimmune phenomena and depression of cellular immunity. The natural history of the condition is not clearly defined since many have been treated as lymphomas. It seems that intensive antitumour chemotherapy and radiotherapy worsen the prognosis, potentiating infection; some are controlled by steroids, perhaps with added cyclophosphamide; many die of severe infections. The lesion

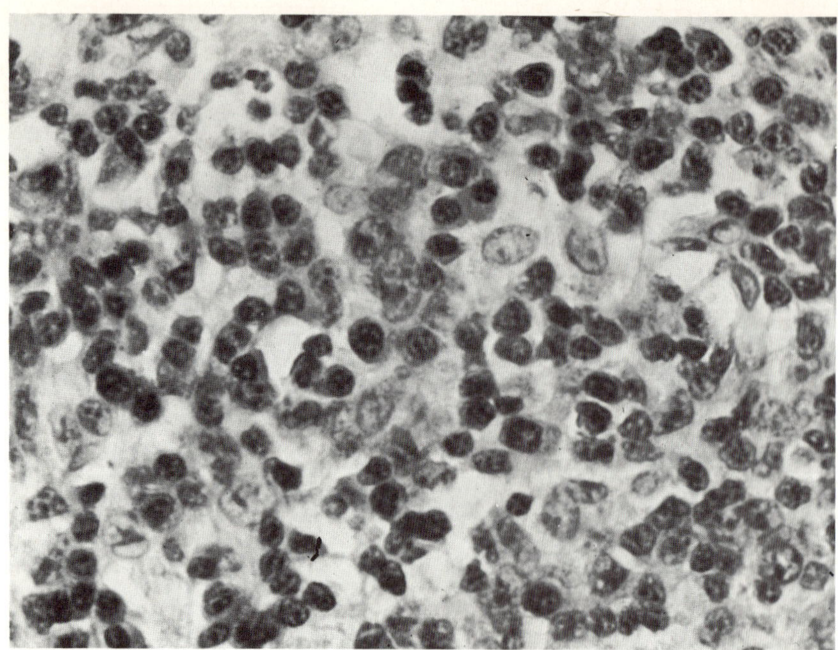

Fig. 3.13. Lymph node from a patient with immunoblastic lymphadenopathy showing infiltration with plasma cells and immunoblastic cells. ×430.

is probably not a neoplasm, although histologically it may bear some relation to Hodgkin's disease and some cases transpose into an immunoblastic sarcoma (Frizzera *et al.* 1974; Lukes and Collins 1975) or into a plasmacytoid malignant lymphoma (Fisher *et al.* 1976). It bears some resemblance to a graft-versus-host reaction; similar changes are described in lymph nodes in lupus erythematosus accompanied by areas of focal necrosis and deposits of haematoxyphil material, presumably nuclear debris (Dorfman and Warnke 1974). The condition may be due to a defect in the regulation of the immune response by suppressor T cells, but the exact aetiology remains to be clarified. A report of ten cases and a review of the literature is given by Cullen *et al.* (1979); survival for more than 2 years is uncommon.

c SINUS HISTIOCYTOSIS WITH MASSIVE LYMPHADENOPATHY

In 1966 Azoury and Reed reported the case of a child aged 2 years presenting with fever and enlargement of the axillary and inguinal lymph nodes. The lymph node showed proliferation of cells in the sinuses and the illustration showed that these were actively phagocytic. Following this, Rosai and Dorfman (1969) recorded four cases showing similar histological changes. They termed the condition 'Sinus histiocytosis

with massive lymphadenopathy' and subsequently published a further 30 cases (Rosai and Dorfman 1972).

The patients tend to be in the younger age group and to present with enlargement of the cervical lymph nodes, often massive. Other groups of nodes are less affected and occasionally there is involvement of the tonsil, testis, orbit and skin. The enlarged nodes are painless and constitutional symptoms are not prominent, although fever and a raised ESR do occur. Anaemia and leucocytosis have been reported and there is a significant degree of hyperglobulinaemia usually involving IgG. The disease runs a benign course with eventual resolution after several months or years.

The lymph nodes show a fibrous thickening of capsule, which may extend somewhat to involve adjacent tissues. The cut surface has an orange-brown colour and the gross architecture is distorted by fibrosis. Histologically there is a dilatation of the sinusoids by histiocytes and this may be so extreme as to distort the architecture. The cells are actively phagocytic and can be shown to have ingested a variety of cells, mostly lymphocytes but occasionally neutrophil polymorphs, plasma cells or erythrocytes. Initially the phagocytosed cells are well-preserved but are eventually broken down, the histiocytes then containing cell debris and lipid material. Mitotic figures are rare in these cells and no organisms can be demonstrated. Lennert *et al.* (1972) consider that there are

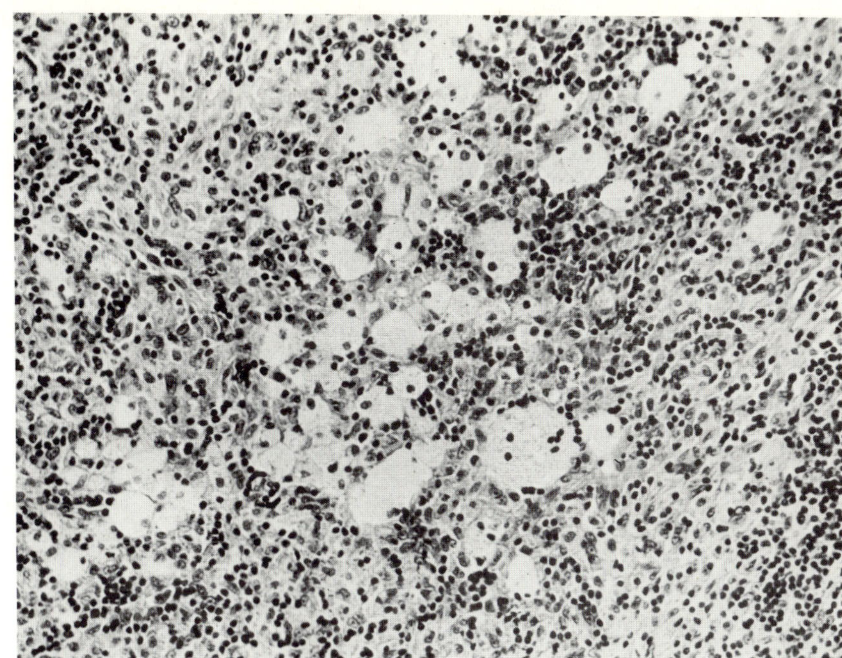

Fig. 3.14. Lymph node from a patient with
sinus histiocytosis with massive
lymphadenopathy (SHML) showing large
foamy macrophages in the sinusoids.
×108.

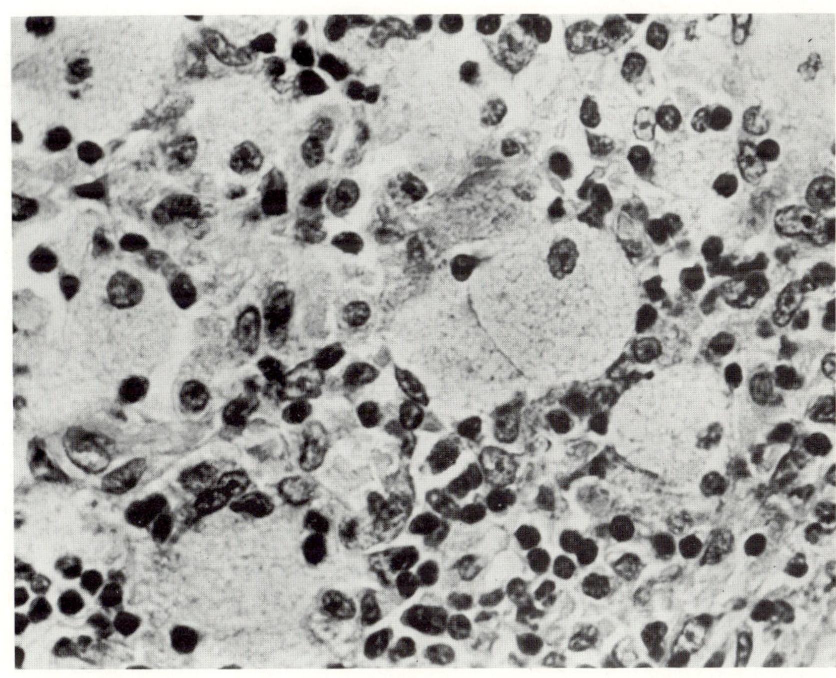

Fig. 3.15. Detail of lymph node in SHML
showing large macrophages. ×430.

two forms of sinus histiocyte, one having a faintly-staining cytoplasm and showing prominent phagocytosis, the other with an eosinophilic cytoplasm and a tendency to giant cell formation, with rather less phagocytic activity. The same authors demonstrated histiocytes in the pulp between the sinuses, probably derived from blood monocytes, the pulp also containing numbers of plasma cells, although eosinophils were rare. Electron microscopy confirms that the cells in the sinusoids are macrophages (Sinclair-Smith *et al.* 1974) (Figs 3.14 and 3.15).

The aetiology of the condition is unknown. It is not neoplastic and no infective agent can be implicated. It is not known whether the basic defect lies in the macrophages which are abnormally stimulated, or in the ingested cells, rendering them more liable to phagocytosis. Beecroft *et al.* (1973) showed a decreased response of lymphocytes to PHA in one case, which returned to normal as the patient improved.

This is therefore a rare condition but one which must be distinguished from lymphoma and malignant histiocytosis.

8 Acute febrile mucocutaneous lymph node syndrome (Kawasaki's disease)

First described by Kawasaki in 1967 in Japan (see Kawasaki *et al.* 1974), in Hawaii (Melish *et al.* 1976) and in other parts of the world, this syndrome consists of fever, congestion of the ocular conjunctiva, lesions on the oral mucosa, erythema and oedema of the extremities, a polymorphic rash and acute non-suppurative enlargement of the cervical lymph nodes. It occurs almost exclusively in children and in fatal cases autopsy has revealed a close resemblance of the disease to infantile polyarteritis nodosa, the coronary arteries being particularly affected. The lymph nodes show a non-specific reactive lymphoid hyperplasia. The condition is of unknown aetiology. A review of the literature is given by Yanagihara and Todd (1980).

9 Lymph node changes in non-lymphoreticular neoplasia

When a neoplasm metastasizes to a lymph node it usually rapidly replaces and destroys it. Evidence of a reaction to the tumour is usually scanty and the reaction almost always ineffectual. Any function which lymph nodes have of delaying the spread of tumours is a very temporary one. Only a few tumour cells if any can be destroyed in a node. The origin of metastatic tumour may be evident or may be demonstrable by immunoperoxidase staining of tissue markers indicating

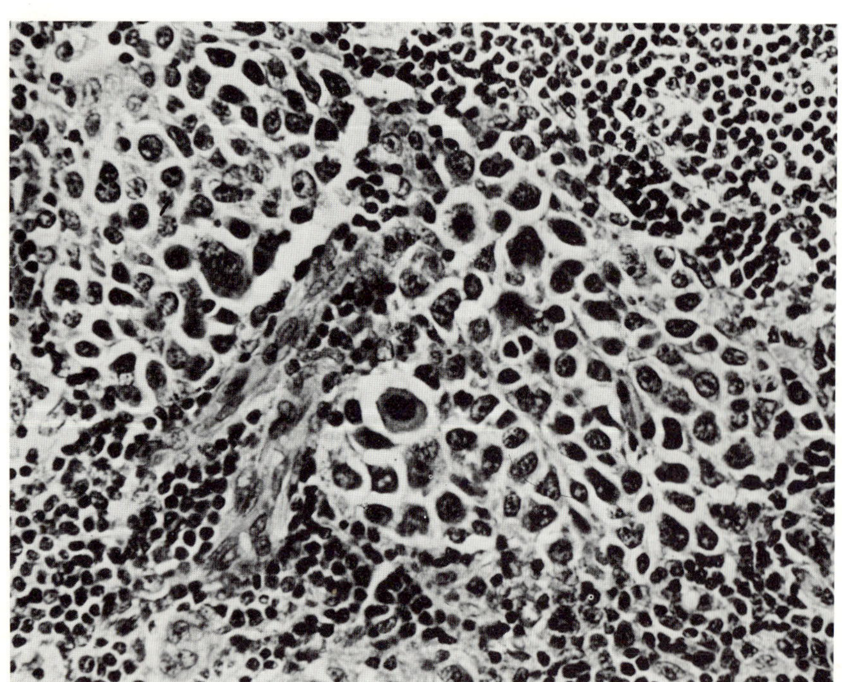

Fig. 3.16. A lymph node showing infiltration by pleomorphic malignant cells; some of these could be confused with malignant lymphoreticular cells. Note the clear line of demarcation between the neoplastic cells and the adjacent lymphoid tissue. ×216.

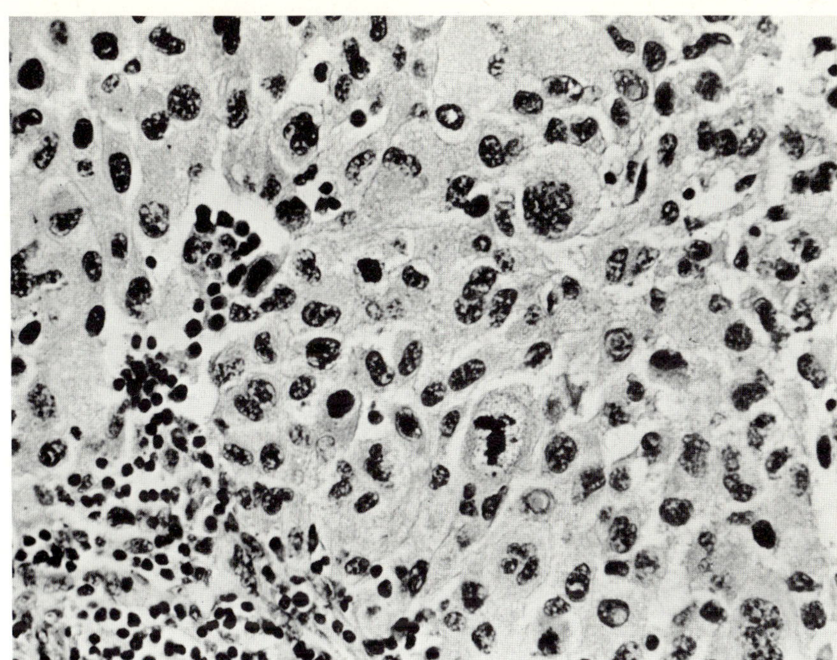

Fig. 3.17. A lymph node showing infiltration by the pleomorphic malignant cells of secondary malignant melanoma. These cells bear a superficial resemblance to malignant histiocytes. ×216.

specifically or less specifically the tissue of origin. The changes seen in lymph nodes carcinoma are:

(*a*)   Obvious replacement with evident neoplasm—usually cancer. Where the sinusoids are packed with large carcinoma or amelanotic melanoma cells, this may rarely cause confusion with the changes of malignant histiocytosis (Figs 3.16 and 3.17).

(*b*)   Small foci of cancer cells in a subcapsular sinus. This is rare. Some such foci appear degenerate and may not survive (Fig. 3.18).

(*c*)   Diffuse intermingling of cancer cells with lymphocytes as in secondary deposits from lymphoepithelioma of the nasopharynx. This can be difficult to identify as secondary neoplasm.

(*d*)   infiltration with small round or oat-shaped cells usually derived from a bronchial primary. This can be hard or impossible to discriminate from small cell lymphoma.

(*e*)   infiltration with large carcinoma cells with some fibrosis, usually from a bronchial or thyroid primary. This can be confused with atypical Hodgkin's disease.

(*f*)   Lymph nodes draining a neoplasm may be enlarged in the absence of metastasis (reviewed by Carr 1980). The best known change is sinus histiocytosis (Black *et al.* 1953) in which the sinuses are filled with large eosinophilic histio-cytes—so-called sinus histiocytosis—probably reflecting hyperplasia and hypertrophy of sinus macrophages and increased traffic through the node. It is commoner in the nodes draining breast cancers in Japanese patients where the disease has a less malignant course (Friedell *et al.* 1974). McDivitt (1978), however, did not regard sinus histiocytosis as a useful prognostic feature. An attempt has been made to relate lymphocyte populations, in lymph nodes draining tumour, to prognosis (Tsakraklides *et al.* 1974 and 1975). Four patterns were described—lymphocyte predominance, where the extrafollicular (T cell) parts of the node are stuffed with lymphocytes, follicular (B cell) reaction, an intermediate, average state, and lymphocyte depletion. In the case of breast, uterus, cervical and upper respiratory carcinoma, lymphocyte predominance is held to be associated with good prognosis and lymphocyte depletion with bad prognosis. The present practical importance of these findings is not clear. Sarcoid reactions occur rarely in nodes draining neoplasms.

An unusual and complex set of changes are seen in lymph nodes in Kaposi's sarcoma. There may be a follicular hyperplasia sometimes of striking vascularity, accompanied by plasma cell infiltration of the medullary cords. The node may also show an angiomatous pattern and spindle cell proliferation in the sinusoids, presumably representing metastasis. The

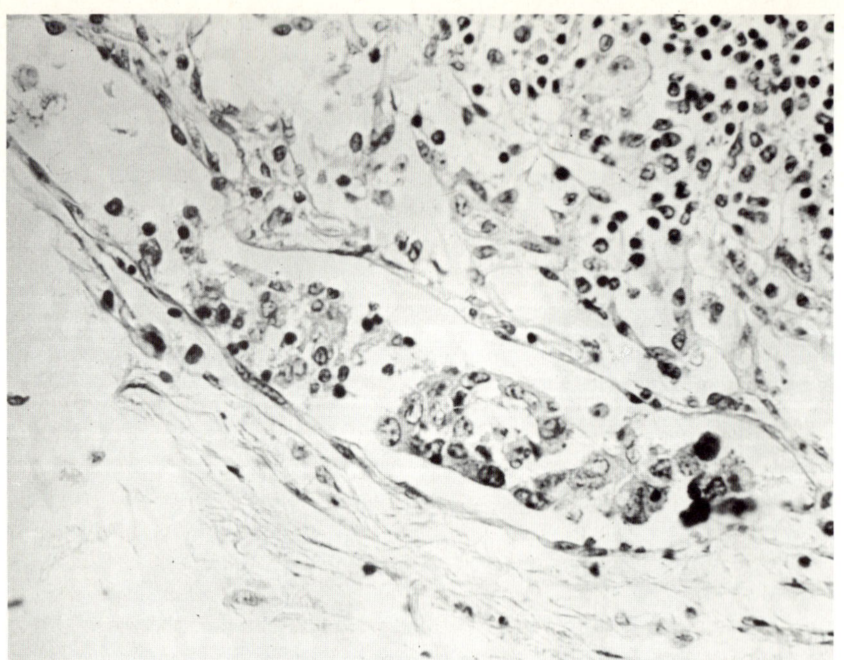

Fig. 3.18. A cluster of carcinoma cells in the subcapsular sinus of an axillary lymph node draining a carcinoma of breast. The primary lesion showed a well marked lymphocytic response; the group of cells in the field illustrated was the only evidence of metastasis in a radical mastectomy specimen. × 335.

lymphadenopathy may be accompanied by hepatosplenomegaly, anaemia and hyperglobulinaemia (Lubin and Rywlin 1971; Dorfman and Warnke 1974). Patients with Kaposi's sarcoma also have an increased incidence of malignant lymphoma.

The rare occurrence of heterotopic mature epithelium in lymph nodes must not be confused with secondary carcinoma.

Congenital heterotopic rests of different cell types may rarely occur in lymph nodes—for instance, rests of squamous epithelium, columnar epithelium, glandular epithelium, melanocytes or thyroid epithelium, either in the capsule or less commonly in the interior of the node. Diagnosis depends on the presence or absence of the usual criteria of malignancy—dedifferentiation, pleomorphism and mitosis. Particular difficulty can occur in the case of rests of melanocytes in a node draining a melanoma and of aberrant thyroid epithelium. Current opinion is that the latter nearly always represent metastasis from occult thyroid carcinoma. There are very rare reports of carcinoma arising from a benign inclusion (Edlow and Carter 1973; Hart 1971; McCarthy *et al.* 1974; Meyer and Steinberg 1969).

INFLAMMATORY CONDITIONS

As noted above, inflammation in a lymph node has banal characteristics but is commonly modified by reactive changes in the node, and also by the progressing immunological status of the host in relation to the causative organism. Some consideration will be given here to the special circumstances of development in lymph nodes of two important granulomas, tuberculosis and leprosy.

The systemic immune response is of importance in determining the histological pattern in several granulomatous lesions. In leprosy in particular the degree of cellular immune response is important (Turk and Waters 1971). Humoral factors may also play a role in development of a granuloma (Chapman 1972). For instance, in histoplasmosis and coccidioidomycosis, circulating antibodies may be present in the first two weeks of infection before cell-mediated immunity (as shown by a positive skin test) develops. Initial immobilization of macrophages in a granuloma may depend on production of macrophage migration inhibition factor by sensitized lymphocytes, and continuation of the granulomatous response may be related to local deposition of antigen–antibody complex. Where high immunoglobulin levels exist in the absence of delayed hypersensitivity, dissemination of infection may occur, e.g. in lepromatous leprosy.

10 Tuberculous lymphadenopathy

In a study of granuloma formation in lymph nodes, Gaafar and Turk (1970) found that soluble antigens injected into the skin produced only reactive changes in the follicles, whereas BCG inoculation resulted in the formation of granulomas. These are formed, in the first instance, by macrophages which have been transported in the lymphatics from the area of inflammation at the site of injection. The macrophages accumulate in the subcapsular sinus for the first few days during which time reactive changes occur in the cortex and medulla. During the next few weeks the macrophages, containing organisms, migrate slowly into the paracortical areas, enlarge, assume an epithelioid appearance and form localized granulomas in which latterly local division of macrophages occurs (Epstein 1967). With the development of delayed hypersensitivity, central necrosis occurs in the granulomas with eventual caseation.

Tuberculous granulomas (Fig. 3.19) are frequently seen in human lymph nodes—tuberculosis presenting in a lymph node accounts for 40% of all cases of non-respiratory

infection (Hooper 1972). The classical histologic appearance of caseating giant cell granulomas present little difficulty and acid-fast bacilli may be demonstrated, although they may be scanty. Lymphadenopathy may also be due to infection with an atypical 'anonymous' mycobacterium and in these the histological pattern may vary slightly. MacKellar *et al.* (1967) observed fewer giant cells and more basophilic nuclear debris in such lesions. Reid and Wolinsky (1969) found that 7 out of 30 cases showed suppuration and granulomatous inflammation without caseation, although they felt that the changes were not sufficiently characteristic to be diagnostic.

The relation of the immune status of the patient to the histological pattern in the node is not entirely clear-cut. In explant cultures, tubercle bacilli can remain for long periods within macrophages in a state of apparent symbiosis (Breiger 1949). The formation of definitive granulomas *in vivo* may depend on the development of delayed hypersensitivity, and central caseation may follow conversion to tuberculin positivity. In the so-called non-reactive form of tuberculosis, large numbers of acid-fast bacilli are found in the lesions, which show areas of necrosis without granuloma formation (O'Brien 1954). In such cases there is usually a haematological abnormality which may be associated with depression of cellular immunity; similar lesions are seen with tuberculosis in patients receiving steroids (Forbes 1961). Occasionally it

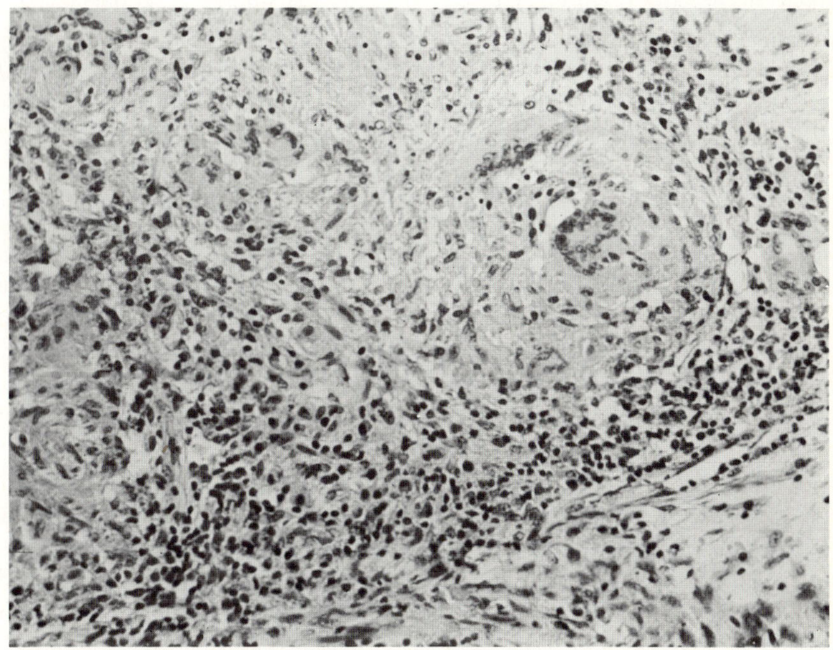

Fig. 3.19. Lymph node showing a tuberculous granuloma with a giant cell system and scanty caseation. × 108.

may be difficult to distinguish tuberculous granulomas from sarcoid granulomas (Drury 1970). Occasionally central necrosis in a sarcoid granuloma may simulate caseation while tuberculous granulomas may be non-caseating at some stage in their evolution (Lewis 1961). The fine structure of the granulomas in these two conditions may show certain similarities (Jones Williams *et al.* 1970) but tubercle bacilli may be ultrastructurally demonstrable. Giant cell granulomas are present in the mesenteric nodes of over one-third of cases of Crohn's disease (Cook 1972) but the condition seldom presents as a lymph node abnormality and diagnostic difficulty is rare.

11 Lymphadenopathy in leprosy

The role of the immune response in the formation of granulomas is clearly seen in the response to infection with *Mycobacterium leprae* (Turk and Waters 1971). The pathological response to this organism ranges from the tuberculoid form in patients with well-developed cell-mediated immunity and a positive lepromin reaction to the lepromatous form with poor cell-mediated immunity and a negative lepromin reaction. Intermediate cases are described as 'borderline' leprosy. Lymph nodes from patients with tuberculoid leprosy show only reactive changes even though granulomatous lesions are present in the tissues of the draining area. Such nodes may show hyperplasia of the paracortical areas with dividing immunoblasts. 'Borderline' cases show less ability to inhibit the spread of the organism and sarcoid-like granulomas develop in and may almost replace the paracortical areas. Acid-fast bacilli are either absent or seen in only small numbers.

In the lepromatous form the lymph nodes are commonly enlarged, the paracortical areas show extensive lymphoid depletion and are infiltrated with large numbers of foamy macrophages containing acid-fast bacilli. The macrophages may tend to coalesce into syncytial clumps and giant cells may be seen but no true granulomas are formed. The cortex of the node may show a follicular reaction with germinal centre formation and abundant plasma cells. Thus, although these patients demonstrate a deficient delayed hypersensitivity, humoral immunity may be normal, although clearly insufficient of itself to eliminate the infection. Turk and Waters (1971) postulate that the immunological deficiency may be genetically determined, since cure of lepromatous leprosy is not accompanied by a return to lepromin positivity. However, other lymphoid organs may be involved in the infection, particularly the thymus, where the multiplication of bacteria may be greater than in the lymph nodes (Gaugas *et al.* 1970), leading to a secondary depression of cell-mediated responses. In leprosy, necrosis is rarely seen in the lymph nodes but an acute necrotizing lymphadenitis may be seen in some patients with lepromatous leprosy and erythema nodosum leprosum. The condition is a manifestation of an acute vasculitis and is probably immunologically mediated, responding to treatment with steroids or ACTH (Karat *et al.* 1968).

12 Sarcoidosis and sarcoid-like reactions

Sarcoidosis is a systemic disease characterized by the presence in many organs of a non-caseating giant cell granulomatous lesion. It may present as an acute febrile illness or as a more chronic respiratory disorder. Lesions are found in skin, joints, lungs, uveal tract, salivary and lacrimal glands and even in the heart and central nervous system. Enlargement of lymph nodes and spleen commonly occurs. The aetiology is unknown and the prognosis good; less than 5% of cases progress to severe disability (see Scadding 1967; Citron 1972 for reviews).

The lymph nodes show diffuse loss of architecture and infiltration by large eosinophilic epithelioid macrophages, characteristically arranged in clusters, with a varying lymphocytic infiltrate and sometimes, notably in the later stages, peripheral fibrosis (Fig. 3.20). The macrophages interlock closely and fuse to form giant cells. Three kinds of inclusion are found usually in the giant cells. Birefringent crystals (3–10 μm) of calcium carbonate are common; much larger basophil bodies with scalloped edges (conchoidal or Schaumann bodies) probably form around these crystals and represent residual bodies, e.g. secondary lysosomes. Acidophilic star shaped ('asteroid') inclusions are much less common (Jones Williams *et al.* 1968 and 1970).

A sarcoid-like reaction is found in lymph nodes in other situations—in berylliosis, rarely in lymph nodes draining neoplasms, and rarely in malignant lymphoma. In the latter situation the presence of a very few malignant histiocytic cells scattered throughout the sarcoid lesion may indicate the need for further biopsy (Fig. 3.21 and 3.22). This will show malignant lymphoma. Giant cell granulomas similar to those of sarcoidosis are demonstrable in the mesenteric nodes of about one third of patients with Crohn's disease (Cook 1972). The disease however seldom presents as a lymph node abnormality and diagnostic difficulty is rare. Similarly granulomatous lesions occur in intestinal lymph nodes in Whipple's

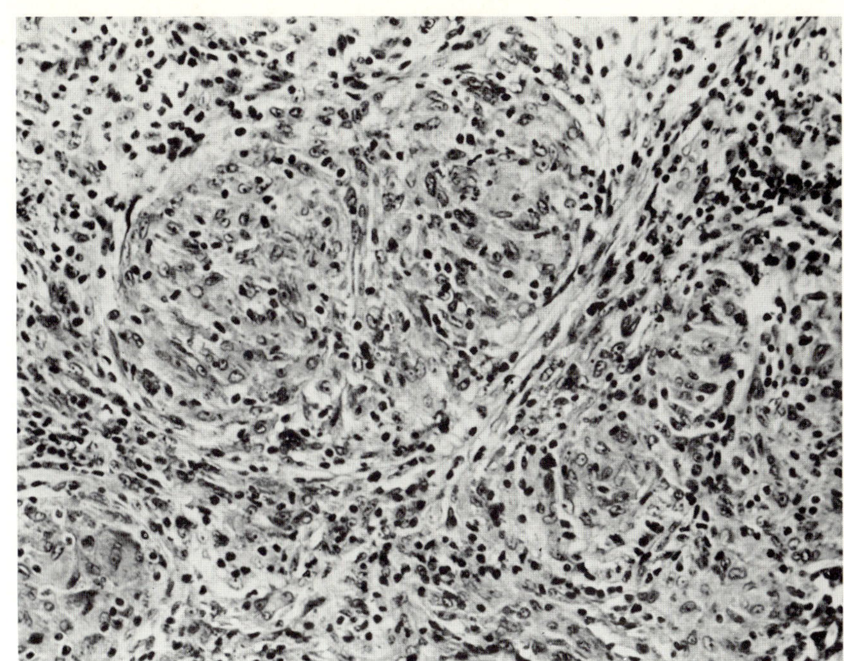

Fig. 3.20. Lymph node showing a non-caseating granuloma with numerous large histiocytes in sarcoidosis. × 108.

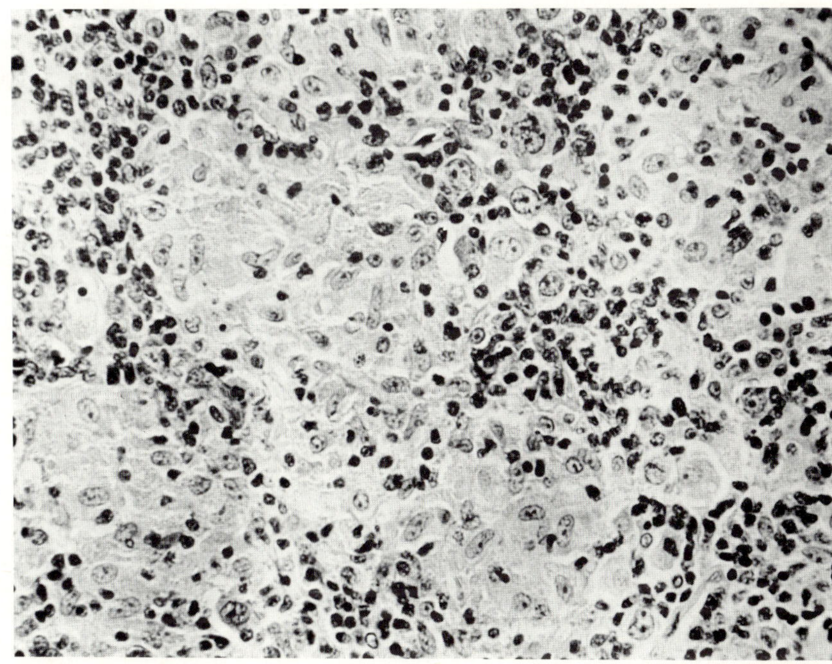

Fig. 3.21. Lymph node showing sarcoid change and a few large atypical histiocytic cells. Repeat biopsy showed classical Hodgkin's disease. This is a typical example of the uncommon sarcoid reaction in malignant lymphoma. × 216.

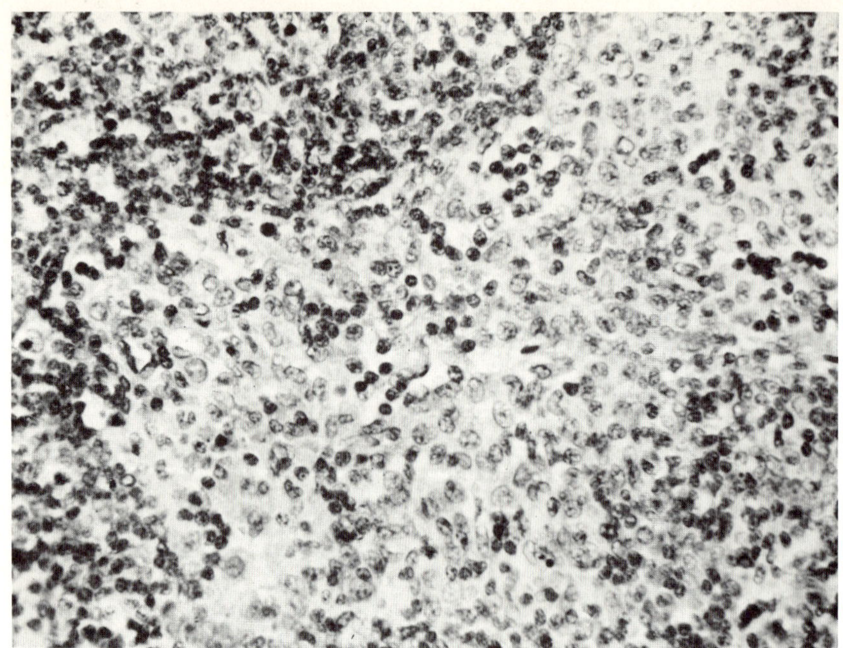

Fig. 3.22. A lymph node showing the sinus hyperplasia which with hyperplasia of paracortical lymphoid tissue occurs in dermatopathic lymphadenopathy. × 216.

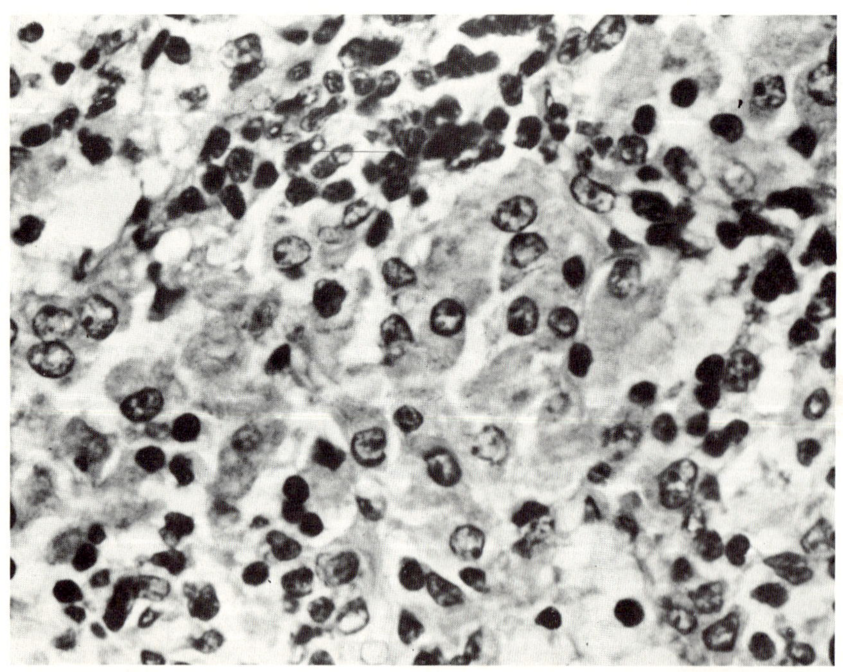

Fig. 3.23. A lymph node showing the changes of Whipple's disease. The node is infiltrated by numerous large mature PAS positive histiocytes which can be demonstrated by EM to contain numerous bacteria. × 430.

disease. The node shows a patchy infiltration with large macrophages which show a striking positive PAS reaction. The diagnosis can be clinched by demonstrating the presence of numerous bacilli; these are well preserved, even in material reclaimed from paraffin blocks (Fig. 3.23).

13 Syphilitic lymphadenitis

Regional or generalized lymphadenitis may occur in patients with syphilis, although it is rare in the tertiary stage. Occasionally the enlarged nodes constitute the presenting feature and a diagnostic lymph node biopsy is undertaken. Such cases are recorded by Hartsock *et al.* (1970) and by Turner and Wright (1973). The lymph nodes show a variety of appearances. There is commonly follicular hyperplasia sometimes very well marked. The paracortical areas tend to be depleted of lymphocytes and infiltrated with macrophages; spirochaetes may be demonstrable by silver stains in the walls of postcapillary venules. There may be especially in the same areas sarcoid-like epithelioid cells and giant cells. Finally there may be diffuse plasma cell infiltration, capsular fibrosis and vasculitis.

14 Brucellosis

Lymph node enlargement can be seen in this condition, but since the diagnosis is usually made by bacteriological or serological means, biopsy is rarely undertaken. Information concerning the histologic changes in the lymph nodes is therefore scanty, but cases have been recorded, e.g. Sharp (1934) and Sprunt and McBryde (1936). The nodes show areas of granulomatous inflammation resembling tuberculosis but with little necrosis, although a degree of caseation and occasional giant cells may be seen. The changes are not diagnostic but should be suggestive of the condition when seen.

15 Chlamydial infections

The chlamydia (formerly Bedsonia) are a group of organisms falling between the bacteria and viruses and are the causative agents of psittacosis, trachoma and lymphogranuloma venereum. It is almost certain that a similar agent also causes cat-scratch fever, although the organism has not been positively identified in this disease. In lymphogranuloma and cat-scratch fever, the regional lymph nodes may be enlarged and show a similar histology (Winship 1953; Wilcox 1963). The nodes are enlarged, soft and adherent to the adjacent tissues. The initial changes are seen at the site of entry of the afferent lymphatics with ill-defined areas of histiocytic cell hyperplasia and clusters of polymorph leucocytes and plasma cells. Small epithelioid cell granulomas may be present. The

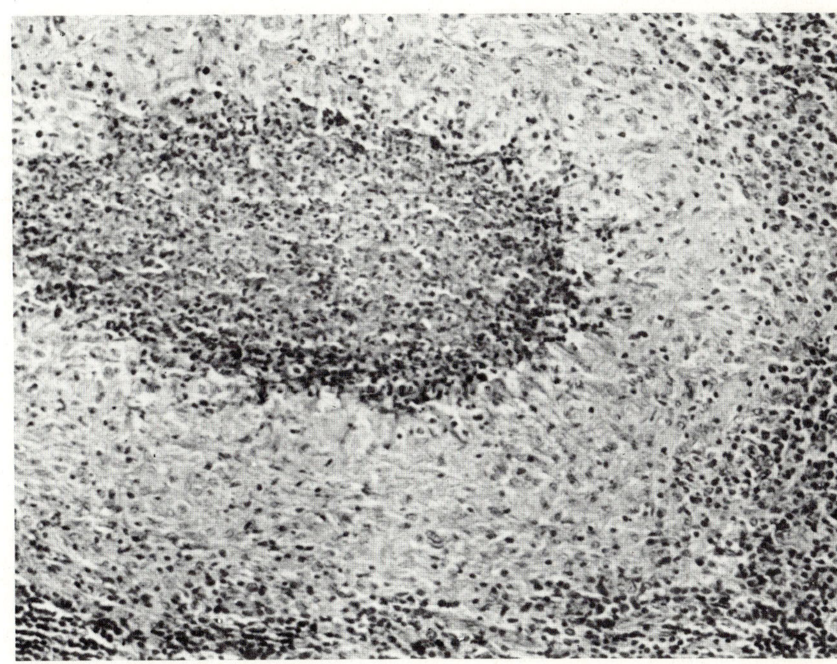

Fig. 3.24. Lymph node showing changes typical of cat-scratch fever. A palisaded rim of macrophages surrounds a central core of neutrophil polymorphs. × 108.

peripheral sinuses are filled with inflammatory cells and the follicles are enlarged with reactive germinal centres. Later characteristic microabscesses form at first in the cortex and then in the medulla (Fig. 3.24). In their fully developed state they have a stellate configuration with a central abscess containing polymorph leucocytes. Epithelioid cells develop at the edge of the abscess and giant cells may be seen. Giemsa stains may show inclusion bodies. The abscesses may coalesce to form gross areas of suppuration which may extend outside the node with local abscess formation. The diagnosis can be confirmed serologically in the case of lymphogranuloma venereum or by a skin test in cat-scratch disease.

16 Yersinial infections

Yersinia enterocolitica (formerly *Pasteurella pseudo-tuberculosis*) is a Gram-negative organism which probably enters the body via the gastrointestinal tract causing acute disease of the ileo-caecal region often simulating acute appendicitis. At operation the mesenteric lymph nodes are enlarged and may be biopsied. The pathological changes were first recorded by Masshoff and Dölle (1953). Later cases were described by Carlsson *et al.* (1964) and by Mair *et al.* (1970). Early changes in the lymph node show non-specific sinus and follicular hyperplasia, but later the unusual feature is seen of accumu-

lation of polymorph leucocytes in the germinal centres of the follicles. These accumulations eventually enlarge to form round microabscesses surrounded by palisaded histiocytes but no giant cells. Gram negative acid-fast diplo-bacilli may be seen in the lesions. Similar changes may occur in the appendix when this is removed (Fig. 3.25).

17 *Pneumocystis carinii*

This is a pulmonary infection caused by a protozoon and lymph nodes are not usually involved unless there is some evidence of immune depression. Three cases of lymphadenitis are reported by Barnett *et al.* (1969) where granulomatous lesions containing the organism were seen.

18 Fungal infections

These seldom present in lymph nodes and usually form part of an infection involving other organs primarily. However, involvement of nodes by *Histoplasma capsulatum* and *Coccidioides immitis* has been recorded by Symmers (1966) and one case of cryptococcal lymphadenitis described by Talerman *et al.* (1970). The lymph node shows a proliferation of large macrophages. Diagnosis depends on demonstration of the

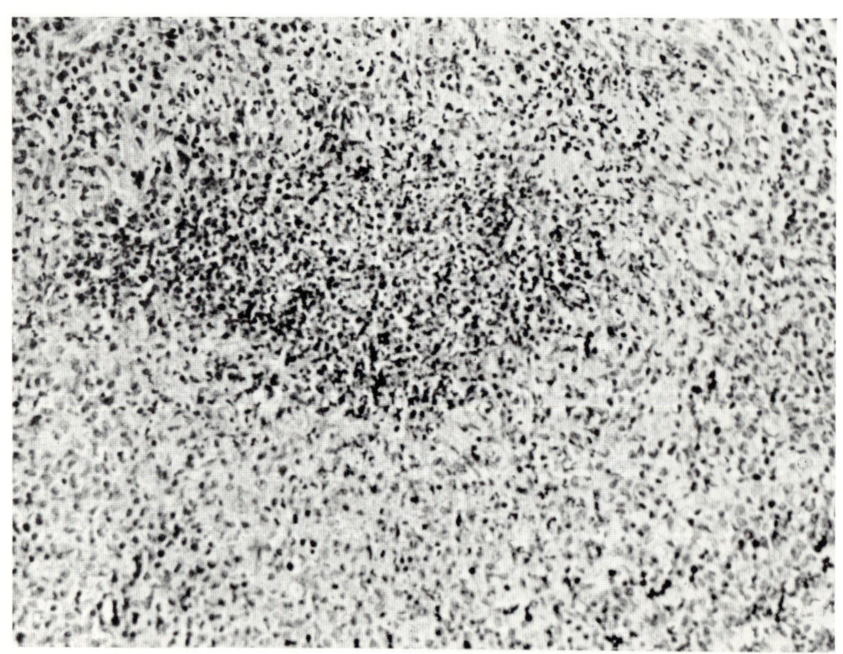

Fig. 3.25. Lymph node showing an abscess with central pus formation surrounded by macrophages. The appearances (rather similar to those seen in Fig. 3.24) are due to infection with *Yersinia enterocolitica* (*Pasteurella pseudo-tuberculosis*).

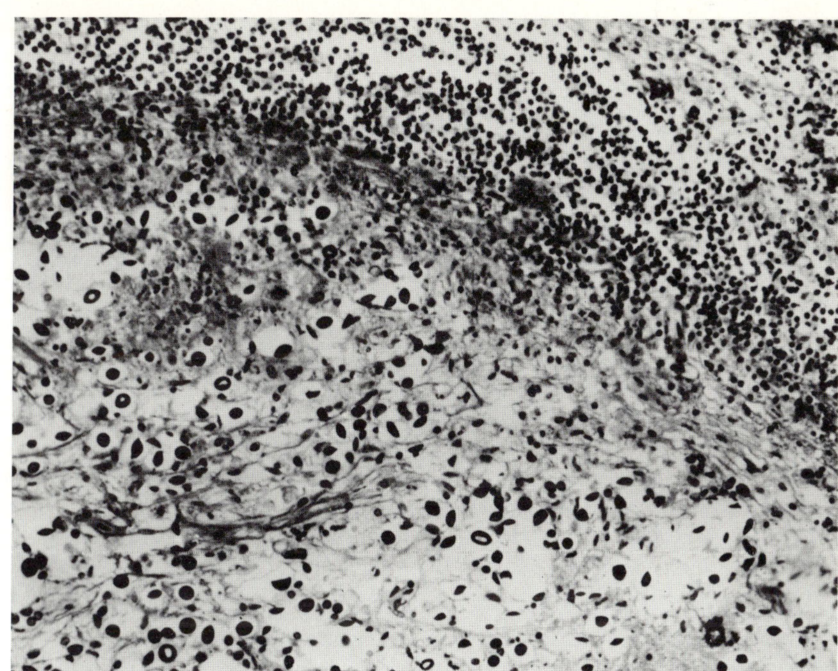

Fig. 3.26. Section of lymph node showing the circular profiles of *Cryptococcus neoformans* in a cryptococcal abscess. Gridley stain (×108).

organism by staining by the periodic acid Schiff or Gridley techniques (Fig. 3.26).

19 Degenerative lesions

Degenerative and ischaemic disease of lymph nodes is rare.

a AMYLOID LYMPHADENOPATHY

While lymph node involvement occurs in up to 37% of cases of amyloidosis (Ko *et al.* 1976) it rarely presents with lymphadenopathy. This was however described by Mackenzie (1963) where there appeared to be a selective involvement of the nodes by amyloid deposition.

b LYMPH NODE INFARCTION

Spontaneous infarction of superficial lymph nodes was reported by Davies and Stansfeld (1972) and by Benisch and Howard (1975). The lymph nodes show almost complete infarction with only a thin rim of surviving lymphoid tissue. The condition appears to be due to thrombosis of pericapsular and hilar veins. More localised areas of infarction due to atheromatous embolism were present in the case of Shah and

Kisilevsky (1978). Infarction may be a warning sign of the presence of lymphoma (Cleary *et al.* 1982).

REFERENCES

ADDIS B.J., ISAACSON P. & BILLINGS J.A. (1980) Plasmacytoma of lymph nodes. *Cancer* **46**, 340–6.

ALLEN M.S., TALBOT W.H. & MCDONALD R.M. (1966) Atypical lymph node hyperplasia after administration of attenuated live measles vaccine. *N. Eng. J. Med.* **274**, 677–8.

ANAGNOSTOU D. & HARRISON C.V. (1972) Angiofollicular lymph node hyperplasia (Castleman). *J. Clin. Path.* **25**, 306–11.

AZOURY F.J. & REED R.J. (1966) Histiocytosis: Report of an unusual case. *N. Eng. J. Med.* **274**, 928–30.

BALLOW M., PARK B.H., DUPONT B., CALDWELL R.R., LONSDALE D. & GOOD R.A. (1974) Benign giant lymphoid hyperplasia of mediastinum with associated abnormalities of the immune system. *J. Pediatr.* **84**, 418–20.

BARNETT R.N., HULL J.G. & VORTEL V. (1969) Pneumocystis carinii in liver and spleen. *Arch. Path. (Chicago)*, **88**, 175–80.

BARTOLI E., MASSARELLI G. & SOGGIA G. (1980) Multicentric giant lymph hyperplasia. *Amer. J. Clin. Path.* **73**, 423–6.

BEECROFT D.M.O., DIX M.R., MCGREGOR B.J.L. & SHAW R.L. (1973) Benign sinus histiocytosis with massive lymphadenopathy. *J. Clin. Path.* **26**, 463–9.

BENISCH B.M. & HOWARD R.G. (1975) Lymph node infarction in two young men. *Amer. J. Clin. Path* **63**, 818–23.

BERG J.W. (1971) Morphological evidence for immune response to breast cancer. An historical review. *Cancer* **28**, 1453–6.

BESWICK I.P. (1955) The spleen in glandular fever. *J. Path. Bact.* **70**, 407–14.

BEVERLEY J.K.A. (1969) Toxoplasmosis in man. *Brit. J. Hosp. Med.* **2**, 645–53.

BICHEL J. (1976) Post vaccinial lymphadenitis developing into Hodgkin's disease. *Acta Med. Scand.* **199**, 523–5.

BLACK M.M., KERPE S. & SPEER F.D. (1953) Lymph node structure in patients with cancer of the breast. *Amer. J. Path.* **29**, 505–22.

BLACK M.M. & LEIS H.P. (1971) Cellular responses to autologous breast cancer tissue. Correlation with stage and lymphoreticu-loendothelial reaction. *Cancer* **28**, 263–73.

BREARLEY R.L., CHAPMAN J., CULLEN M.H., HORTON M.A., STANSFELD A.G. & WATERS A.H. (1979) Haematological features of immunoblastic lymphadenopathy with dysproteinaemia. *J. Clin. Pathol.* **32**, 356–60.

BREIGER E.M. (1949) Host-parasite relationships in tuberculous infection. *Tubercle* **30**, 227–36 and 242–53.

BUTLER J.J. (1968) Non-neoplastic lesions of lymph nodes of man to be differentiated from lymphomas. *Nat. Cancer Inst. Monog. No. 32*, 233–55.

CARLSSON M.G., RYD H. & STERNBY N.H. (1964) A case of human infection with pasteurella pseudotuberculosis. x. *Acta. Path. Microbial. Scand.* **62**, 128–32.

CARR I. (1980) The Pathologist's role in interpreting metastatic lymph node disease. In *Lymphatic System Metastasis* (Eds Weiss L., Gilbert H.A., Ballon S.C. & Hall G.K.) Boston.

CARR I. & McGINTY F. (1974) Lymphatic metastasis and its inhibition: an experimental model. *J. Path.* **113**, 85–95.

CARTER R.L. & PENMAN H.G. (1969) *Infectious mononucleosis.* Blackwell Scientific Publications, Oxford.

CASTLEMAN B. & TOWNE V.W. (1954) Hyperplasia of mediastinal lymph nodes. *N. Eng. J. Med.* **250**, 26–30.

CASTLEMAN B., IVERSON L. & PARDO MENENDEZ V. (1956) Localised mediastinal lymph node hyperplasia resembling thymoma. *Cancer* **9**, 822–30.

CHAPMAN J.S. (1972) A review of early events in tubercle formation. *Acta Path. Microbial. Scand. (A) Suppl.* **233**, 189–94.

CITRON K.M. (1972–4) Sarcoidosis. *Medicine (London)* **14**, 896–903.

CLEARY K.R., OSBORNE B.M. & BUTLER J.J. (1982) Lymph node infarction foreshadowing malignant lymphoma. *Amer. J. Surg. Path* **6**, 435–42.

COOK M.G. (1972) The size and histological appearances of mesenteric lymph nodes in Crohn's disease. *Gut* **13**, 970–2.

CRUICKSHANK B. (1958) Lesions of lymph nodes in rheumatoid disease and DLE. *Scot. Med. J.* **3**, 110–19.

CULLEN M.H., STANSFELD A.G., OLIVER R.T.D., LISTER T.A. & MALPAS J.S. (1979) Angioimmunoblastic lymphadenopathy. Report of ten cases and review of the literature. *Quar. J. Med.* **48**, 151–77.

CUSTER R.P. & SMITH E.B. (1948) Pathology of infectious mononucleosis. *Blood* **3**, 830–57.

DAVIES J.D. & STANSFELD A.G. (1972) Spontaneous infarction of the superficial lymph nodes. *J. Clin. Pathol.* **25**, 689–96.

DORFMAN R.F. & WARNKE R. (1974) Lymphadenopathy simulating the malignant lymphomas. *Hum. Path.* **5**, 519–50.

DRURY R.A.B. (1970) Problems in histological interpretation in sarcoidosis. *Postgrad. Med. J.* **46**, 478–83.

DOWNEY H. & STASNEY J. (1936) The pathology of the lymph nodes in infectious mononucleosis. *Fol. Haemat.* **54**, 417–38.

EDLOW D.W. & CARTER D. (1973) Heterotopic epithelium in axillary lymph node. Report of a case and review of the literature. *Am. J. Clin. Pathol.* **59**, 666–73.

EMSON H.E. (1973) Extrathoracic angiofollicular lymphoid hyperplasia with coincidental myasthenia gravis. *Cancer* **31**, 241–5.

EPSTEIN W.L. (1967) Granulomatous hypersensitivity. *Prog. Allerg.* **11**, 36–88.

FINKELDEY W. (1931) Uber Riesenzellbefunde in den Gaumenmandeln, zugleich ein Beitrag zur Histopathologie der Mandelveranderungen in Maserninkubationsstadium. *Virchows Arch.* **281**, 323–9.

FIRAT D., STUTZMAN L., STUDENSKI E.R. & PIEKREN J. (1965) Giant follicular lymph node disease. Clinical and pathological review of 64 cases. *Amer. J. Med.* **39**, 252–9.

FISHER R.I., JAFFE E.S., BRAYLAN R.C., ANDERSEN J.C. & TAN H.K. (1976) Immunoblastic lymphadenopathy: Evolution into a malignant lymphoma with plasmacytoid features. *Amer. J. Med.* **61**, 553–9.

FORBES G.B. (1961) Non-reactive tuberculosis in a cortisone-treated patient. *Tubercle* **42**, 233–40.

FRENKEL J.K. (1967) Adoptive immunity to intracellular infection. *J. Immunol.* **98**, 1309–19.

FRIEDELL G.H., SOTO E.A., KUMAOKA S., ABE O., HAYWARD J.L. & BULBROOK R.D. (1974) Sinus histiocytosis in British and Japanese patients with breast cancer. *Lancet* **2**, 1228–9.

FRIZZERA G., MORAN E.M. & RAPPAPORT H. (1974) Angioimmunoblastic lymphadenopathy with dysproteinaemia. *Lancet* **1**, 1070–3.

GAAFAR S.M. & TURK J.L. (1970) Granuloma formation in lymph nodes. *J. Pathol.* **100**, 9–20.

GALL E.A. & STOUT H.A. (1940) The histological lesion in the lymph nodes in infectious mononucleosis. *Amer. J. Path.* **16**, 433–48.

GAMS R.A., NEAL J.A. & CONRAD F.G. (1968) Hydantoin-induced pseudolymphoma. *Ann. Intern. Med.* **69**, 557–68.

GAUGAS J.M., PAYNE S. & WHARTON F.P. (1970) Association of macrophage lipids with Mycobacterium lepraemurium in the mouse thymus and lymph node. *Brit. J. Exp. Path.* **51**, 87–91.

HAFERKAMP O., ROSENAU W. & LENNERT K. (1971) Vascular transformation of lymph node sinuses due to venous obstruction. *Arch. Path.* **92**, 81–3.

HANNA M.G., SZAKAL A.K. & TYNDALL R.L. (1970) Histoproliferative effect of Rauscher Leukaemia virus on lymphatic tissue: histological and ultrastructural studies of germinal centres and their relation to leukemogenesis. *Cancer Res.* **30**, 1748–63.

HARRISON C.V. (1960) In *Recent Advances in Pathology*, 7th edn. (Ed. Harrison C.V.) Churchill, London.

HARRISON C.V. (1966) In *Recent Advances in Pathology*, 7th edn. (Ed. Harrison C.V.) Churchill, London.

HARRISON E.G. & BERNATZ P.E. (1963) Angiofollicular mediastinal lymph node hyperplasia resembling thymoma. *Arch. Path. (Chicago)*, **75**, 284–92.

Hart W.R. (1971) Primary nevus of a lymph node. *Am. J. Clin. Path.* **55**, 88–92.

Hartsock R.J. (1968) Post vaccinial lymphadenitis. Hyperplasia of lymphoid tissue that simulates malignant lymphomas. *Cancer* **21**, 632–49.

Hartsock R.J., Halling L.W. & King F.M. (1970) Luetic lymphadenitis: a clinical and histological study of 20 cases. *Amer. J. Clin. Path.* **53**, 304–14.

Henry L., Beverley J.K.A., Shortland J.R. & Coup A.J. (1973) Experimental toxoplasmic lymphadenopathy in rabbits. *Brit. J. Exp. Path.* **54**, 312–21.

Hooper A.A. (1972) Tuberculous peripheral lymphadenitis. *Brit. J. Surg.* **59**, 353–9.

Hyman G.A. & Sommers S.C. (1966) The development of Hodgkin's disease and lymphoma during anticonvulsant therapy. *Blood* **28**, 416–27.

Iverson L. (1956) Thymoma; review and classification. *Amer. J. Path.* **32**, 695–719.

James D.G., Anderson R., Langley D. & Ainslie D. (1964) Ocular sarcoidosis. *Brit. J. Ophthalmol.* **48**, 461–70.

Jones Williams W. & Williams D. (1968) The properties and development of conchoidal bodies in sarcoid and sarcoid-like granulomas. *Postgrad. Med. J.* **46**, 496–500.

Jones Williams W., Erasmus D.A., James E.M.V. & Davies T. (1970) The fine structure of sarcoid and tuberculous granulomas. *Postgrad. Med. J.* **46**, 496–500.

Kahn L.B., Ranchod M., Stables D.P., King H. & Yudelman I. (1973) Giant lymph node hyperplasia with haematological abnormalities. *S. Afr. Med. J.* **47**, 811–16.

Karat A.B., Karat S., Job C.K. & Sudarsanam D. (1968) Acute necrotizing lepromatous lymphadenitis. An erythema nodosum leprosum-like reaction in lymph nodes. *Brit. Med. J.* **4**, 223–34.

Kawasaki T., Kosaki F., Okawa S., Shigematsu I. & Yanagawa H. (1974) A new acute febrile mucocutaneous lymph node syndrome (MLNS) prevailing in Japan. *Pediatrics* **54**, 271–76.

Keller A.R., Hochholzer L. & Castleman B. (1972) Hyaline-vascular and plasma cell types of giant lymph node hyperplasia of the mediastinum and other locations. *Cancer* **29**, 670–83.

Ko H.S., Davidson, J.W. & Pruzanski W. (1976) Amyloid lymphadenopathy. *Ann. Int. Med.* **85**, 763–4.

Krasznai G. & Gyory G. (1968) Hydantoin lymphadenopathy. *J. Path. Bact.* **95**, 314–17.

Lattes R. & Pachter M.R. (1962) Benign lymphoid masses of probable hamartomatous nature. Analysis of 12 cases. *Cancer* **15**, 197–214.

Lennert K., Niedorf H.R., Blumcke S. & Hardmeier T. (1972) Lymphadenitis with massive haemophagocytic sinus histiocytosis. *Virchow's Arch. (Z. Path.)* **10**, 14–29.

Lewis J.G. (1961) The evolution of sarcoidosis into caseating tuberculosis of the lungs and skin. *Tubercle* **42**, 95–100.

Litt M. (1972) Studies in experimental eosinophilia IX. Inhibition by puromycin of the eosinophil response which hemocyanin elicits in guinea-pig lymph nodes. *J. Immunol.* **109**, 222–6.

Lubin J. & Rywlin A.M. (1971) Lymphoma-like lymph node changes in Kaposi's sarcoma. *Arch. Path. Derm.* **93**, 554–61.

Lukes R.J. & Collins R.D. (1975) A functional classification of malignant lymphomas. In *The Reticuloendothelial System* (Eds Rebuck J.W., Berard C.W. & Abell M.R.). Williams and Wilkins, Baltimore.

Lukes R.J. & Tindle B.H. (1975) Immunoblastic lymphadenopathy. *New Eng. J. Med.* **292**, 1–8.

Luscieti P., Mubschmid T., Cottier H., Hess M.W. & Sobin L.H. (1980) Human lymph node morphology as a function of age and site. *J. Clin. Path.* **33**, 454–61.

MacKellar A., Hilton H.B. & Masters P.L. (1967) Mycobacterial lymphadenitis in childhood. *Arch Dis. Child.* **42**, 70–4.

Mackenzie D.H. (1963) Amyloidosis presenting as lymphadenopathy. *Brit. Med. J.* **4**, 1449–50.

Mair N.S., White G.D. & Schubert F.K. (1970) Yersinia enterocolitica infection in the bush-baby (Galago). *Vet. Rec.* **86**, 69–71.

Masshoff W. & Dölle W. (1953) Uber eine besondere form der sog mesenteralien lymphadenopathie 'Die abseendivende reticulocytaire lymphadenitis'. *Arch. Path. Anat.* **323**, 664–84.

McCarthy S.W., Palmer A.A., Bale P.M. *et al.* (1974) Naevus cells in lymph node. *Pathology* **6**, 351–8.

McDivitt R.W. (1978) Breast carcinoma. *Hum. Path.* **9**, 3–21.

Mehrotra R. (1978) Histological and ultrastructural changes in experimentally produced post-vaccinial lymphadenitis in rabbits. *J. Pathol.* **126**, 39–44.

Melish M.E., Hicks R.M. & Larson E.J. (1976) Mucocutaneous lymph node syndrome in the United States. *Amer. J. Dis. Child.* **130**, 599–607.

Metcalf D., Furth J. & Buffet R.F. (1969) Pathogenesis of mouse leukaemia caused by Friend virus. *Cancer Res. (Chicago)* **19**, 52–8.

Meyer J.S., Steinberg L.S. (1969) Microscopically benign thyroid follicles in cervical lymph nodes. *Cancer* **24**, 302–11.

Motulsky A.G., Weinberg S., Saphir O. & Rosenberg E. (1952) Lymph nodes in rheumatoid arthritis. *Arch. Intern. Med.* **90**, 660–76.

Nairn R.C. & Anderson T.E. (1955) Erythrodermia with lipomelanic reticulum-cell hyperplasia of lymph nodes (Dermatopathic lymphadenitis). *Brit. Med. J.* **1**, 820–24.

Nosanchuk J.S. & Schnitzer B. (1969) Follicular hyperplasia in lymph nodes from patients with rheumatoid arthritis. A clinicopathologic study. *Cancer* **24**, 243–54.

O'Brien J.R. (1954) Non-reactive tuberculosis. *J. Clin. Path.* **7**, 216–25.

Patterson S.D., Larson E.B. & Corey L. (1980) Atypical generalised zoster with lymphadenitis mimicking lymphoma. *New Engl. J. Med.* **302**, 848–51.

Pautrier L.M. & Woringer F. (1937) Contribution a l'étude de l'histophysiologie cutanée a propos d'un aspect histopathologique nouveau du ganglion lymphatique; la reticulose lipomélanique accompagnant certaine dermatoses généralisées, les échanges entre la peau et le ganglion. *Ann. Derm. Syph. (Paris)* **8**, 257–73.

Pemberton J., Broders A.C. & Maino V.J. (1950) Giant haemolymph nodes. Report of 2 cases. *Surg. Clin. N. Amer.* **30**, 1147–53.

Piringer-Kuchinka A., Martin I. & Thalhammer O. (1958) Über die vorzuglich cervico-nuchale Lymphadenitis mit kleinhardiger

Epitheloidzellwucherung. *Virchow's Arch. Path. Anat.* **331**, 522–35.

PURTILO D.T., DeFLORIO D., HUTT L.M., BHAWAN J., YANG J.P.S., OTTO R. & EDWARDS W. (1977) Variable phenotypic expression of an X-linked recessive lymphoproliferative syndrome. *N. Eng. J. Med.* **297**, 1077–80.

PURTILO D.T., SZYMANSKI I., BHAWAN J., YANG J.P.S., HUTT L.M., BOTO W., DENICOLA L., MAIER R. & THORLEY-LAWSON D. (1978) Epstein–Barr infections in the X-linked recessive lymphoproliferative syndrome. *Lancet* **1**, 798–801.

RAPPAPORT H., WINTER W.J. & HICKS E.B. (1956) Follicular lymphoma. *Cancer* **9**, 792–821.

REE H. & FANGER H. (1975) Paracortical alteration in lymphadenopathic and tumour-draining lymph nodes. A histologic study. *Human Pathol.* **6**, 363–72.

REID J.D. & WOLINSKY E. (1969) Histopathology of lymphadenitis caused by atypical mycobacteria. *Amer. Rev. Resp. Dis.* **99**, 8–12.

ROSAI J. & DORFMAN R.F. (1969) Sinus histiocytosis with massive lymphadenopathy. A newly recognised benign clinico-pathological entity. *Arch. Path.* **87**, 63–70.

ROSAI J. & DORFMAN R.F. (1972) Sinus histiocytosis with massive lymphadenopathy: a pseudolymphomatous benign disorder. Analysis of 34 cases. *Cancer* **30**, 1174–88.

ROSENFELD S., SWILLER A.I., SHENOY Y.M.V. & MORRISON A.N. (1961) Syndrome simulating lymphosarcoma induced by diphenyl hydantoin sodium. *J. Amer. Med. Ass.* **176**, 491–3.

SABIN A.B. & FELDMAN H.A. (1948) Dyes as microchemical indicators of a new immunity phenomenon affecting a protozoon parasite (Toxoplasma). *Science (N.Y.)* **108**, 660–3.

SALTZSTEIN S.L. (1962) Lymphoma or drug reaction occurring during Hydantoin therapy for epilepsy. *Amer. J. Med.* **32**, 286–97.

SALTZSTEIN S.L. (1965) The fate of patients with non-diagnostic lymph node biopsies. *Surg.* **58**, 659–62.

SALTZSTEIN S.L. & ACKERMAN L.V. (1959) Lymphadenopathy induced by anticonvulsant drugs and mimicking clinically and pathologically malignant lymphomas. *Cancer* **12**, 164–82.

SAXEN E. & SAXEN L. (1959) The histological diagnosis of glandular toxoplasmosis. *Lab. Invest.* **8**, 386–94.

SCADDING J.G. (1967) *Sarcoidosis.* Eyre and Spottiswoode, London.

SCHROER K.R. & FRANSSILA K.O. (1979) Atypical hyperplasia of lymph nodes. *Cancer* **44**, 1155–63.

SHAH K.H. & KISILEVSKY R. (1978) Infarction of the lymph nodes. *Human Pathol.* **9**, 597–9.

SHARP W.B. (1934) Pathology of undulant fever. *Arch Path.* **18**, 72–108.

SIEGLER R., LANE I., FROSCH Y. & MORAN S. (1973) Early response to lymph node cells to Abelson leukaemia virus. *Lab. Invest.* **29**, 273–7.

SILVERBERG S.G., FRABLE W.J. & BROOKS J.W. (1973) Sinus histiocytosis in non-diagnostic scalene lymph node biopsies. *Cancer* **32**, 177–80.

SINCLAIR-SMITH C.C., KAHN L.B. & UYS C.J. (1974) Sinus histiocytosis with massive lymphadenopathy. Report of two additional cases with ultrastructural observations. *S. Afr. Med. J.* **48**, 451–4.

SPAIN D.M. (1957) Sex differences in incidence and severity of lymph node lipogranulomatosis. *Arch. Path.* **64**, 54–7.

SPRUNT D.M., McBRYDE A. (1936) Morbid anatomic changes in cases of brucella infection in man with report of necropsy. *Arch. Path.* **21**, 217–26.

STANSFELD A.G. (1961) The histological diagnosis of toxoplasmic lymphadenitis. *J. Clin. Path.* **14**, 565–73.

STANTON M.F. & PINKERTON H. (1953) Benign acquired toxoplasmosis with subsequent pregnancy. *Amer. J. Clin. Path.* **23**, 1199–1207.

SYMMERS D. (1921) Primary haemangiolymphoma of the haemal nodes. An unusual variety of malignant tumour. *Arch. Intern. Med.* **28**, 467–74.

SYMMERS W. ST. C. (1966) Deep-seated fungal infections currently seen in the histopathologic service of a medical school laboratory in Britain. *Amer. J. Clin. Path.* **46**, 514–37.

TALERMAN A., BRADLEY J.M. & WOOLAND B. (1970) Cryptococcal lymphadenitis. *J. Med. Microbiol.* **3**, 633–8.

THORBURN J.D., STEPHENS H.B. & GRIMES O.F. (1952) Benign thymoma in the hilus of the lung, case report. *J. Thoracic Surg.* **24**, 540–3.

TSAKRAKLIDES V., OLSEN P., KERSEY J.H. & GOOD R.A. (1974) Prognostic significance of the regional lymph node histology in cancer of the breast. *Cancer* **34**, 1259–67.

TSAKRAKLIDES V., WANEBO H.J., STEINBERG S.S., STEARNS M. & GOOD R.A. (1975) Prognostic evaluation of regional lymph node morphology in endorectal cancer. *Am. J. Surg.* **129**, 174–80.

TUNG K.S.K. & McCORMACK L.J. (1967) Angiomatous lymphoid hamartoma. Report of five cases with a review of the literature. *Cancer* **20**, 525–36.

TURK J.L. & WATERS M.F.R. (1971) Immunological significance of changes in the lymph nodes across the leprosy spectrum. *Clin. Exp. Immunol.* **8**, 363–76.

TURNER D.R. & WRIGHT D.J.M. (1973) Lymphadenopathy in early syphilis. *J. Path.* **110**, 305–8.

VAN DEN BERG F.W.T., KAISERLING E. & LENNERT K. (1976) Glomus-Zellnester des Lymphknotens. *Virchows. Arch. Pathol. Anat.* **371**, 27–34.

WARNER N.E. & FRIEDMAN N.B. (1956) Lipogranulomatous pseudo-sarcoid. *Ann. Intern. Med.* **45**, 662–73.

WARTHIN A.S. (1931) Occurrence of numerous large giant cells in the tonsils and pharyngeal mucosa in the prodromal stage of measles. Report of 4 cases. *Arch. Path.* **11**, 864–74.

WILCOX P.H. (1963) Cat-scratch disease. *Brit. Med. J.* **2**, 541–2.

WINSHIP T. (1953) Pathological changes in so-called cat-scratch fever. *Amer. J. Clin. Path.* **23**, 1012–18.

WOOD W.G. & HARKINS M.M. (1979) Nephropathy in angio-immunoblastic lymphadenopathy. *Amer. J. Clin. Path.* **71**, 58–63.

WORK K. & HUTCHISON W.M. (1969) A new cystic form of Toxoplasma gondii. *Acta. Path. Microbiol. Scand.* **75**, 191–2.

YANAGIHARA R. & TODD J.K. (1980) Acute febrile mucocutaneous lymph node syndrome. *Amer. J. Dis. Child.* **134**, 603–14.

ZETTERGREN L. (1961) Probably neoplastic proliferation of lymphoid tissue (follicular lympho-reticuloma). Report of 4 cases with a survey of the literature. *Acta. Path. Microbiol. Scand.* **51**, 113–26.

Hodgkin's disease is the most common malignant lymphoma in most countries. Thomas Hodgkin (1832) reported seven cases in whom gross enlargement of the lymph nodes and, with one exception, spleen, was found during autopsy. The histological appearances were reported by Greenfield (1878) and the characteristic giant cells were described by Sternberg (1898) and Reed (1902). The literature has been summarized in more recent reviews (Butler 1975; Ioachim 1975; Kaplan 1976, 1980 and 1981; Lacher 1976).

THE LESION OF HODGKIN'S DISEASE

Both grossly (Fig 4.1) and histologically the lymph node may be completely replaced by tumour, or show discrete nodules, leaving areas of the nodal architecture intact. Partial involvement, when present, conveys a better prognosis in some types of the disease (Henry 1971). Histologically there is an infiltrate of malignant 'Hodgkin' cells 20 μm or more in diameter, with large nuclei containing prominent and often eosinophilic nucleoli. The cytoplasm is amphophilic and its edges often irregular, or with fine processes. Ultrastructurally these cells vary; many contain considerable amounts of endoplasmic reticulum and numerous lysosomes and have some resemblance to macrophages. Others are less well differentiated (Fig 4.2). The Reed–Sternberg cell (R–S cell) is very large (20–40 μm) and either binucleate, or with such a deeply indented single nucleus that it appears binucleate on section; the two nuclei or heminuclei form a mirror image (Figs 4.3 and 4.4). The ultrastructure of the cytoplasm contains scattered profiles of endoplasmic reticulum and small vacuoles (Fig 4.5), and sometimes several profiles of lysosomes are present. Characteristically closely related lymphocytes at the periphery invaginate their processes into the Reed–Sternberg cell.

The above features are fairly constant but the many histologic variations from case to case have led to various schemes for subclassification. That of Jackson and Parker (1947) has been superseded by the Rye classification, itself arising from an earlier scheme proposed by Lukes and Butler (1966). This draws on an observation by Rosenthal in 1936 that prognosis was related to the degree of lymphocytic infiltration present in the lesion, the greater the number of lymphocytes, the better the prognosis. The Rye classification (Lukes *et al.* 1966) delineates two extreme varieties, lymphocytic predominance and lymphocytic depletion. To these are added the classical 'mixed-cellularity' Hodgkin's disease, and the more recently described nodular sclerosing type.

Lymphocyte predominance

The affected architecture is replaced by a diffuse or nodular proliferation of small lymphocytes. Reed–Sternberg cells may be difficult to demonstrate but malignant cells of the same series—Lukes' 'L and H cells'—may be seen (Fig 4.6). These have a characteristically folded lobate nucleus with a small amount of acidophilic cytoplasm. Reactive epithelioid histiocytes occur in varying numbers and in some cases may form a very obvious feature of the histology (Fig 4.7).

Lymphocyte depletion

The architecture of the node is usually totally replaced by a proliferation of neoplastic Hodgkin and Reed–Sternberg cells. The degree of both cellular and nuclear pleomorphism may be striking (Fig 4.8) and areas of necrosis are common, in contrast to the lymphocyte predominance variety. Lymphocytes are present in only small numbers and these may be concentrated in localised areas, leaving sheets of neoplastic tissue totally free of lymphocytes. Some cases may show a fine deposition of fibrous tissue which is not doubly refractile, as in the nodular sclerosing variety, and may be associated with intercellular hyaline material.

Mixed cellularity

There is infiltration of the affected areas by varying propor-

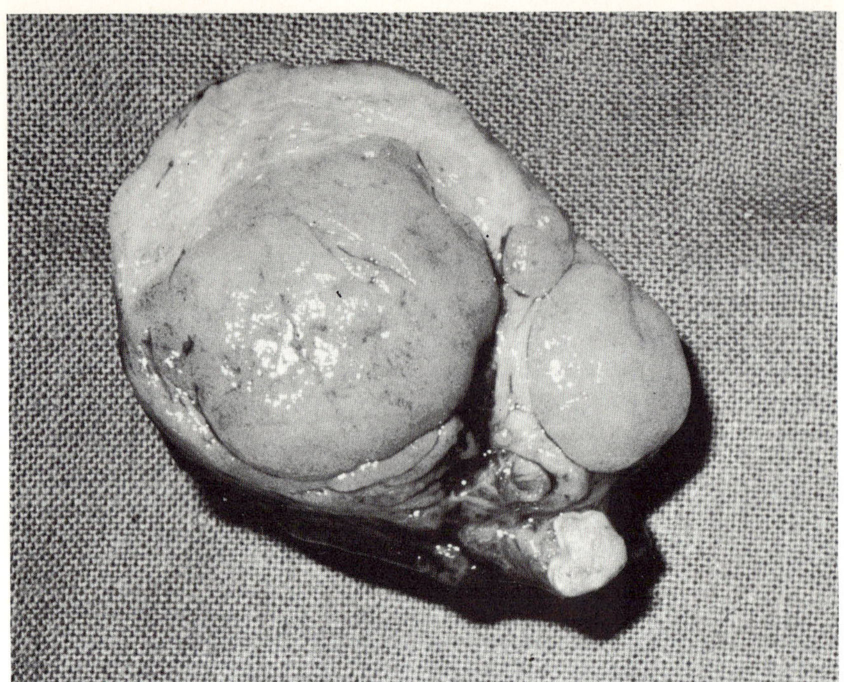

Fig. 4.1. Gross picture of an enlarged
cervical lymph node from a patient with
classical Hodgkin's disease. The node is
grey, firm and bulges slightly over its
capsule. ×1.

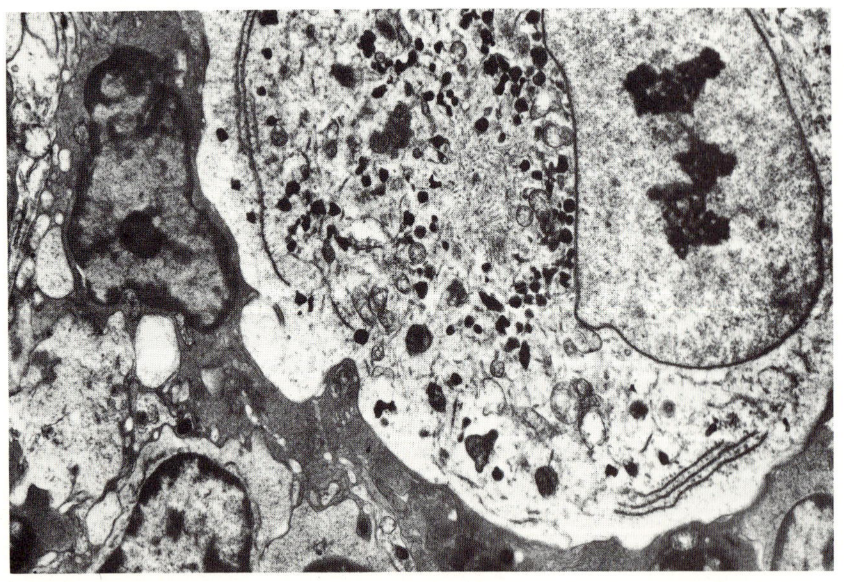

Fig. 4.2. Electron micrograph of Hodgkin
cell. The nucleolus is prominent; the
cytoplasm contains strands of granular
endoplasmic reticulum and numerous
lysosomes. ×7,500.

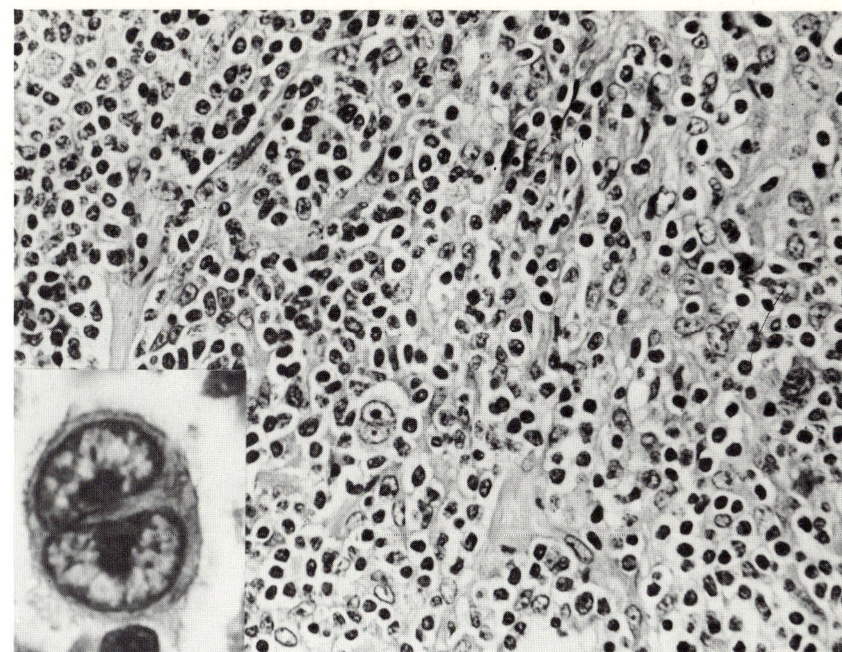

Fig. 4.3. Lymph node showing the changes of classical Hodgkin's disease-fibrosis, malignant histiocytic cells, binucleate (Reed-Sternberg) cells and a moderate infiltrate of lymphocytes, eosinophils and a few plasma cells. ×215.

Fig. 4.4. (*inset*) Detail of Reed-Sternberg cell in a lymph node in classical Hodgkin's disease. ×1,075.

tions of lymphocytes, eosinophils, plasma cells, histiocytes and fibroblasts. Neoplastic Hodgkin cells are prominent, and classical Reed–Sternberg cells are not difficult to find. A nodular arrangement may be detectable but there are no broad bands of fibrosis. Occasionally, sections will be examined showing large numbers of predominantly lymphocytes, eosinophils or plasma cells, but the 'mixed' pattern of cells will always be present. Small areas of necrosis may be seen.

Nodular sclerosing

This variety was described by Smetana and Cohen (1956) and given the name by Lukes and Butler (1966). In its fully developed form the affected node shows nodules of tumour surrounded by intersecting bands of birefringent collagenous fibrous tissue, producing either focal or complete destruction of the normal nodal architecture (Fig 4.9). The histology of the tumour nodules may resemble any of the three other subtypes. A characteristic cell described by Lukes and Butler (1966) is the 'lacunar' cell thought to be a variant of the Reed–Sternberg cell (Fig 4.10, 4.11). This contains a small, hyperlobed nucleus and clear cytoplasm which may show shrinkage after formalin fixation. The presence of this cell in

the absence of significant fibrosis may allow a diagnosis of a cellular phase of the nodular sclerosing type. Nodular sclerosing Hodgkin's disease classically occurs more commonly in young adult females with a localised presentation in the neck or superior mediastinum.

Hodgkin's disease with granulomas

In some 10% of cases, sarcoid-like, non-caseating, giant cell epithelioid granulomas may be found, either in association with the neoplastic tissue or in organs such as liver and spleen which are not directly involved by tumour. In view of the incidence of infection in Hodgkin's disease, tuberculosis and fungal infections in particular should be excluded. In some cases, sarcoidosis and Hodgkin's disease may co-exist (Brincker 1972). Cases where the granulomas are a manifestation of the disease itself may show a better response to treatment (Sacks *et al.* 1978).

THE REED–STERNBERG CELL

Although this cell has long been regarded as being binucleate, ultrastructural studies indicate that it is often mononuclear with an excessively folded nucleus. The cytoplasm contains

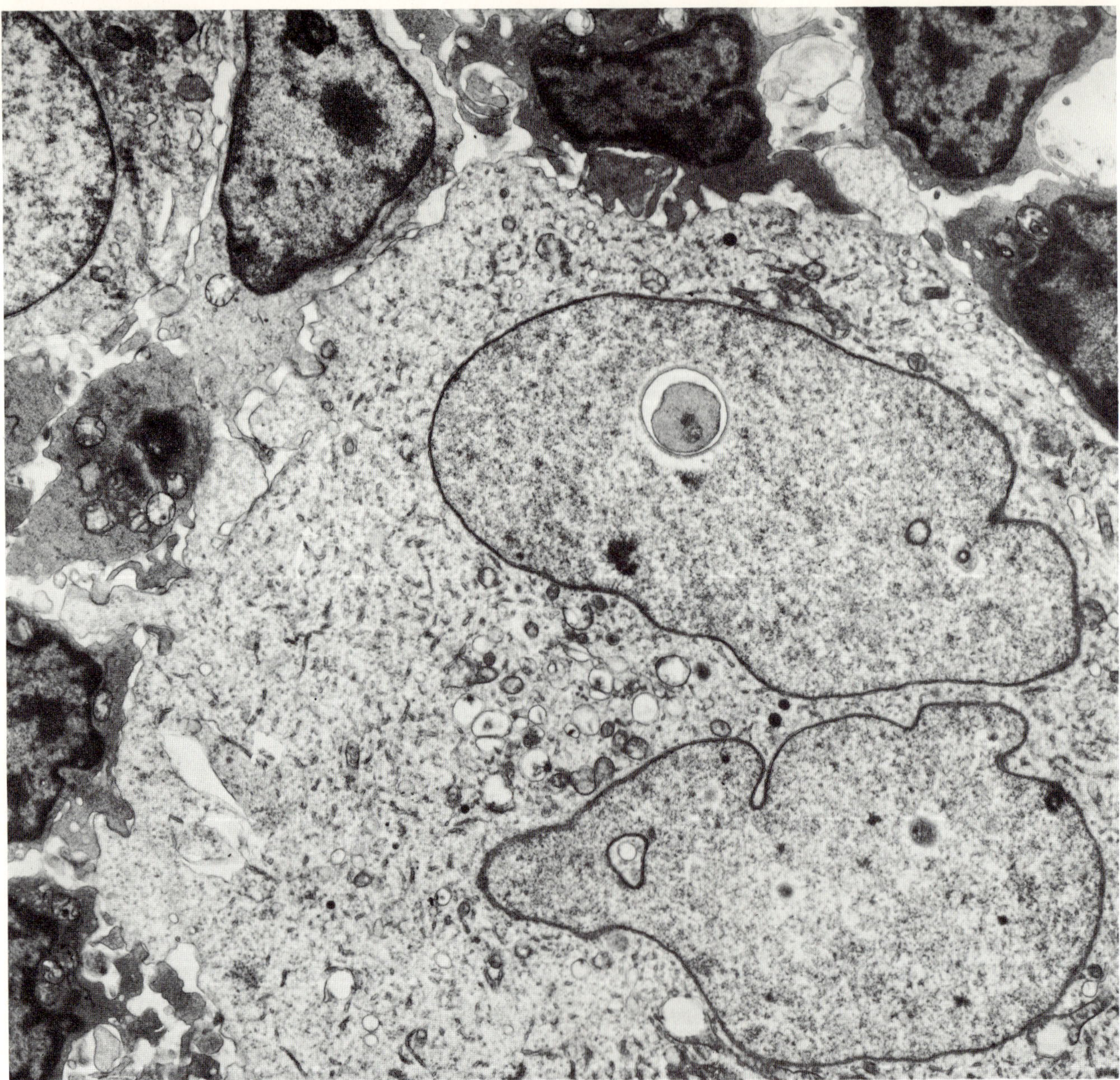

Fig. 4.5. Electron micrograph of Reed–Sternberg cell in Hodgkin's disease. Note the closely related lymphocytes at the periphery with cytoplasmic processes invaginating the cytoplasm of the tumor cell. × 10,000.

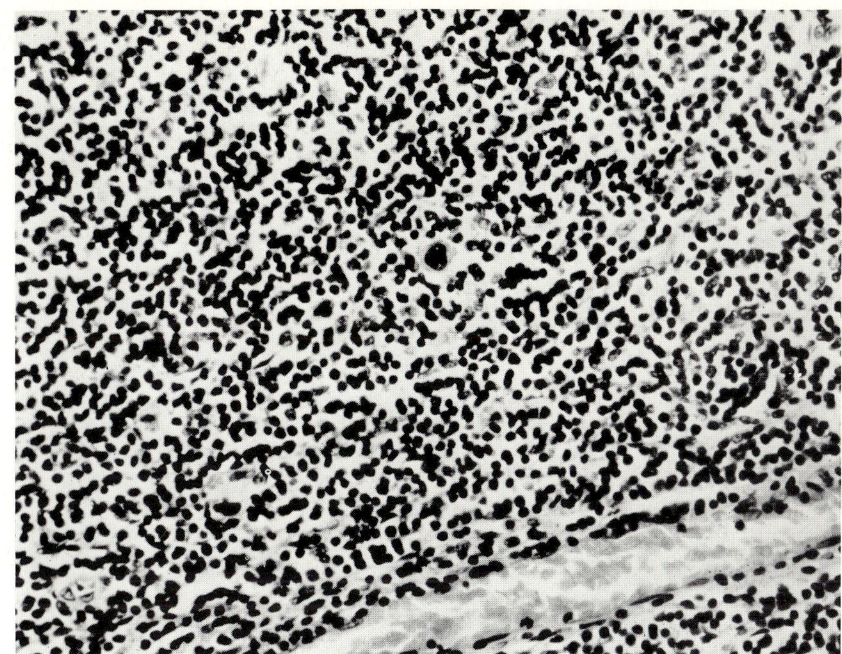

Fig. 4.6. Lymph node showing the changes of lymphocyte predominant Hodgkin's disease. The lymph node structure is lost, being diffusely over-run with lymphocytes. A single malignant histiocytic cell lies in the middle of the field. Such cells can be hard to find and it can be difficult to distinguish this lesion from a diffuse small lymphocytic non-Hodgkin's lymphoma. ×215.

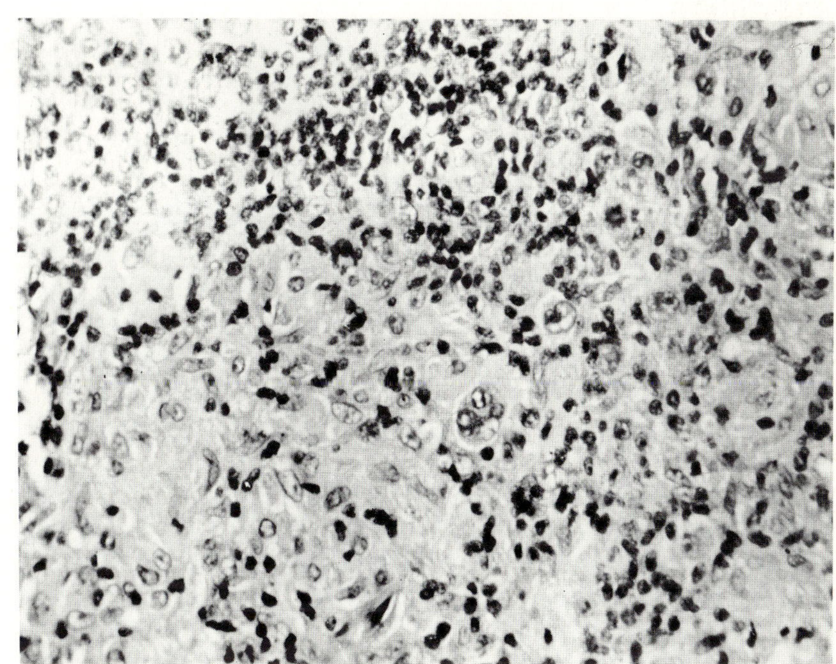

Fig. 4.7. Lymph node showing the changes of the histiocytic variant of lymphocytic predominant Hodgkin's disease (lymphocytic–histiocytic HD). Two malignant histiocytic cells are present and a considerable infiltrate of reactive, non-neoplastic histiocytes. ×215.

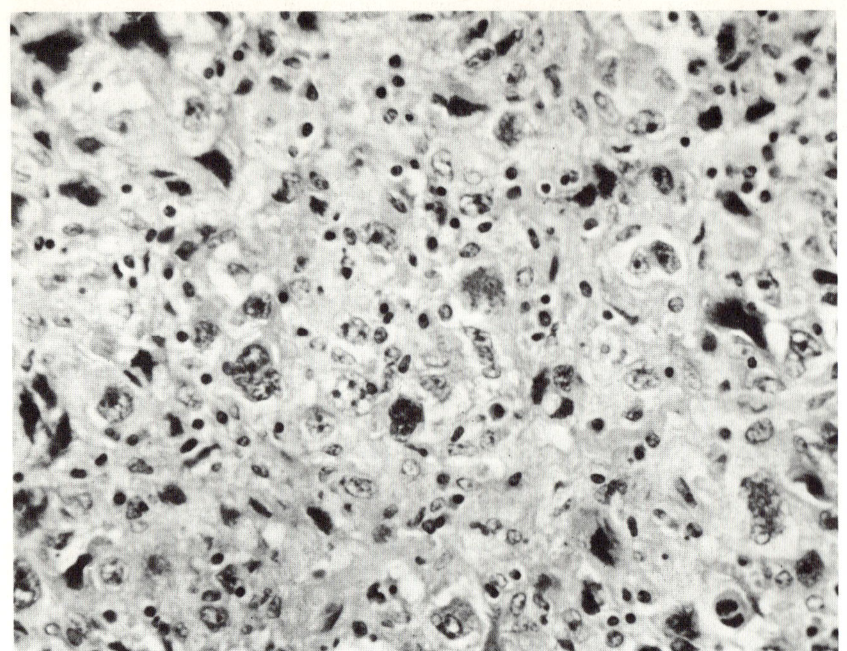

Fig. 4.8. Lymph node showing diffuse infiltration with pleomorphic malignant histiocytic cells and fibrosis and a few scattered lymphocytes. The heterogeneity of the picture suggests that this is lymphocytic depletion Hodgkin's disease, rather than malignant lymphoma, histiocytic cell type. ×215.

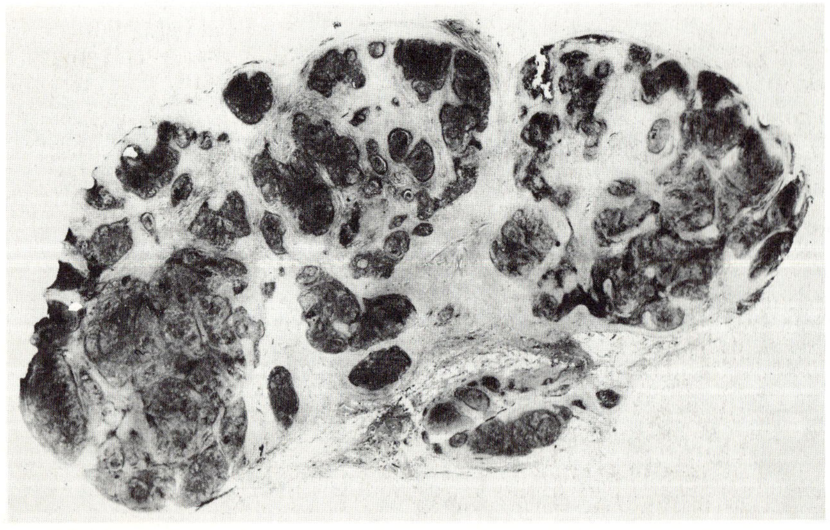

Fig. 4.9. Low power micrograph of a lymph node showing the gross intersecting bands of fibrous tissue characteristic of nodular sclerosing Hodgkin's disease. ×2.4.

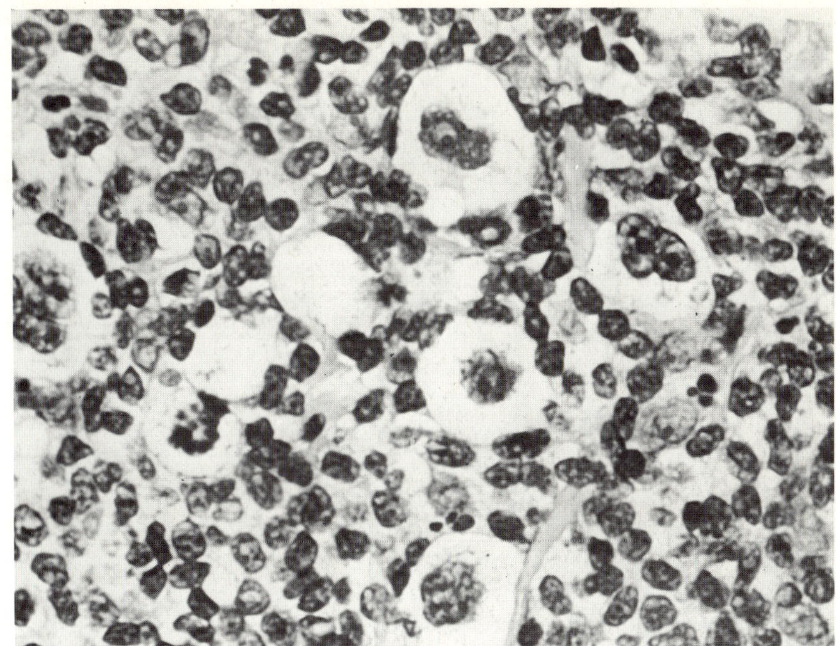

Fig. 4.10. Group of lacunar cells showing the gross cytoplasmic vacuolation characteristic of this variant of the malignant histiocytic cell seen in nodular sclerosing Hodgkin's disease. This is probably a fixation artefact. × 432.

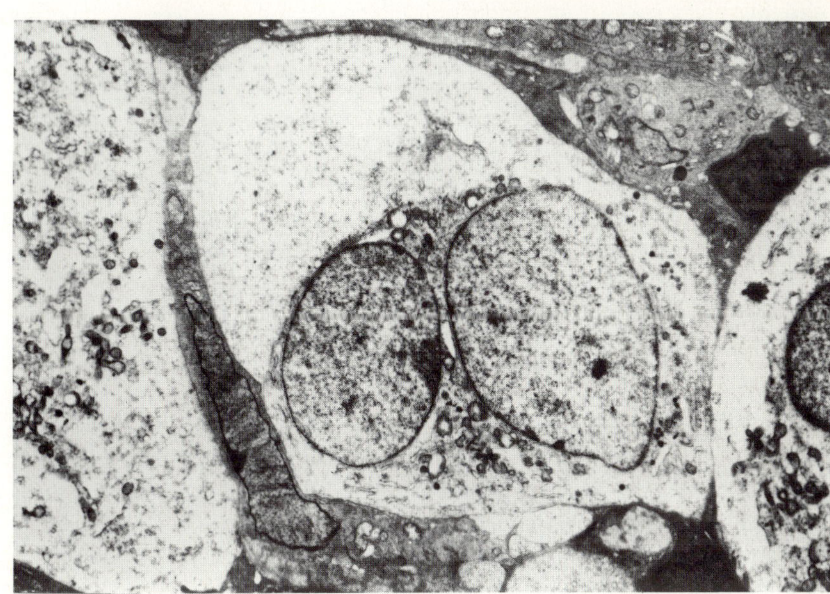

Fig. 4.11. Electron micrograph of lacunar cell in nodular sclerosing Hodgkin's disease. There is a large area of highly hydrated cytoplasm. × 6,000.

scattered mitochondria and profiles of endoplasmic reticulum and is surrounded by a ring of T-lymphocytes, which often protrude cytoplasm processes into the larger cell (Fig 4.5). It is probable that the R–S cell represents an end-stage variant of the neoplastic 'Hodgkin' cell. The characteristic R–S cell is easy to recognise but its identification is not always straightforward. There are usually prominent acidophilic nucleoli and a clear perinuclear area. Reed (1902) stated that the nucleus is always large in proportion to the overall size of the cell, may be single or multiple, bean-shaped or irregularly indented and have up to an 8–10 nuclei (a historical survey is given by Rather 1972). Reed noted the absence of mitosis in these cells, confirmed by Peckham and Cooper (1969), who showed that while uptake of tritiated thymidine could be shown in the 'Hodgkin' cells, it was not demonstrable in the R–S cells. Other studies have shown that R–S cell can take up thymidine after long periods of incubation, but their capacity to divide is still in doubt. Spriggs (1971) studied the chromosome pattern and found similar abnormalities in each 'Hodgkin' cell examined, suggesting a process of 'clonal' proliferation from an abnormal precursor cell. It is now realised that the Reed–Sternberg cell is not necessarily specific for Hodgkin's disease. Strum *et al.* (1970) and other authors have described them in a variety of other conditions, the most interesting of which are infectious mononucleosis and Burkitt's lymphoma, both associated with the Epstein–Barr virus. Similar cells may be seen in cases of measles, thymoma, mycosis fungoides and in certain carcinomas. Reed–Sternberg cells are only significant in the diagnosis of Hodgkin's disease if the rest of the histological appearances are appropriate. Lukes (1971) notes three variants of the R–S cell;

a   the lacunar cell of the nodular sclerosing type;

b   the polyploid 'L and H' cell found in the lymphocyte predominance variety;

c   the pleomorphic variant of the lymphocyte depletion type.

The nature of the Reed–Sternberg cell is still in doubt. There is conflicting ultrastructural evidence of macrophage origin (Carr 1975; Kay 1975) and of T-lymphocyte origin (Dorfman *et al.* 1973). The demonstration of immunoglobulin in these and 'Hodgkin' cells supports B-lymphocytic origin (Taylor 1974; Azar 1975; Glick 1976) and similar conclusions were reached by Anagnostou *et al.* (1977), concerning the lacunar cell. Curran and Jones (1978) suggest that Hodgkin and Reed–Sternberg cells derive from dendritic cells. Kaplan (1981) in a review of the subject, noted, for instance, that binucleate cells label with tritiated thymidine in culture, that giant cells may contain both κ and λ light chains which they must have absorbed rather than produced, and that the way in which these cells cluster in tissue culture is quite unlike the behaviour of lymphocytes. Kaplan's conclusion is that Reed–Sternberg cells are neoplastic, not end-stage cells and probably of macrophage lineage.

THE HISTOLOGICAL DIAGNOSIS OF HODGKIN'S DISEASE

The diagnosis of Hodgkin's disease may be difficult. In a review of 600 cases originally diagnosed as Hodgkin's disease, Symmers (1968) found that only 317 cases (53%) actually had the disease, while 85 cases diagnosed as other conditions eventually proved to have Hodgkin's disease. The difficulties in diagnosis fall into two categories:

1   Is the condition Hodgkin's disease at all?

2   If so, to what histological sub-type should it be allocated?

The most common conditions wrongly diagnosed as Hodgkin's disease were non-specific reactive lymphadenopathy, infectious mononucleosis, toxoplasmosis, dermatopathic lymphadenopathy and drug-induced lesions. These have been discussed in Chapter 3. In these conditions the basic architecture of the node is retained, although it may be severely distorted. Difficulties may still arise, however, since Hodgkin's disease may show partial involvement of the lymph node, leaving areas of normal structure intact. Hodgkin's disease may also occur in follicular forms. In view of the diverse histological appearances presented by Hodgkin's disease, it is advisable that Reed–Sternberg cells should be identified. These may be atypical and in the lymphocytic forms so difficult to find that the search has to be abandoned, but adherence to this rule will prevent errors. Conversely, R–S cells may be found in reactive conditions and the supporting histological changes must be in evidence before a diagnosis of Hodgkin's disease is made on the presence of R–S cells alone. This latter is obviously somewhat of a circular argument, but highlights the difficulty occasioned by some cases. In the absence of a local panel of pathologists, a second opinion on such sections should be sought.

Criteria for the classification of Hodgkin's disease have been given (Lukes 1971) and the difficulties discussed (Neiman 1978). In a survey of 176 cases reviewed by three pathologists, complete agreement was possible in only 120 of the cases, although all three disagreed in only two instances. Problems may arise where different histological appearances are seen in biopsies from different areas taken at the same time or even in areas within the same lymph node; Custer and Bernhard (1948) noted that 384/700 cases showed such differences. Similarly, progression in time to a 'worse' histological picture may occur as was described by Jackson and Parker (1947). This tendency to progression, however, varies with the histological subtype. Strum and Rappaport (1971a) found that in cases with two or more biopsies 44/48 (91.7%) cases of nodular sclerosing Hodgkin's disease remained unchanged, whereas this was true in only 5/13 (38.5%) cases of the lymphocytic variety, transposition being possible to any of the other three types. The mixed cellularity type may progress to the lymphocytic depletion form but reversion to a 'better' type does not seem to occur.

Thomas and Berard (1973) state that in 345 patients 17% were of the lymphocyte predominance type, 30% mixed cellularity, 12% lymphocytic depletion, 37% nodular sclerosing and 3% unclassified. All except the nodular sclerosing type were commoner in the male. When ranked by histological type and clinical stage on presentation, Stage I had a poor prognosis in only the lymphocyte depletion type, in Stage II and III, prognosis follows the histological type, while Stage IV only has a good prognosis in the lymphocyte predominance type. However, histological progression to a worse type found at necropsy occurred frequently; at autopsy, almost all initially lymphocytic predominance cases showed this feature, more than half of the nodular sclerosing cases and about a quarter of the mixed cellularity type. Progression occurs more commonly in the male, accounting for the worse prognosis.

The lymphocytic predominance form of Hodgkin's disease may show such an intense proliferation of lymphocytes as to resemble a lymphocytic variety of a non-Hodgkin lymphoma or chronic lymphocytic leukaemia. The latter can be excluded by blood and marrow examination. In a non-Hodgkin lymphoma, macrophages containing cell debris may be present (the starry-sky appearance) and occasional epithelioid histiocytes occur, but the presence of large numbers of the latter is a pointer to Hodgkin's disease and should initiate a search for Reed–Sternberg cells. The lymphocytic forms of Hodgkin's disease may show a follicular pattern, mimicking other follicular lymphomas. These are not true follicles and should be distinguished from the true follicular hyperplasia seen in reactive conditions.

In the extreme form of the lymphocyte depletion type, no lymphocytes are present, the tumour consisting of a diffuse proliferation of pleomorphic neoplastic cells, among which Reed–Sternberg cells should be identified. There may be some confusion with the less well-differentiated forms of non-Hodgkin's lymphoma, but the latter do not often show the extreme cellular and nuclear pleomorphism seen in Hodgkin's disease and will not demonstrate the diffuse fibrosis sometimes seen in the latter. When the cells have abundant eosinophilic cytoplasm, however, distinction may be difficult from a malignant lymphoma (histiocytic type).

The mixed cellularity type presents few difficulties, although forms with large numbers of eosinophils or of plasma cells may produce an initially puzzling appearance. However, classical Reed–Sternberg cells are usually prominent, and once found, the diagnosis becomes apparent.

The nodular sclerosing variety is unmistakable in its fully developed form but when the fibrosis is less, some pathologists make a diagnosis of a 'cellular' phase of the type, largely on a basis of the presence of lacunar cells. In the review of Strum and Rappaport (1971a) 5/7 such cases eventually transposed into the typical nodular sclerosing pattern. In the series of Lukes and his co-workers, nodular sclerosing types account for a fairly high percentage of all cases—149/377 cases in one study (Lukes 1963). This may be caused by undue weight being placed on the presence of birefringent collagen as a feature in its own right. The biological potential of the cellular types may represent a valid observation, but it makes for confusing terminology and many pathologists including Butler (1975) and Marshall *et al.* (1976) are reluctant to diagnose nodular sclerosing Hodgkin's disease in the absence of both sclerosis and nodule formation.

It is probable that Hodgkin's disease represents a spectrum of change; cases will be encountered of overlap between the sub-types of the Rye, or any other classification. Thus, eosinophils and plasma cells may be found in cases of lymphocytic predominance and cases of this type 'with too many R–S cells' may represent a more aggressive type. The number of lymphocytes in the mixed cellularity types varies between wide limits as does the number of obviously neoplastic cells. Areas of frankly lymphocytic depletion type may be seen, and conversely, sometimes helpfully, lymphocytic depletion forms may show focal areas of more classical mixed cellularity appearance. It is wise, therefore, in addition to reporting the histology of the case in terms of the Rye Classification to include a more extended description of the findings and an assessment of the biological potential of the tumour.

The relationship of Hodgkin's disease to the non-Hodgkin lymphomas is not entirely clear. Occasional cases of a follicular lymphoma developing into Hodgkin's disease have been reported and the latter has been followed by both acute and chronic leukaemia, but such cases are rare and it is best to regard Hodgkin's disease as a separate entity neither developing from nor transposing into the other lymphomas.

THE RELATIONSHIP OF SUBCLASSIFICATION TO PROGNOSIS

The prognosis of cases of Hodgkin's disease has been dramatically improved by recent advances in treatment, based on accurate staging of the disease and on histological assessment. As a result, prognosis is less clearly related to the histological subtype than was seen with older methods of treatment. Thus in one series (Fuller *et al.* 1977) the survival rates of the lymphocytic predominance, nodular sclerosing and mixed cellularity types were all similar, although there was a tendency for the tumour in nodular sclerosing cases to spread to the lung and pleura. Even cases of extensive disease responded well. However, examination of former series of cases shows that the histological appearance does reflect biological behaviour.

Even the Jackson and Parker (1947) classification was of some use in estimating prognosis, though 80% of 5-year survivors were in the 'granuloma' group and were not prognostically identified (Butler 1973). In the series of Jelliffe and Thomson (1955) the cases of 'paragranuloma' showed a 50% 10-year survival and 'granuloma' 6% whereas no cases of 'sarcoma' survived for 10 years. This variation in histological pattern and its relationship to prognosis elicited some interest in those cases of Hodgkin's disease surviving for long periods of time (Harrison 1952; Dawson and Harrison 1961; Wright 1960). These did not all fit into the category 'paragranuloma' and were described as 'benign' Hodgkin's disease by Dawson and Harrison (1961) who record a 10-year survival rate of 85% in these cases. In some cases 20-year survivals were recorded, leading Easson and Russell (1963) to speak of the 'cure' of Hodgkin's disease, the survival pattern of such cases thereafter reverting to that of the general population.

The Rye classification gives somewhat more precise prognostic information. In general lymphocytic predominance and nodular sclerosing varieties have an excellent prognosis, the lymphocytic depletion group a poor outcome, with the mixed cellularity type occupying an intermediate position. Thus Franssila *et al.* (1967) in a study of 97 cases, found 5-year survivals as follows: lymphocytic predominance (9

cases) 55%, nodular sclerosing (45 cases) 47%, mixed cellularity (32 cases) 3% and lymphocytic depletion (11 cases) 0%. The corresponding figures of Gough (1970) were 58%, 45%, 18% and 8% respectively. In a study of 10-year survivors Henry (1970) showed a figure of 70% for the lymphocytic forms 46% in the nodular sclerosing group and 19% for the mixed cell forms. No case of lymphocytic depletion survived for this length of time, only 25% were alive at the end of one year and all had died before three years had elapsed. However in the cases of Marshall *et al.* (1976), the outcome of the nodular sclerosing type tended to be worse than in other recorded series.

Butler (1973) made a comparative analysis of the usefulness of the Rye classification in 8 large series. Usually the lymphocyte predominant form implied the best prognosis followed in diminishing order by the nodular sclerosis, the mixed and the lymphocytic depletion types, but in 2 of the 8 series the nodular sclerosing form implied the best prognosis, and in 2 of the 8 series the mixed cell and lymphocyte depleted forms had an equally bad prognosis. The nodular sclerosing type was the easiest and the lymphocytic type the hardest to identify histologically without equivocation. There was at least 10% disagreement among groups of 3 pathologists. These difficulties point out the need for review of such lesions by more than 1 pathologist.

Incomplete replacement of the lymph node by neoplasm was noted by Rosenthal (1936) and many subsequent authors. In a study of long survivals in Hodgkin's disease Henry (1970) found this feature in 18/27 cases surviving for over 10 years. In a subsequent review of 166 cases partial involvement was found in 61 (Henry 1971). In general, this carried a better prognosis than in those cases where the architecture was completely destroyed, although this was only significant in the nodular sclerosing and mixed cell varieties. In the lymphocytic forms the prognosis was so good and in the lymphoid depletion type so bad, that the effect of partial involvement did not become manifest.

There is some correlation between disease staging and histological type (Gough 1970). The lymphocytic and nodular sclerosing types tend to grow slowly in clinical stage I and to remain localized. The lymphocytic depletion cases usually spread rapidly and widely. In Henry's series (1971) only 12 of 58 cases of the lymphocytic or nodular sclerosing types presented as Stage III or IV. However 9/12 cases of lymphocytic depletion were in Stage I when first seen. The mixed-cellularlity cases showed a wider spread with 52 cases in Stage I, 20 Stage II, 15 Stage III and 8 Stage IV.

THE MANNER OF SPREAD

The simplest explanation of the manner of spread of Hodgkin's disease is that it originates in a single lymph node or group of nodes, probably in the paracortical areas and spreads to contiguous nodes, even against the direction of the flow of lymph (Rosenberg and Kaplan 1966). Later, spread occurs by the blood stream to give disseminated extranodal lesions. Smithers (1974) however, believes that spread occurs between nodes with the lymphatic flow, with blood stream spread to other sites modified by their susceptibility to tumour induction. Neoplastic lymphoreticular cells may indeed follow the migration paths of their normal counterparts (Pilgrim 1972). Malignant Hodgkin cells may be found in thoracic duct lymph but curiously are rarely found in the sinuses of lymph nodes. Invasion of blood vessels is not uncommon in affected lymph nodes, though it can easily be missed unless elastic stains are used to delineate the remains of destroyed arteries. R–S cells can be found in the circulation if sought with sufficient care, and it is probable that the presence of vascular invasion accounts for the haematogenous dissemination of the disease. Rappaport and Strum (1970) and Naeim *et al.* (1974) believe that this implies a worse prognosis, notably in the lymphocyte depletion cases. Lamoureux *et al.* (1973) however, comment on the lack of vascular invasion in many patients with widespread extranodal dissemination and Kirschner *et al.* (1974) suggest that while vascular invasion in lymph nodes is not prognostically significant, it is of evil omen when seen in splenectomy specimens. The current balance of evidence would suggest that vascular invasion does imply a worse prognosis.

To obtain accurate information on the spread of disease it has become the practice to perform a laparotomy in cases of Hodgkin's disease—to remove the spleen for pathological examination, take a wedge liver biopsy and remove a certain number of abdominal lymph nodes for section. In a study of 65 patients (Glatstein *et al.* 1969) 19 patients had only spleen involvement, 21 both liver and spleen involved and 25 showed involvement of neither organ. No patient showed liver involvement without the spleen being affected. In a large subsequent series Kadin *et al.* (1971) and Rosenberg (1972), the preoperative clinical assessment of splenic involvement was inaccurate in one third of the 117 cases studied. 51 cases showed abdominal involvement, unsuspected clinically in 11 (21%) and equivocal in 10 (20%). The converse also applied, 50% patients with clinically enlarged spleens had no evidence of Hodgkin's disease when the excised spleen was examined pathologically, the enlargement being due to congestion, hyperplasia or granuloma formation. In 8% of patients the spleen was the only organ involved below the diaphragm, and in most patients with abdominal lymph node involvement, the spleen was affected also. In our experience if splenomegaly ($\geqslant 220$ g) is present, whatever the pathologic cause, there is a high incidence of abdominal lymph node involvement (Hancock *et al.* 1979a).

The technique was also adopted in British centres (Jelliffe *et al.* 1970; Farrer-Brown *et al.* 1971; Farrer-Brown *et al.* 1972; reviewed by Gazet 1973). In 22 patients the preoperative diagnosis of splenic involvement was correct in only 10, but although clinical enlargement was not a good guide in general, involved spleens were heavier than those not affected, an average of 304 g as against 192 g for the latter. 20/44 patients had a biopsy of the abdominal lymph nodes. Of these 14 were positive and in turn 11 of these had splenic involvement. There is some correlation of the findings with clinical staging arrived at before operation. Thus Brunk *et al.* (1970) obtained results according to the Table 4.1.

From these figures it seemed that laparotomy might only be performed in cases presenting in Stages III and IV, since in Stages I and II abdominal involvement was unlikely to be present. Aisenberg *et al.* (1971) gave the following indications for laparotomy and splenectomy. Systemic symptoms, a positive abdominal lymphangiogram and a palpable spleen were absolute indications, or two or more of the following criteria:

1 Doubtful lymphangiogram
2 Enlarged spleen on X-ray
3 Palpable liver
4 Elevated B.S.P. retention
5 Elevated alkaline phosphatase
6 Histological typing of mixed cellularity or lymphocytic depletion.

Others have pointed out that for the effective treatment of truly localised disease by radiotherapy an accurate assessment by diagnostic laparotomy and splenectomy is essential (Sut-

Table 4.1

Preoperative clinical stage	Operative findings	
	Spleen +ve	Liver +ve
I	1/13	0/13
II	2/5	0/5
III	10/14	8/14
IV	2/2	1/2

cliffe *et al.* 1976) since a significant number of patients do have the clinical staging altered as a result of this operation. It is now generally accepted that about 25% of patients with clinical Stage I or II are at risk from abdominal involvement (Aisenberg 1978).

Our own policy until recently was to perform laparotomy and splenectomy in selected patients, i.e. those staged clinically as IA IIA (mixed cell or lymphocyte depletion histology type) and IB IIB and IIIA (all histology types). In our reported series (Hancock *et al.* 1979a) of 52 patients selected from a total of 147, 21 showed more extensive disease than was clinically evident; this includes 8 of the 10 patients initially staged IIB. Two patients from the group of 25 staged IA IIA (lymphocyte predominant or nodular sclerosis histology) not selected for laparotomy have so far relapsed outside the primary mantle treatment field, a recurrence rate fortunately lower than that seen in many other centres. We have had four deaths from septicaemia (with little or no Hodgkin's disease evident) in our splenectomy group, compared with only one in the non-splenectomy group. The risks of infection, therefore, have to be balanced against the benefits of better staging of the Hodgkin's disease. Our current policy with regard to diagnostic laparotomy, in line with current British National Lymphoma Investigation protocols, is given in Chapter 13.

The relationship of splenic involvement to histology is not exact. In our experience involvement with lymphocyte predominant/nodular sclerosis types is less frequent than with mixed cell and lymphocyte depletion types. In the series of Kadin *et al.* (1971), however, 46% of the cases of lymphocyte predominance, 30% of nodular sclerosing and 63% of mixed cellularity showed abdominal involvement, and in a series of 44 cases Farrer-Brown *et al.* (1971) found splenic involvement as follows: lymphocytic forms 6/7 cases, nodular sclerosing 11/23 and mixed cellularity 5/14. The splenic histology may differ from that seen in the original lymph node biopsy. Although no cases of lymphocytic depletion were included in the latter series, the spleens contained areas of the lymphocytic depletion variety in two cases from each group, and the histologic appearance can vary even in different areas of the same spleen. The spleen must be closely examined; in some cases only minute foci of the disease may be present. Three cases in the series of Farrer-Brown *et al.* (1972) showed only slight prominence of the Malpighian bodies grossly and on histological examination only the follicles were involved; the disease appeared to begin in the periarteriolar regions, raising the question once more of haematogenous spread or multifo-

cal origin of the disease. The histology of the liver biopsy also needs careful assessment. The usual criteria for the diagnosis of Hodgkin's disease must be rigorously applied, including the finding of Reed–Sternberg cells. In a proportion of cases the liver shows non-specific portal inflammatory changes, fibrosis or granulomas, which should be ignored for staging purposes, even though such changes may be of importance in the assessment of the case as a whole.

INCIDENCE

The cause of Hodgkin's disease is unknown. It is not even known whether it is one disease or several, or whether it is neoplastic or not—though it seems likely that it is one neoplastic process.

In most communities, the curve of age incidence is bimodal, with a peak in early and another in late adult life. From birth to 10 years the male:female incidence is 3:1, but in early adult life the two sexes are equally affected. In the elderly, males again predominate by a factor of 2:1 (MacMahon 1957 and 1966). MacMahon advanced the theory that Hodgkin's disease might in fact be two diseases, inflammatory in nature in young adults, becoming neoplastic in older age. In certain States in the Southern USA, mortality from Hodgkin's disease in the elderly is the same as in the country as a whole but young adults show only half the national death rate from the disease (Cole *et al.* 1968). The early peak is due to the occurrence of the nodular sclerosing variety, which tends to occur in the younger patient, is more common in females, presents more often as localised disease and has a better prognosis. Thus, Hodgkin's disease may well be one neoplastic entity showing a spectrum of histological patterns with corresponding differences in sex incidence, presentation and response to treatment, the disease in the elderly having a 'worse' prognosis. The variation of histology with age was studied by Newell (1970) who analysed the occurrence of 23 histological features. In the older age groups, there was a high score for the incidence of atypical mitoses and for initial disseminated presentation of the disease. In the young, the disease tended to be more localised with more R–S cells, less atypical mitoses, more fibroses, more eosinophils and a greater incidence of partial involvement of the node. Newell felt that these findings supported the dual nature of the disease.

There are also geographic variations in incidence. The bimodal distribution with age is notably absent in Japan. In affluent countries, the disease is more frequent in the higher socio-economic groupings and occurs less commonly in children, although when the latter are affected, they tend to have the 'better' histologic gradings with a higher incidence in females. In under-developed countries, children are more affected and with 'worse' histological gradings. In tropical countries the disease is more aggressive in adults (Vianna *et al.* 1971a; Olweny *et al.* 1971; Correa and O'Connor 1973). Nodular sclerosing Hodgkin's disease is commoner in the USA than in Britain and rare in Japan—where Hodgkin's disease as a whole is relatively uncommon in relation to other lymphomas (Kageyama *et al.* 1973).

EPIDEMIOLOGY

There is some evidence for the 'spread' of Hodgkin's disease in the community. There is a 2–3 times increased chance of occurrences in the relatives of a case, and cases have been reported in twins, husbands and wives and infants and mothers (Razis *et al.* 1959). Some 100 such events have now been recorded. Time-space clustering has also been reported (Vianna *et al.* 1972; Davies 1972). Epidemiological evidence of case to case transmission was found in a group of 31 cases; it was noted that in 5 of 8 schools in which a case of Hodgkin's disease was reported, further cases occurred, whereas none was reported in 8 other matched schools. The incubation period suggested by these studies was 3–8 years, but in a recent Dutch case study a much shorter incubation period of 2–6 months was suggested (Wagener and Haanen 1975). Although several clusters of Hodgkin's disease have now been reported the statistical evaluation of their significance is extremely difficult and the conclusions have come under criticism (Grufferman 1977). Although Vianna and Polan (1973) have extended their studies, clustering is not common, and in view of possible misinterpretation of such findings, both by patients and by the community in general, it should be emphasised that hasty conclusions concerning an infective aetiology should not be drawn from a rare event, occurring in a disease that is itself rare (roughly 4 cases per 100 000 population per annum overall).

Gutensohn and Cole (1981) in a thorough investigation of the epidemiology, drew an analogy between the natural histories of Hodgkin's disease and poliomyelitis, and concluded that a delayed and infrequent infection by a common virus, e.g. the Epstein–Barr virus, was a probable aetiological factor in Hodgkin's disease. In their study of childhood environmental factors it was noted that cases of Hodgkin's disease had a smaller family size, fewer playmates, better educated mothers and an increased rate of infectious mononucleosis.

AETIOLOGY

It is postulated from the above evidence that Hodgkin's disease may be due to a low-virulence virus which enters by the oral or respiratory route, is held up in gut-associated lymphoid tissue releasing immune complexes into the circulation (Brown *et al.* 1978), which may then reach the systemic lymphoid tissues and produce the changes of Hodgkin's disease (Vianna *et al.* 1971a). This would fit the alleged increase in frequency of the disease in patients who have had tonsillectomy or appendicectomy in early life (Vianna *et al.* 1971b) though this was not confirmed by Ruuskanen (1971). The evidence for the infectious aetiology of the disease is reviewed by Vianna (1976) and Kinlen (1977). There is, as yet, no unequivocal evidence for a viral aetiology and certainly in a locally observed cluster of nine cases occurring in 1972–75 in an area of less than 1 km^2 (Evans *et al.* 1977) there was no suggestion of patient contact before the onset of the disease. Even were viruses to be convincingly isolated, it would be hard to prove them other than a passenger virus. However, there are indirect observations which stimulate the search for possible causative agents. There have been reports of either sequential or concurrent infectious mononucleosis and Hodgkin's disease (Smithers 1967) and the Paul–Bunnell reaction may be positive in the latter. Antibody titres against the Epstein–Barr virus tend to be high in patients with Hodgkin's disease, particularly the more malignant variants (Johansson *et al.* 1970; Levine 1971) but efforts to grow the virus have been unsuccessful (Hirshaut *et al.* 1974). However, cells containing EBV nuclear antigen have been cultured from affected spleens. Oncorna and papova (SV 40) virus have also been implicated, and structures resembling mycoplasma have been identified. High molecular weight RNA and reverse transcriptase are present in Hodgkin's tissue but this may be only a further example of secondary infection, abundant evidence of which has come to light in the past.

One current hypothesis is that the disease is basically a viral infection of thymus-derived (T) lymphocytes which undergo an alteration of their surface antigens. These are then regarded as foreign by normal immunocompetent T cells which react against the altered lymphocytes. This has the effect of inducing an autoimmune type of reaction resulting in the production of neoplastic 'Hodgkin' cells and the end-stage R–S cells (Order and Hellman 1972). This theory may explain the initial sites of involvement in Hodgkin's disease, the lymph nodes, spleen and thymus, wherein the majority of T-lymphocytes are to be found. The T-cell involvement may produce depletion of these cells with depression of cellular immunity; replacement by B cells take place leading to the formation of fibrous tissue. The lymphocytic type of the disease would represent a preponderance of reactive normal T cells and the lymphocytic depletion forms an extensive neoplastic change in the presence of depressed cellular immunity. This would be supported by the finding of increased numbers of T-lymphocytes in affected lymph nodes, and the demonstration of lymphocytes surrounding the malignant cells (Archibald and Frenster 1973). Such a theory would, however, have to take into account the depression of cellular immunity commonly seen in the disease.

As Kaplan and Smithers (1959) suggest, Hodgkin's disease in man bears some relation to a chronic graft-versus-host reaction seen in the experimental animal. When such a reaction is induced, malignant lymphomas may develop (Gleichmann *et al.* 1972). This depends on an immune response since unless the graft actually reacts against the host tissue, such neoplasms do not occur. However, an additional factor of virus activation is also involved since cell-free filtrates of the spleens produced lymphomas when injected into newborn mice. These authors view the production of lymphomas as activation of an oncogenic virus by an immune response. It must be admitted, however, that these animal lymphomas do not resemble Hodgkin's disease.

Sinkovics and Schullenberger (1975) postulate a fusion, possibly virus-induced, of a neoplastic T cell and a B cell, with a subsequent immunological reaction. If suppressor T cells are eliminated, then autoreactive B cell clones could become established. Thus, most recent theories combine an infective and an immunological component in the aetiology of the neoplasm but at the moment this cannot be considered proven.

Antigenic typing of leucocytes has also been undertaken in patients with Hodgkin's disease (Zervas *et al.* 1970) and an increased frequency of certain HLA antigens (HLA-A1, B_5 and B8 particularly) is found (Simons and Amiel 1977). It may be, therefore, that a certain antigenic grouping may affect both the antibody response (Sybesma 1972) of the body or the susceptibility to oncogenic viruses. It is also likely that patients with certain HLA types (e.g. B_8) have better survivals (Falk and Osoba 1971).

Although the putative neoplastic cell in Hodgkin's disease (the Reed–Sternberg cell) has been grown in culture and characterised (Kaplan and Gartner 1977), viral studies have not so far been possible. However, some current long term cell cultures (believed to be Reed–Sternberg in type) may provide the answer (Gallo and Gelmann 1981).

CLINICAL MANIFESTATIONS

Hodgkin's lymphoma has a bimodal age incidence, one peak occurring at 15–34 years and the other after 55 years. The disease is commoner in males, except in the case of the nodular sclerosis type which has a predilection for young females. In general lymphocyte predominant histology is seen in young adults, whereas lymphocyte depletion occurs more frequently in older age groups. Mixed cellularity histology is seen in all age groups. In Sheffield, England we see over 50 new cases each year, from a population of about $1\frac{1}{2}$ million; this is about 5% of malignant disease in the population.

The clinical features of many large series of patients have been reported (Ultmann *et al.* 1966; Tubiana *et al.* 1971; Kaplan 1972 and 1980; Smithers 1973; Butler 1973; Lacher 1976) and we have recently reported on experiences with 278 patients treated from 1971–76 (Hancock *et al.* 1979a) (updated to 1979 in Table 4.2).

Painless firm mobile lymph node enlargement is the commonest presenting symptom. In the initial stages the cervical (60–80%), axillary (6–20%) and inguinal nodes (6–12%) are found to be involved. Other groups of nodes,

Table 4.2 Presenting features of 403 patients treated in Sheffield (1970–1979)

Age	≤ 35 years	48%
	≥ 36 years	52%
Sex	male	62%
	female	38%
Clinical presentation	Neck nodes	60%
	Axillary/groin nodes	17%
	Other sites	8%
	Systemic symptoms	15%
Presenting stage	I	27%
	II	29%
	III	24%
	IV	20%
Symptom status	A	59%
	B	41%
Histology type	Lymphocyte predominant	20%
	Nodular sclerosis	20%
	Mixed cellularity	47%
	Lymphocyte depleted	13%

e.g. mediastinal, abdominal, are less frequently involved initially but become enlarged as the disease progresses. The spleen is involved pathologically in about 33% of cases at presentation, but this rises to over 75% in the later stages. In the more advanced stages of the disease almost any organ may be involved but isolated extranodal presentation of Hodgkin's disease is uncommon, particularly since it is now generally appreciated that the disease may be far more widespread than is clinically suspected.

The presence of constitutional symptoms should also be noted, i.e. fever, occasionally of the Pel–Ebstein variety, abnormal sweating and loss of weight. Such symptoms together with non-specific complaints such as pruritus, alcohol intolerance and generalised malaise may be the presenting features in some patients.

SPLEEN

Isolated involvement of the spleen is rare, although it will be involved in about 30% of cases at the time of presentation, is frequently involved in later stages of the disease, and probably always if death is due to Hodgkin's disease. The mixed cellularity histological type is frequently associated with splenic (together with intra-abdominal lymph node) involvement (Dorfman 1971). It is notable, however, that evidence of splenic enlargement is not diagnostic of splenic lymphomatous infiltration. Splenomegaly may also be due to reactive hyperplasia or granuloma formation. Conversely, the clinically normal spleen may be histologically involved by disease (Kadin *et al.* 1971).

HAEMOPOIETIC SYSTEM

Anaemia is frequently seen in Hodgkin's disease and may result from a number of factors.

Hypochromic microcytic anaemia occurs commonly at the start of the disease. The serum iron and iron binding capacity are reduced. The serum ferritin is usually elevated and there is adequate stainable iron in the bone marrow. The basic defect here appears to be a mal-utilization of haemoglobin iron (Haurani *et al.* 1963) as in the anaemia of infection and inflammation. This type of anaemia improves with treatment of the Hodgkin's disease and the serum iron is often used as a parameter of disease activity.

Macrocytosis (with a megaloblastic bone marrow) usually results from abnormalities in folate metabolism, partly from conditioned deficiency due to rapid cell turnover, partly from dietary deficiency in the very ill patient, and partly as an accompaniment of haemolytic anaemia. Rarely vitamin B_{12} and/or folate deficiency may arise due to small bowel infiltration by the lymphoma.

Haemolytic anaemia is usually a late feature of Hodgkin's disease (Dacie 1967) and is less common in this lymphoma than in the non-Hodgkin's types. Haemolysis has been variously ascribed to increased red cell osmotic fragility (Verloop 1955), and to the non-specific effects of fever (Ranlov and Videback 1963); the best understood explanation is the development of red cell auto-antibodies where the Coombs' antiglobulin test is positive in the presence of a reduced red cell survival time. Reticulocytosis, reduced haptoglobin level and acholuric jaundice may be present.

Bone marrow involvement with Hodgkin's disease is best diagnosed by trephine or open biopsy. Rarely the peripheral blood will show a leucoerythroblastic picture. Marrow suppression by radiotherapy and particularly chemotherapy is common, and may also occur in terminal disease from uraemia. Haemorrhage is an occasional consequence of thrombocytopenia.

Hypersplenism may occur later in the disease with peripheral pancytopenia but usually in the presence of an active marrow. Haemodilution may be another important factor in the genesis of the anaemia of Hodgkin's disease (Wrigley *et al.* 1973).

Leukaemia is rare in Hodgkin's disease (Gill and McCall 1943; Wrigley *et al.* 1973) but should be considered as a cause of resistant anaemia in the patient not responding to therapy. Three of a group of 1095 patients (Sahakian *et al.* 1974) and nine of a group of 764 patients (Valagussa *et al.* 1980) developed non-lymphoblastic leukaemia, probably related to intensive chemotherapy.

In the peripheral blood, leucocytosis, eosinophilia and thrombocytosis may occur, particularly with widespread disease and especially when intra-abdominal lymph nodes are involved. Lymphopenia commonly occurs in lymphocyte depleted Hodgkin's disease and where the disease is disseminated. Hodgkin cells and Reed–Sternberg cells are sometimes found in the peripheral blood (Bouroncle 1966).

ALIMENTARY SYSTEM

At autopsy nearly 30% of patients have alimentary involvement of stomach, pancreas and intestines. Peritoneal involvement may also occur and may be responsible for ascites during life. Primary lymphomas of the bowel are usually of the non-Hodgkin's variety but occasionally these may be seen as the initial manifestation of Hodgkin's disease (Naqvi *et al.* 1969) and may be accompanied by evidence of malabsorption (Brunt *et al.* 1969). In generalized disease the bowel is involved either from lymphatic or haematogenous spread or by infiltration of abdominal lymph node masses.

CARDIOVASCULAR SYSTEM

There are only isolated case reports of Hodgkin's disease presenting initially with cardiac disease. Hagans (1950) reports a patient presenting with signs and symptoms of pericarditis with effusion. In widespread disease the heart is involved in 10–15% of cases (Richmond *et al.* 1962; Roberts *et al.* 1968). Signs of cardiac dysfunction are seen when the parietal pericardium is involved by large mediastinal glands. Radiotherapy to this region may then cause pericardial adhesions and fibrosis perhaps with cardiac constriction (Roberts *et al.* 1968). We have seen only one patient with clinical and radiological evidence of pericardial effusion at the time of presentation with Hodgkin's disease and he remained asymptomatic throughout therapy.

GENITO-URINARY SYSTEM

Involvement of the genito-urinary system is a common finding at autopsy. Over half the 272 cases reviewed by Richmond *et al.* (1962) had some involvement. 13% of these cases had renal parenchymal infiltration but none of them had clinical evidence of renal involvement during life. We have recently treated a 16-year old male with Hodgkin's disease who had evidence of renal impairment at the time of presentation and eventually died in renal failure as a result of bilateral diffuse renal lymphomatous infiltration (Champion *et al.* 1976).

Renal function is most commonly impaired by obstruction from enlarged retroperitoneal lymph nodes. Uric acid nephropathy can be a serious complication particularly in the early stages of therapy during induction of remission. Hypercalcaemia and amyloidosis occur rarely (Kiely *et al.* 1969). There also appears to be an increased incidence of nephrotic syndrome in active Hodgkin's disease (Plager and Stutzman 1971) and the syndrome may remit following treatment of the lymphoma.

In an extensive review of the literature Chorlton *et al.* (1974) discussed 4 cases of Hodgkin's disease presenting with involvement of the female reproductive tract (all involving the uterine cervix). In the study of Richmond *et al.* (1962) 25% of their cases had evidence of involvement at autopsy. Involvement of the male reproductive system however was seen in only 2% of their cases.

LIVER

Isolated hepatic involvement has been reported (Symmers 1944) but this must be exceedingly rare. With disseminated disease the liver is involved in over half of cases though this may not be detected clinically or by liver function studies (Rosenberg 1971). Involvement is usually found only in the presence of splenic disease and is rarely found with lymph node disease restricted to above the diaphragm. Jaundice in Hodgkin's disease occurs with extensive hepatic infiltration and cellular destruction, with obstruction of the biliary tree by lymph nodes in the porta hepatis or as a result of haemolysis, seen usually in later stages of the disease (Dacie 1967).

BONE

The incidence of bony deposits in Hodgkin's disease is about 5–15% (Granger and Whitaker 1967; MacDonald 1973), but primary involvement is very rare (Willis 1967). Bony lesions develop either from haematogenous spread or by direct spread from involved nodes. They are detected radiologically or by isotope scanning often after arousal of clinical suspicion if the patient presents with bone pain or with the signs or symptoms of nerve compression. On radiological examination the lesions may appear osteolytic, osteosclerotic or of mixed type. The osteolytic type of lesion is the commonest found. Ferrant *et al.* (1975) detected bone lesions in 14 of 38 patients, 11 of these being proved histologically.

LUNG

Infiltration of the pleura may give rise to pleural effusions in up to one third of patients with Hodgkin's disease (Ultmann *et al.* 1966). At autopsy nearly two thirds have pleural effusions.

Intra-thoracic lymph node involvement is common, particularly in nodular sclerosing Hodgkin's disease. It is usually detected on chest radiography but occasionally gives rise to local symptoms by compression of major bronchi. Paratracheal and anterior mediastinal lymph nodes are commonly involved—a distinguishing feature from sarcoidosis, infections and primary lung neoplasms.

Primary lung parenchymal involvement is exceedingly rare (Kern *et al.* 1961 reviewed by Peckham 1973) but may be present in patients with more generalized disease. At autopsy more than 40% of cases have lung involvement (Richmond *et al.* 1962). Such involvement usually occurs, particularly in patients with nodular sclerosing Hodgkin's disease, as a result of extension of the tumour from involved intra-thoracic lymph nodes, probably by retrograde spread along lymphatic channels. Haematogenous spread also occurs, accounting for the occasional finding of discrete lung deposits.

The radiological appearance may be of diffuse pulmonary infiltration, discrete deposits, or more rarely of miliary mottling (often indistinguishable from tuberculosis, a very important clinical point bearing in mind the increased incidence of this infection in Hodgkin's disease).

A rare finding with intra-thoracic disease particularly in young adults and children is hypertrophic osteoarthropathy (Shapiro and Zvaifler 1973). We have recently treated a 16 year old female with intra-thoracic (nodular sclerosing) Hodgkin's disease who presented with clinical and radiographical features of hypertrophic osteoarthropathy including gross digital clubbing. The features regressed markedly after chemotherapy of her lymphoma (Hancock *et al.* 1976).

SKIN

The skin manifestations of Hodgkin's disease (Bluefarb 1959) may be specific or non-specific. Specific cutaneous involvement usually occurs by direct lymph node infiltration or occasionally by retrograde lymphatic spread. The manifestations which include infiltrations, nodules, plaques, ulcers and erythroderma are almost invariably associated with disease elsewhere in the body, primary skin involvement being extremely uncommon (Szur *et al.* 1970). The non-specific skin manifestations of Hodgkin's disease are pruritus (often with production of prurigo-like lesions), ichthyosis, hyper-pigmentation and herpes infections.

NERVOUS SYSTEM

Primary Hodgkin's disease of the brain has been reported (Sparling and Adams 1946) but, in general, infiltration of neurological tissue is uncommon. Even at autopsy there is involvement in only 5% of cases. Occasionally a patient may present with neurological signs from the pressure effects of extraneural deposits.

Peripheral neuropathy usually results from compression of nerves and nerve plexuses by neighbouring neoplastic tissue, but direct nerve infiltration can occur. Vincristine neurotoxicity is a common complication of chemotherapy. The lesion may be either a peripheral or an autonomic neuropathy (Hancock and Naysmith 1975). *Herpes zoster* 'neuritis' can occur at any stage of the disease.

Intra-cranial deposits may arise from discrete lymphomatous lesions (Burstein *et al.* 1963) or from direct extension of meningeal or bony deposits (Todd 1967). These lesions can cause all the signs and symptoms of a space occupying lesion with neurological sequelae and evidence of raised intracranial pressure.

Spinal cord lesions may give a clinical pattern varying from back and root pain to fully developed quadriplegia. Such pressure effects result from epidural or vertebral deposits or from collapse of an involved vertebral body.

Remote neurological effects of Hodgkin's disease are seen less commonly than with other malignancies. Nevertheless multifocal leucoencephalopathy (Ästrom *et al.* 1958) subacute cerebellar degeneration (Brain & Wilkinson 1965), peripheral neuropathy (Hutchinson *et al.* 1958) and subacute poliomyelitis (Walton *et al.* 1968) have all been reported. The familiar condition of malignant cachexia can occur in advanced Hodgkin's disease. Together with the great loss of subcutaneous fat there is diffuse wasting of muscles with symmetrical weakness.

Whenever unexplained intra-cranial symptoms occur the possibility of torulosis, cryptococcosis or other bizarre opportunistic infections should be investigated (Williams *et al.* 1959). In our series of patients, seven have developed neurological complications attributable to the lymphoma. One man presented with quadriplegia as the first manifestation of the disease—he had extensive epidural lymphomatous infiltration. Three other patients have developed epidural deposits as part of generalized disease. One man developed epilepsy as a manifestation of cerebral lymphoma deposits and another has cerebellar ataxia as a remote effect of the disease.

OTHER ORGANS

The thymus is a extranodal primary site (Katz and Lattes 1969). Involvement of the breast (Adair *et al.* 1945) and thyroid (Smithers 1970) have rarely been encountered. Hodgkin's disease of Waldeyer's ring is exceedingly uncommon (Todd and Michaels 1974) and even at autopsy there is only about 1% involvement.

SYSTEMIC SYMPTOMS

Systemic symptoms are usually indicative of widespread disease (Tubiana *et al.* 1971). Fever may be undulant in type (Pel-Ebstein) or irregular. Drenching night sweats may be an accompanying feature as well as other symptoms such as general malaise (often exacerbated by co-existent anaemia) weight loss and pruritus.

Pain in the lymph nodes after taking even small quantities of alcohol occurs in about one in six of patients with Hodgkin's disease; it is non-specific and may occur more commonly in other malignancies (Brewin 1966).

CHILDHOOD HODGKIN'S DISEASE

Hodgkin's disease in children (Hays 1975; Jenkin *et al.* 1975) usually presents with cervical adenopathy; systemic manifestations are less common than in adults. The histological type is usually nodular sclerosis, less commonly mixed cell or lymphocyte predominant and rarely lymphocyte depleted. Accurate staging is particularly important in children because of the more deleterious effects of radiotherapy and chemotherapy in this age group.

IMMUNE RESPONSES IN
HODGKIN'S DISEASE

In studies on immune responses in lymphomatous patients due allowance must always be made for the immunosuppressive effects of treatment. Even so there is frequently a depression in cellular immunity in patients with Hodgkin's disease as measured, e.g. by the tuberculin reaction, the skin reaction to such antigens as candida or mumps or the rejection of homografts (Schier *et al.* 1956; Aisenberg 1962; Kelly *et al.* 1960). Skin test reactivity to multiple antigens is depressed mainly in patients with disseminated disease and a more malignant histological picture (Young *et al.* 1972).

In vitro studies of lymphocyte function in Hodgkin's disease are numerous. The ability of the peripheral lymphocyte to undergo transformation after stimulation with plant mitogens (such as phytohaemagglutinin) may be depressed (Hersh and Oppenheim 1965) particularly in more advanced stages of the disease; these changes may revert to normal after successful treatment (Jackson *et al.* 1970).

The ability of the T-lymphocytes to form rosettes with sheep red cells may also be depressed (Cohnen *et al.* 1973);

this may be a qualitative rather than a quantitative T cell defect (Bobrove *et al.* 1975).

We studied cellular immunity in untreated patients using several methods of assessment (Hancock *et al.* 1977). Total depression was seen in only 10% of patients, all with disseminated disease. We found a generally elevated level of all serum immunoglobulin classes confirming that antibody responses remain relatively well preserved until the disease is far advanced (Aisenberg and Leskowitz 1963).

In follow up studies (Hancock *et al.* 1977 and 1982b) we found that treatment, particularly with cytotoxic drugs, depressed cellular immunity, and that this depression was still evident after five years of remission. Progressive falls in serum immunoglobulins were noted with low values of IgG and IgM being particularly a feature of patients having had splenectomy and chemotherapy. Although we were able to demonstrate defects in cellular immunoreactivity on *in vitro* tests there was no excess of infections in this group of patients. Defects in immune function have been found in other long term survivors of Hodgkin's disease in remission (Fuks *et al.* 1976; Fisher *et al.* 1980). The reason for these persistent defects is uncertain. It may be that certain aspects of T cell function are depressed by the presence of soluble factors or by the presence of suppressor T cells or suppressor monocytes (Fisher *et al.* 1981). These studies do, however, suggest that the immunological defect in Hodgkin's disease may be constitutional rather than just a disease and/or treatment mediated defect.

No defect in so-called reticuloendothelial (Sheagren *et al.* 1967) or peripheral neutrophil function is found in Hodgkin's disease. Neutrophil phagocytosis may in fact be enhanced particularly in patients with disseminated disease (Hancock *et al.* 1976).

Lymphopenia occurs commonly in Hodgkin's disease. It is partly related to the poor cellular immune response and usually indicates a bad prognosis. Aisenberg (1965) found that only 4 of 50 patients with advanced disease had a normal lymphocyte count in the peripheral blood. The pre-treatment peripheral lymphocyte count was related to prognosis in 328 cases of Hodgkin's disease by Swan and Knowelden (1971). Three groups emerged; those with a count of less than 1,000/μl had the worst prognosis (5-year survival 12%); those with a count between 1,000 and 1,500/μl were intermediate (5-year survival 26%); those with a count above 1,500/μl had the best prognosis (5-year survival 35%). These findings correlated well with histology in the 247 cases where biopsy material and pre-treatment counts were available. The lymphocytic predominance group had the highest mean count

(2,250/μl) and the lymphocytic depletion group the lowest (1,276/μl); the means of the mixed and nodular sclerosing varieties were intermediate. No patient in the lymphocytic predominance group had an initial count of less than 1,000/μl and only 6.7% had counts of less than 1,500/μl. In the lymphocytic depletion group these figures were 36.8% and 71.1% respectively. Brown *et al.* (1967) failed to find any statistical correlation between the lymphocyte count and histology but did show lower counts in Stage III and IV cases. He also found an initial lymphocytopenia ($<1,500/\mu$l) in 80% of cases who were subsequently unreactive to treatment.

A recent British National Lymphoma Investigation Study of 1100 patients confirmed the adverse effect of low lymphocyte count on prognosis (MacLennan *et al.* 1981). In our own prospective study of 181 consecutive untreated patients (Hancock *et al.* 1982a) lymphocyte counts did not correlate with histology type but were lower in Stage IV disease. Survival at 5 years was significantly worse in patients with counts less than 1500/μl than for those with normal counts (56 versus 79%).

The lymphocytes in the peripheral blood also show qualitative variations. There are more large lymphocytes with a high content of cytoplasmic RNA and PAS positive material and an increased uptake of tritiated thymidine *in vitro*. These cells are immunologically active rising from a value of $<0.5\%$ to 4% 5–7 days after the original stimulus. After treatment the percentage of such cells fell in patients who responded to treatment and rose in those who did not (Crowther *et al.* 1969a and b). Lymphopenia may be associated with a reduction in absolute T-lymphocyte counts (Stiehm *et al.* 1972) but most studies of the immune function in Hodgkin's disease suggest that whilst the total lymphocyte count may correlate with T- and B-lymphocyte numbers, it does not necessarily correlate with other parameters of immune function, e.g. lymphocyte transformation, leucocyte migration inhibition, skin test reactivity, immunoglobulin levels (Bobrove *et al.* 1975; Hancock *et al.* 1976; Hancock *et al.* 1980).

HODGKIN'S TISSUE 'ANTIGENS'

The immunological derangement seen in Hodgkin's disease and the varying prognosis seen in relationship to the lymphocytic response in tissue biopsies suggest the possibility of an immunological response in the host against the tumour. In any such discussion distinction must be made between true tumour-associated antigens, which are immunogenic in the tumour bearing host, and substances which are detectable by hetero-antisera raised in other species, perhaps best described as tumour-associated substances.

Two tumour-associated substances demonstrated in Hodgkin's tissue by Order *et al.* (1972) have been shown to be a ferritin and an α_1-globulin (Eshhar *et al.* 1974). A radionuclide-linked immunoglobulin against the ferritin antigen has been prepared and shown to bind to Hodgkin's tissue *in vivo* (Order *et al.* 1975). Sensitization to a crude extract of tumour tissue from Hodgkin's spleen has recently been demonstrated using a leucocyte migration technique. The sensitizing substance is probably ferritin in an abnormal form (Hancock *et al.* 1976 and 1979b).

AUTOIMMUNE DISEASE

It is well recognized that autoimmune phenomena may complicate the course of Hodgkin's disease and other lymphomas and may wax and wane with the activity of the disease.

It is thought that B cell capacity to produce antibodies against exogenous antigens and against the individuals own tissues is kept in check by thymus dependent T-lymphocytes (Allison *et al.* 1971). It would follow that autoantibodies could develop in patients with depressed cellular immunity and that this may account for the incidence of autoimmune disease in association with the lymphomas. Haemolytic anaemia (Dacie 1967) collagen-vascular disorders (Miller 1967) and pemphigus (Sood and Pasricha 1974; Naysmith and Hancock 1976) have all been reported in Hodgkin's disease.

SECOND NEOPLASMS

There is now good evidence that both acute leukaemia and non-Hodgkin's lymphoma may arise in patients treated with radiotherapy and combination chemotherapy, and that there is an increased incidence of solid tumours in such patients. The overall incidence of such events is difficult to estimate, but 2–5% is probably a conservative estimate (Arsenau *et al.* 1977; Coleman *et al.* 1977; Krikorian *et al.* 1979; Valagussa *et al.* 1980; Nelson *et al.* 1981). In the Sheffield series the incidence in patients treated since 1970 is 2%, but this may, of course, increase with time.

The theory of depressed immune surveillance is only one possible explanation for the occurrence of second neoplasms. This could equally well be blamed on the mutagenic effects of immunosuppressive therapy and of course the lowered resistance to oncogenic viral infection.

INFECTIONS

Immunosuppressed patients with disseminated Hodgkin's disease who undergo therapy often suffer infections with bacteria, viruses, fungi and parasites (Casazza *et al.* 1966; Gowing 1973). Usually the cause is one of the common pathogenic organisms—staphylococcus or streptococcus, often in hospital practice antibiotic resistant, but sometimes the organisms involved are opportunistic (e.g. cryptococcus, pneumocystis, aspergillus) and rarely cause trouble in patients with normal immune status. Other organisms causing minor infection in normal individuals (e.g. Candida, herpes viruses, vaccinia) can prove severe or even fatal in immunodepressed patients, e.g. Hancock and Henry 1977. The most common offender is *Herpes zoster* which occurs in up to 25% of patients with Hodgkin's disease (Schimpff *et al.* 1972). Tuberculosis may complicate immunosuppressive therapy; some authorities would recommend giving prophylactic antituberculous therapy to those patients on immunosuppressive therapy with evidence of old tuberculosis.

In any patient who becomes pyrexial it is important to exclude infection as a cause of the fever before attributing this to the disease process. This is particularly important in the immunodepressed patient on cytotoxic chemotherapy where granulopenia (as well as immunodepression) may be an added factor in the genesis of the infection.

PARANEOPLASTIC (NON-METASTATIC) SYNDROMES

NEUROLOGICAL DISORDERS

Non-metastatic neurological disorders of obscure origin occur in about 2% of patients with lymphoma—both Hodgkin's and non-Hodgkin's (Currie *et al.* 1970) and are therefore less common than in patients with other forms of cancer. Encephalopathies (including progressive multifocal leuco-encephalopathy and cerebellar degeneration), neuropathies (including peripheral sensorimotor neuropathy), myelopathies and myopathies (including polymyositis) have all been described. The aetiology of such syndromes is unknown though opportunistic infections and autoimmunity have been suggested.

ENDOCRINE DISORDERS

Ectopic hormone production is extremely rare in malignant lymphoma; isolated cases of inappropriate ADH secretion, hypercalcaemia (without osteolytic deposits) and hyperthyroidism have been reported (Ross 1972; Hobbs and Miller 1966).

MISCELLANEOUS DISORDERS

Skin manifestations are discussed elsewhere; dermatomyositis and *Acanthosis nigricans* have been described in Hodgkin's disease (Smithers 1973b). There is an increased incidence of nephrotic syndrome in Hodgkin's disease (Plager and Stutzman 1971). The cause of the syndrome is uncertain but may be related to the deposition of immune complexes in the glomerular basement membrane.

THE MANNER OF DEATH IN HODGKIN'S DISEASE

The two commonest patterns of death in Hodgkin's disease are of severe infection and disseminated neoplasm (Table 4.3). The infection may, as discussed earlier, be unusual

Table 4.3 Autopsy findings in Sheffield patients

Hodgkin's disease + pneumonia	50%
+ septicaemia	12%
+ opportunistic infection	5%
+ second neoplasm	5%
+ other complications	10%
Septicaemia, no Hodgkin's disease	8%
Second neoplasm, no Hodgkin's disease	5%
Other disease, no Hodgkin's disease	5%

opportunistic infections but most commonly in our experience are the ordinary pyogenic infections, usually bronchopneumonia, or lobar pneumonia, sometimes in the presence of marrow failure induced by chemotherapeutic agents. At necropsy, in our experience and in the series of Gowing

(1973), the lymph nodes are usually involved by neoplasm, the liver and spleen in about 70% of patients and the lungs, pleura and bone in 40%; many other sites may be involved but less frequently.

INVESTIGATION AND MANAGEMENT

This topic is discussed fully in Chapter 13. It depends on meticulous diagnostic evaluation and staging and involves intensive investigation including blood analyses, radiology (including lymphography) bone marrow examination, radio-isotopic scans and possibly laparotomy with splenectomy and biopsy of abdominal lymph nodes, liver and bone marrow. The patient is therefore first clinically and then pathologically assessed to allow the selection for appropriate treatment (megavoltage radiotherapy and/or multidrug combination chemotherapy).

As a guide to progress and treatment, therefore, schemes of staging have been evolved. One of the earliest schemes was that devised by Peters (1950) who introduced three stages based on initial clinical spread of the disease: I Localized disease, II Intermediate, III Widespread disease. The subject of clinical staging was also discussed at the Rye Conference (Rosenberg 1966) and the scheme devised there has subsequently been modified to that presently accepted at the Ann Arbor Conference (Carbone *et al.* 1971).

Each stage is sub-divided into A (asymptomatic) or B (symptomatic) categories according to the presence of weight loss (of greater than 10% of body weight in 6 months prior to presentation), unexplained fever (above 38°C) or night sweats. Pruritus, and short febrile illnesses associated with infection are not categorized as B symptoms.

This staging procedure is assessed first according to clinical and investigative criteria. It is then modified according to the further pathological findings of diagnostic laparotomy.

If clinical staging is used as a guide to treatment, certain difficulties arise, particularly in the assessment of involvement of abdominal organs. Both the spleen and liver may be affected without being clinically enlarged, and while lympho-angiography does give some indication of para-aortic lymph node involvement the method is not sufficiently precise to give an exact result.

Most centres now select patients for staging laparotomy on the basis of the clinical findings.

STAGE I

Involvement of a single lymph node region (I) or single extralymphatic organ or site (I_E).

STAGE II

Involvement of two or more lymph node regions on the same side of the diaphragm (II) or localized involvement of extralymphatic organ or site and of one or more lymph node regions on the same side of the diaphragm (II_E).

STAGE III

Involvement of lymph node regions on both sides of the diaphragm (III) which may be accompanied by localized involvement of extralymphatic organ (III_E) spleen (III_S) or both (III_{SE}).

STAGE IV

Diffuse involvement of one or more extralymphatic organs with or without associated lymph node involvement. Sites of involvement are denoted by symbols:

N—Lymph nodes		S—Spleen	
H—Liver		L—Lung	
M—Marrow		O—Bone	
P—Pleura		D—Skin	

PROGNOSIS

There has been a dramatic improvement in the prognosis of Hodgkin's lymphoma due to the application of recent diagnostic and therapeutic advances. A disease which was considered inevitably fatal 20 years ago is now within the realms of clinical cure, a fact which is doubly rewarding since many of the patients are young. The investigation and therapy is therefore best managed in specialised centres.

The prognosis in Hodgkin's disease depends upon:
1   the stage of the disease at presentation
2   the histology
3   the efficiency with which the disease is staged and treated (Hamilton Fairley 1974).

In our experience (Hancock *et al.* 1979a) unfavourable features are male sex, older age, widespread and symptomatic disease, lymphocyte depletion histology and high ESR; better survival figures are evident for younger age, female sex, localised disease and absence of symptoms, lymphocyte predominance and nodular sclerosing histology and low ESR.

Many of these indices were interdependent, for example lymphocyte predominance was associated with Stage I, asymptomatic disease, with low ESR and with remission. Nodular sclerosis was associated with good response, Stage II (usually neck and thoracic nodes) and was commoner with female sex. Mixed cellularity occurred in all stages and had intermediate prognosis, whereas lymphocyte depletion was associated with clinical Stage IV, B symptoms and non-response to treatment. Details of the therapeutic regimes available for Hodgkin's disease are given more fully in Chapter 13.

Radiotherapy is the mainstay of the management of localised Hodgkin's disease. For disseminated disease chemotherapy is appropriate. The estimated chances of being cured of Hodgkin's disease regardless of the extent of the disease at presentation have risen from 5% at the beginning of the century to at least 75% (Hamilton Fairley 1975). Radical radiotherapy using super-voltage wide field techniques has improved the 5-year survival in Stage I and IIA disease to above 90%.

For disseminated disease (Stages IIIB and IV) cyclical combination chemotherapy is the correct treatment; remission rates of 75–85% are possible (DeVita *et al.* 1970; Nicholson *et al.* 1970; McElwain 1971; DeVita *et al.* 1972). Previous therapy with local ionising irradiation does not significantly affect the response to combination chemotherapy, but previous single agent therapy and extensive irradiation lower remission rates to 45%. The 5-year survival of previously untreated patients with disseminated disease is above 70% with complete maintained remission in over half of these patients.

The overall 5-year survival rate for unselected patients treated by the Sheffield group in the 1970's is 64% (85% for local disease treated with radiotherapy and 47% for those with widespread or recurrent disease treated with chemotherapy). Our figures are not as good as those reported by others, but this may be partly explained by the higher proportion of older patients, of unfavourable histology and of Stage IV disease in our series compared with others. In our experience

(a)   failure to obtain complete remission within three months of starting treatment is a bad sign;

(b)   relapse of Hodgkin's disease after more than 3 years of apparent complete remission is only occasionally seen though it is recognised that Hodgkin's disease tissue can remain dormant for many years (Henry 1970; Strum and Rappaport 1971b); this must be taken into account when assessing clinical cure.

Nevertheless the disease-free survival for all patients regardless of histology or extent of disease flattens out at 10 years to about 50% (Kaplan and Rosenberg 1975), and it is reasonable to assume that this figure may represent the minimum cure rate in a previously inevitably fatal disease.

REFERENCES

ADAIR F.E., CRAVER L.F. & HERRMANN J.B. (1945) Hodgkin's disease of the breast. *Surg. Gyn. Obstet.* **80**, 205–10.

AISENBERG A.C. (1965) Lymphocytopaenia in Hodgkin's disease. *Blood* **25**, 1037–42.

AISENBERG A.C. (1962) Studies on delayed hypersensitivity in Hodgkin's disease. *J. Clin. Invest.* **41**, 1964–70.

AISENBERG A.C. (1978) The staging and treatment of Hodgkin's disease. *N. Eng. J. Med.* **299**, 1228–32.

AISENBERG A.C., GOLDMAN J.M., RAKER J.W. & WANG C.C. (1971) Spleen involvement at the onset of Hodgkin's disease. *Ann. Intern. Med.* **74**, 544–47.

AISENBERG A.C. & LESKOWITZ S. (1963) Antibody formation in Hodgkin's disease. *N. Eng. J. Med.* **268**, 1269–72.

ALLISON A.C., DENMAN A.M. & BARNES R.D. (1971) Co-operating and controlling functions of thymus derived lymphocytes in relation to auto-immunity. *Lancet* **ii**, 135–40.

ANAGNOSTOU D., PARKER J.W., TAYLOR C.R., TINDLE B.H. & LUKES R.J. (1977) Lacunar cells of sclerosing Hodgkin's disease. *Cancer* **39**, 1032–43.

ARCHIBALD R.B. & FRENSTER J.H. (1973) Quantitative ultrastructural analysis of *in vivo* lymphocyte-Reed-Sternberg Cell interactions in Hodgkin's disease. *Natl. Cancer Inst. Monogr.* **36**, 239–45.

ARSENEAU J.C., SPONZO R.W., LEVIN D.L., SCHNIPPER L.E., BONNER H., YOUNG R.C., CANELLOS G.P., HOHNSON R.E. & DeVITA V.T. (1972) Non-lymphomatous malignant tumours complicating Hodgkin's disease. Possible association with intensive therapy. *N. Eng. J. Med.* **287**, 1119–22.

ARSENAU J.C., CANELLOS G.P., JOHNSON R. & DeVITA V.T. (1977) Risk of new cancers in patients with Hodgkin's Disease. *Cancer* **40**, 1912–16.

ÄSTROM K.E., MANCALL E.L. & RICHARDSON E.P. (1958) Progressive multifocal leukoencephalopathy. A hitherto unrecognised complication of chronic lymphatic leukaemia and Hodgkin's disease. *Brain* **81**, 93–111.

AZAR H.A. (1975) Significance of the Reed-Sternberg cell. *Hum. Path.* **6**, 479–84.

BLUEFARB S.M. (1959) *Cutaneous Manifestations of the Malignant Lymphomas*, pp. 240–94. Charles C. Thomas, Springfield, Illinois.

BOBROVE A.M., FUKS Z., STROBER S. & KAPLAN H.S. (1975)

Quantitation of T and B lymphocytes and cellular immune function in Hodgkin's disease. *Cancer* **36**, 169–79.

BOURONCLE B.A. (1966) Sternberg-Reed cells in the peripheral blood of patients with Hodgkin's disease. *Blood* **27**, 544–56.

BRAIN LORD & WILKINSON M. (1965) Subacute cerebellar degeneration associated with neoplasms. *Brain* **88**, 465–78.

BREWIN T.B. (1966) Alcohol intolerance in neoplastic disease. *Brit. Med. J.* **2**, 437–41.

BRINKER H. (1972) Sarcoid reactions and sarcoidosis in Hodgkin's disease and other malignant lymphomata. *Brit. J. Cancer* **26**, 120–8.

BROWN C.A., HALL C.L., LONG J.C., CAREY K., WEITZMAN S.A. & AISENBERG A.C. (1978) Circulating immune complexes in Hodgkin's disease. *Amer. J. Med.* **64**, 289–94.

BROWN R.S., HAYNES H.A., FOLEY H.T., GODWIN H.A., BERARD C.W. & CARBONE P.P. (1967) Hodgkin's disease; immunologic, clinical and histologic features of 50 untreated patients. *Ann. Intern. Med.* **67**, 291–302.

BRUNK S.F., GULESSERIAN H.P., HASS A.C. & GIVLER R.L. (1970) Exploratory laparotomy and splenectomy in staging lymphomas. *Clin. Res.* **18**, 470.

BRUNT P.W., SIRCUS W. & MACLEAN N. (1969) Neoplasia and the coeliac syndrome in adults. *Lancet* **1**, 180–4.

BURSTEIN S.D., KERNOHAN J.W. & UIHLEIN A. (1963) Neoplasms of the reticuloendothelial system of the brain. *Cancer* **16**, 289–305.

BUTLER J.J. (1973) Relationship of histologic findings to survival in Hodgkin's disease. *Gann. Monogr. on Cancer Res.* **15**, 275–86.

BUTLER J.J. (1975) The natural history of Hodgkin's disease and its classification. In *The Reticuloendothelail System*, pp. 184–212 (Eds Rebuck J.W., Berard C.W. & Abell M.R.). Williams and Wilkins, Baltimore.

CARBONE P.P., KAPLAN H.S., MUSSHOFF K., SMITHERS D.W. & TUBIANA M. (1971) Report of the committee on Hodgkin's disease. Staging classification symposium. *Cancer Res.* **31**, 1860–1.

CARR I. (1975) The ultrastructure of the abnormal reticulum cells in Hodgkin's disease. *J. Path.* **115**, 45–50.

CASAZZA A.R., DUVALL C.P. & CARBONE P.P. (1966) Summary of infectious complications occurring in patients with Hodgkin's disease. *Cancer Res.* **26**, 1290–6.

CHAMPION A., COUP A.J. & HANCOCK B.W. (1976) Hodgkin's disease and chronic renal failure. *Cancer* **38**, 1867–8.

CHORLTON I., KARNEI R.F., KING F.M. & NORRIS H.J. (1974) Primary malignant reticuloendothelial disease involving the vagina, cervix and corpus uteri. *Obstet. Gyn.* **44**, 735–48.

COHNEN J., AUGENER W., BRITTINGER J. & DOUGLAS S.D. (1973) Rosette forming lymphocytes in Hodgkin's disease. *N. Eng. J. Med.* **289**, 863.

COLE P., MACMAHON B. & AISENBERG A.C. (1968) Mortality from Hodgkin's disease in the United States. Evidence for the multiple aetiology hypothesis. *Lancet* **2**, 1371–6.

COLEMAN C.N., WILLIAMS C.J., FLINT A., GLATSTEIN E.J., ROSENBERG S.A. & KAPLAN H.S. (1977) Hematologic neoplasia in patients treated for Hodgkin's disease. *N. Engl. J. Med.* **297**, 1249–452.

CORREA P. & O'CONNOR G.T. (1973) Geographic pathology of lymphoreticular tumours. Summary of survey from the geographic pathology committee of the international union against cancer. *J. Natl. Cancer Inst.* **50**, 1609–17.

CROWTHER D., HAMILTON FAIRLEY G. & SEWELL R.L. (1969a) Significance of the changes in the circulating lymphoid cells in Hodgkin's disease. *Brit. Med. J.* **2**, 473–7.

CROWTHER D., HAMILTON FAIRLEY G. & SEWELL R.L. (1969b) The periodic-acid Schiff reaction on lymphocytes in human malignant disease. *Brit. J. Haematol.* **16**, 389–96.

CURRAN R.C. & JONES E.L. (1978) Hodgkin's disease. An immuno-histochemical and histological study. *J. Pathol.* **125**, 39–51.

CURRIE S., HENSON R.A., MORGAN H.G. & POOLE A.J. (1970) The incidence of the non-metastatic neurological syndromes of obscure origin in the reticuloses. *Brain* **93**, 629–38.

CUSTER R.P. & BERNHARD W.G. (1948) The inter-relationship of Hodgkin's disease and other lymphatic tumours. *Amer. J. Med. Sci.* **216**, 625–42.

DACIE J.V. (1967) Secondary or symptomatic haemolytic anaemias I Haemolytic anaemias associated with Hodgkin's disease, leukaemia reticulosarcoma and myelosclerosis. In *The Haemolytic Anaemias*, Part III Chapter 13, pp. 721–726. J.A. Churchill Ltd., London.

DAVIES J.N.P. (1972) Hodgkin's disease in the community. *Hum. Path.* **3**, 297–9.

DAWSON P.J. & HARRISON C.V. (1961) A clinicopathological study of benign Hodgkin's disease. *J. Clin. Path.* **14**, 219–31.

DEVITA V.T., CANELLOS G.P. & MOXLEY J.H. (1972) A decade of combination chemotherapy of advanced Hodgkin's disease. *Cancer* **30**, 1495–1504.

DEVITA V.T., SERPICK A.A. & CARBONE P.P. (1970) Combination chemotherapy in the treatment of advanced Hodgkin's disease. *Ann. Intern. Med.* **73**, 881–95.

DORFMAN R.F. (1971) Relationship of history to site in Hodgkin's disease. *Cancer Res.* **31**, 1786–93.

DORFMAN R.F., RICE D.F., MITCHELL A.D., KEMPSON R.L. & LEVINE G. (1973) Ultrastructural studies of Hodgkin's disease. *Natl. Cancer Inst. Monogr.* **36**, 221–38.

EASSON E.C. & RUSSELL M.H. (1963) The cure of Hodgkin's disease. *Brit. Med. J.* **1**, 1704–7.

ESHHAR Z., ORDER S.E. & KATZ D.H. (1974) Ferritin, a Hodgkin's disease associated antigen. *Proc. Natl. Acad. Sci. USA* **71**, 3956–60.

EVANS A.R., HANCOCK B.W., BROWN M.J. & RICHMOND J. (1977) A small cluster of Hodgkin's disease. *Brit. Med. J.* **1**, 1033–57.

FALK T. & OSOBA D. (1971) HL-A antigens and survival in Hodgkin's disease. *Lancet* **2**, 1118–22.

FARRER-BROWN G., BENNETT M.H., HARRISON C.V., MILLETT Y. & JELLIFFE A.M. (1971) The pathological findings following laparotomy in Hodgkin's disease. *Brit. J. Cancer* **25**, 449–57.

FARRER-BROWN G., BENNETT M.H., HARRISON C.V., MILLETT Y. & JELLIFFE A.M. (1972) The diagnosis of Hodgkin's disease in surgically excised spleens. *J. Clin. Path.* **25**, 294–300.

FERRANT A., RODHAIN J., MICHAUX J.L., PIRET L., MALDAGUE B. & SOKAL G. (1975) Detection of skeletal involvement in Hodgkin's disease: a comparison of radiography, bone scanning and bone marrow biopsy in 38 patients. *Cancer* **35**, 1346–53.

FISHER R.I., DeVITA V.T., BOSTIK F., VanHAELAN C., HOWSER D.M., HUBBARD S.M. & YOUNG, R.C. (1980) Resistant immunologic abnormalities in long term survivors of advanced Hodgkin's disease. *Ann. Int. Med.* **92**, 595–9.

FISHER R.I., VAN HAELAN C. & BOSTIK F. (1981) Increased sensitivity to normal adherent suppressor cells in untreated advanced Hodgkin's disease. *Blood* **57**, 830–5.

FRANSSILA K.O., KALIMA T.V. & VOUTILAINEN A. (1967) Histologic classification of Hodgkin's disease. *Cancer* **20**, 1594–1601.

FRIEND C., MAROVITZ W., HENLE G., TSUEI D., HIRSCHHORN K., HOLLAND J.G. & CUTTNER J. (1978) Observations on cell lines derived from a patient with Hodgkin's disease. *Cancer Res.* **38**, 2581–91.

FUKS Z., STROBER S., BOBROVE A.M., SASAZUKI T., McMICHAEL A. & KAPLAN H.S. (1976) Long term effects of radiation on T and B lymphocytes in peripheral blood of patients with Hodgkin's disease. *J. Clin. Invest.* **58**, 803–14.

FULLER L.M., MADOC-JONES H., GAMBLE J.F., BUTLER J.J., SULLIVAN M.P., FERNANDEZ C.H. & GEHAN E.A. (1977) Prognostic significance of histopathology in Hodgkin's disease. *Cancer* **39**, 2174–82.

GALLO R.C. & GELMANN E.P. (1981) In search of the Hodgkin's disease virus. *N. Eng. J. Med.* **304**, 169–70.

GAZET J.C. (1973) Laparotomy and splenectomy in Hodgkin's disease. In *Hodgkin's Disease*, pp. 190–200 (Ed Smithers D.W.). Churchill Livingstone, Edinburgh.

GILL W. & McCALL A.J. (1943) Lymphadenoma and leukaemia. *Brit. Med. J.* **1**, 284–6.

GLATSTEIN E., GUERNSEY J.M., ROSENBERG S.A. & KAPLAN H.S. (1969) The value of laparotomy and splenectomy in the staging of Hodgkin's disease. *Cancer* **24**, 709–18.

GLEICHMANN E., GLEICHMANN H. & SCHWARTZ R.S. (1972) Immunologic induction of malignant lymphoma: genetic factors in the graft-versus host model. *J. Natl. Cancer Inst.* **49**, 793–804.

GLICK A.D. (1976) An ultrastructural study of Reed-Sternberg cells. *Amer. J. Path.* **85**, 195–208.

GOUGH J. (1970) Hodgkin's disease; a correlation of histopathology with survival. *Inter. J. Cancer* **5**, 273–81.

GOWING N.F.C. (1973) Modes of death and post-mortem studies. In *Hodgkin's Disease*, Chapter 17, pp. 163–6 (Ed Smithers D.W.). Churchill Livingstone, Edinburgh.

GRANGER W. & WHITAKER R. (1967) Hodgkin's disease in bone, with special reference to periosteal reaction. *Brit. J. Radiol.* **40**, 939–48.

GREENFIELD W.S. (1878) Specimens illustrative of the pathology of lymphadenoma and leucocythaemia. *Trans. Path. Soc. Lond.* **29**, 272.

GRUFFERMAN S. (1977) Clustering and aggregation of exposures in Hodgkin's disease. *Cancer* **39**, 1829–33

GUTENSOHN N. & COLE P. (1981) Childhood social environment and Hodgkin's disease. *N. Eng. J. Med.* **304**, 135–40.

HAGANS J.A. (1950) Hodgkin's granuloma with pericardial effusion. Unusual case of Hodgkin's disease presenting initially signs and symptoms of pericarditis with effusion. *Amer. Heart J.* **40**, 624–9.

HAMILTON FAIRLEY G. (1972–74) Lymphoproliferative diseases. *Medicine (Lond.)* **24**, 1412–20.

HAMILTON FAIRLEY G. (1975) New trends in cancer II The treatment of the lymphomas and leukaemias. *Health Trends* **7**, 1–5.

HANCOCK B.W., AITKEN M., MARTIN J.F., DUNSMORE I.R., ROSS C.M.D., CARR I. & EMMANUEL I.G. (1979a) Hodgkin's disease in Sheffield (1971–1976): with computer analysis of variables. *Clin. Oncol.* **5**, 283–97.

HANCOCK B.W., BRUCE L., DUNSMORE I.R., WARD A.M. & RICHMOND J. (1977) Follow-up studies of immune status of patients with Hodgkin's disease after splenectomy and treatment, in relapse and remission. *Brit. J. Cancer.* **36**, 347–54.

HANCOCK B.W., BRUCE L., MAY K. & RICHMOND, J. (1979b) Ferritin, a sensitising substance in the leucocyte migration inhibition test in patients with malignant lymphoma. *Brit. J. Haematol.* **43**, 223–33.

HANCOCK B.W., BRUCE L. & RICHMOND J. (1976) Neutrophil function in lymphoreticular malignancy. *Brit. J. Cancer* **33**, 496–500.

HANCOCK B.W., BRUCE L. & RICHMOND J. (1976) Cellular immunity to Hodgkin's disease splenic tissue as measured by leucocyte migration inhibition. *Brit. Med. J.* **1**, 556–7.

HANCOCK B.W., BRUCE L., SUGDEN P., WARD A.M. & RICHMOND J. (1977) Immune status in untreated patients with lymphoreticular malignancy—a multifactorial study. *Clin. Oncol.* **3**, 57–63.

HANCOCK B.W., BRUCE L., WHITHAM M.D., DUNSMORE I.R., WARD A.M. & RICHMOND J. (1982a) Immunity in Hodgkin's disease after 5-years remission. *Brit. J. Cancer* **46**, 593–600.

HANCOCK B.W., DUNSMORE I.R. & SWAN H.T. (1982b) Lymphopenia, a bad prognostic factor in Hodgkin's disease. *Scand. J. Haematol.* **29**, 193–9.

HANCOCK B.W. & HENRY L. (1977) Renal papillary necrosis associated with renal candidiasis in a patient with Hodgkin's disease. *Cancer* **40**, 2309–11.

HANCOCK B.W., MAY K., BRUCE L., DUNSMORE I.R., CLARK A. & WARD A.M. (1980) Haematological and immunological markers in malignant lymphoma. *Tumor Diagnostik* **1**, 140–4.

HANCOCK B.W. & NAYSMITH A. (1975) Vincristine induced autonomic neuropathy. *Brit. Med. J.* **3**, 207.

HANCOCK B.W., POWELL T. & EMMANUEL I.G. (1976) Intrathoracic Hodgkin's disease presenting as hypertrophic osteoarthropathy. *Brit. J. Radiol.* **49**, 647–9.

HARRISON C.V. (1952) Benign Hodgkin's disease (Hodgkin's paragranuloma). *J. Path. Bact.* **64**, 513–18.

HAURANI F.I., YOUNG K. & TOCANTINS L.M. (1963) Reutilization of iron in anaemia complicating malignant neoplasms. *Blood* **22**, 73–81.

HAYS D.M. (1975) The staging of Hodgkin's disease in children. *Cancer*, **35**, 973–8.

HEATH C.W. (1971) Clusters of leukaemia and Hodgkin's disease. *N. Eng. J. Med.* **285**, 1146–7.

HEATH C.W., ROSENSTOCK J.G. & LOBDELL G. (1971) An epidemic of Hodgkin's disease. *Lancet* **2**, 426–7.

HENRY L. (1970) Long survival in Hodgkin's disease. *Clin. Radiol.* **21**, 203–10.

HENRY L. (1971) Partial involvement of the lymph node in Hodgkin's disease. *Clin. Radiol.* 22, 405–10.

HERSH E.M. & OPPENHEIM J.J. (1965) Impaired *in vitro* lymphocyte transformation in Hodgkin's disease. *N. Eng. J. Med.* 273, 1006–12.

HIRSHAUT Y., REAGAN R.L., PERRY S., DE VITA V. & BARILE M.F. (1974) The search for a viral agent in Hodgkin's disease. *Cancer* 34, 1080–9.

HOBBS C.B. & MILLER A.L. (1966) Review of endocrine syndromes associated with tumours of non-endocrine origin. *J. Clin. Path.* 19, 119–27.

HODGKIN T. (1832) On some morbid appearances of the lymphatic glands and spleen. *Med. Chir. Trans.* 17, 68–114.

HUTCHINSON E.C., LEONARD B.J., MAUDSLEY C. & YATES P.O. (1958) Neurological complications of the reticuloses. *Brain* 81, 75–92.

IOACHIM H.L. (1975) New vistas in Hodgkin's Disease. *Pathology Annual*, Vol 10, pp. 419–59 (Ed Sommers S.C.). Appleton-Century-Crofts, New York.

JACKSON S.M., GARRETT J.V. & CRAIG A.W. (1970) Lymphocyte transformation changes during the clinical course of Hodgkin's disease. *Cancer* 25, 843–50.

JACKSON H. & PARKER G. (1947) *Hodgkin's Disease and Allied Disorders.* Oxford University Press, New York.

JELLIFFE A.M., MILLETT L., MARSTON J.A., BENNETT N.H., FARRER-BROWN G., KENDALL B. & KEELING D.H. (1970) Laparotomy and splenectomy as routine investigations in the staging of Hodgkin's disease before treatment. *Clin. Radiol.* 21, 439–45.

JELLIFFE A.M. & THOMSON A.D. (1955) The prognosis in Hodgkin's disease. *Brit. J. Cancer* 9, 21–36.

JENKIN R.D.T., BROWN T.C., PETERS M.D. & SONLEY M.T. (1975) Hodgkin's disease in children. A retrospective analysis 1958–1973. *Cancer* 35, 979–90.

JOHANSSON B., KLEIN G., HENLE W. & HENLE G. (1970) Epstein–Barr virus (EBV) associated antibody patterns in malignant lymphoma and leukaemia I. Hodgkin's disease. *Int. J. Cancer* 6, 450–62.

KADIN M.E., GLATSTEIN E. & DORFMAN R.F. (1971) Clinicopathological studies of 117 untreated patients subjected to laparotomy for the staging of Hodgkin's disease. *Cancer* 27, 1277–94.

KAGEYAMA K., MIKATA A. & WATANABE S. (1973) Hodgkin's disease in Japan. *Gann. Monogr. on Cancer Res.* 15, 239–51.

KAPLAN H.S. (1976) Hodgkin's disease and other human malignant lymphomas. Advances and prospects. *Cancer Res.* 36, 3863–78.

KAPLAN H.S. (1980) *Hodgkin's Disease*, 2nd edn. Harvard University Press, Cambridge, Mass.

KAPLAN H.S. (1981) Hodgkin's disease: biology, treatment, prognosis. *Blood* 57, 813–22.

KAPLAN H.S. & GARTNER, S. (1977) "Sternberg-Reed" giant cells of Hodgkin's disease cultivation in vitro, heterotransplantation and characterisation as neoplastic macrophages. *Int. J. Cancer* 19, 511–25.

KAPLAN H.S. & SMITHERS D.W. (1959) Autoimmunity in man and homologous disease in mice in relation to the malignant lymphomas. *Lancet* 2, 1–4.

KAPLAN H.S. & ROSENBERG S.A. (1975) The management of Hodgkin's disease. *Cancer* 36, 796–803.

KATZ A. & LATTES R. (1969) Granulomatous lymphoma or Hodgkin's disease of thymus, a clinical and histologic study of reevaluation. *Cancer* 23, 1–15.

KAY M.M.B. (1975) Surface characteristics of Hodgkin's cells. *Lancet* ii, 459–60.

KELLER A.R., KAPLAN H.S., LUKES R.J. & RAPPAPORT H. (1968) Correlation of histopathology with other prognostic indicators in Hodgkin's disease. *Cancer* 22, 487–99.

KELLY W.D., LAMB D.L., VARCO R.L. & GOOD R.A. (1960) An investigation of Hodgkin's disease with respect to the problem of homotransplantation. *Ann. N.Y. Acad. Sci.* 87, 187–202.

KERN W.H., GREPEAU A.G. & JONES J.C. (1961) Primary Hodgkin's disease of the lung. Report of 4 cases and review of the literature. *Cancer* 14, 1151–65.

KHOO S.K., WARNER N.L., LIE J.T. & MACKAY L.R. (1973) Carcino-embryonic antigenic activity of tissue extracts: a quantitative study of malignant and benign neoplasms, cirrhotic liver, normal adult and foetal organs. *Int. J. Cancer* 11, 681–7.

KIELY J.M., WAGONER R.D. & HOLLEY K.E. (1969) Renal complications of lymphoma. *Ann. Intern. Med.* 71, 1159–75.

KINLEN L.J. (1977) The epidemiology of leukaemias and lymphomas: a review. *Proc. Roy. Soc. Med.* 70, 553–6.

KIRSCHNER R.H., ABT A.B., O'CONNELL M.J., SKLANSKY B.D., GREEN W.H. & WIERNIK P.H. (1974) Vascular invasion and haematogenous dissemination of Hodgkin's disease. *Cancer* 31, 824–5.

KRIKORIAN J.G., BURKE J.S., ROSENBERG S.A. & KAPLAN H.S. (1979) The occurrence of non-Hodgkin's lymphoma following therapy for Hodgkin's disease. *N. Eng. J. Med.* 300, 452–8.

LACHER M.J. (ED) (1976) *Hodgkin's Disease*. Wiley-Biomedical, New York.

LAMOUREUX K.B., JAFFE E.S., BERARD C.W. & JOHNSON R.E. (1973) Lack of identifiable vascular invasion in patients with extranodal dissemination of Hodgkin's disease. *Cancer* 31, 824–5.

LANCET (1975) Editorial. Blind alleys in the Hodgkin's maze. *Lancet* i, 556–7.

LANCET EDITORIAL (1977) Risk Factors in Hodgkin's disease. *Lancet* I, 888–9.

LAURENCE D.J.R. & NEVILLE A.M. (1972) Foetal antigens and their role in the diagnosis and clinical management of human neoplasm. A review. *Brit. J. Cancer* 26, 335–55.

LAWLER S.D. (1973) Cytogenetic studies. In *Hodgkin's Disease*, pp. 55–63 (Ed Smithers D.W.). Churchill Livingstone, Edinburgh.

LEVINE P.H., ABLASHI D.V., BERARD C.W., CARBONE P.P. & WAGGONER D.E. (1971) Elevated antibody titres to Epstein–Barr virus in Hodgkin's disease. *Cancer* 27, 416–21.

LUKES R.J. (1963) Relationship of histologic features to clinical stages in Hodgkin's disease. *Amer. J. Roentgenol.* 90, 944–55.

LUKES R.J. (1971) Criteria for involvement of lymph node, bone marrow, spleen and liver in Hodgkin's disease. *Cancer Res.* 31, 1755–64.

LUKES R.J. & BUTLER J.J. (1966) The pathology and nomenclature of Hodgkin's disease. *Cancer Res.* 26, 1063–83.

Lukes R.J., Craver L.F., Hall T.C., Rappaport H. & Rubin P. (1966) Report of the Nomenclature Committee. *Cancer Res.* **26,** 131.

MacDonald J.S. (1973) Bone Involvement. In *Hodgkin's Disease,* Chapter 13, pp. 128–136 (Ed Smithers D.W.). Churchill Livingstone, Edinburgh.

McElwain T.J. (1971) Combination chemotherapy of Hodgkin's disease. *Brit. J. Haematol.* **21,** 362.

MacMahon B. (1957) Epidemiological evidence on the nature of Hodgkin's disease. *Cancer* **10,** 1045–54.

MacMahon B. (1966) The epidemiology of Hodgkin's disease. *Cancer Res.* **26,** 1189–1201.

MacLennan K.A., Vaughan Hudson B., Jelliffe A.M., Haybittle J.L. & Vaughan Hudson G. (1981) The pre-treatment peripheral blood lymphocyte count in 1100 patients with Hodgkin's disease: the prognostic significance and relationship to the presence of systemic symptoms. *Clin. Oncol.* **7,** 333–9.

Marshall A.H.E., Matilla A. & Pollock D.J. (1976) A critique and case study of nodular sclerosing Hodgkin's disease. *J. Clin. Path.* **29,** 923–30.

Miller D.G. (1967) The association of immune disease and malignant lymphoma. *Ann. Intern. Med.* **66,** 507–21.

Naeim F., Waisman J. & Coulson W.J. (1974) Hodgkin's disease: the significance of vascular invasion. *Cancer* **34,** 655–62.

Naqvi M.S., Burrows L. & Kark A.E. (1969) Lymphoma of the gastrointestinal tract—prognostic guides based on 162 cases. *Ann. Surg.* **170,** 221–31.

Naysmith A. & Hancock B.W. (1976) Hodgkin's disease and pemphigus. *Brit. J. Derm.* **94,** 695–6.

Neiman R.S. (1978) Current problems in the histopathologic diagnosis and classification of Hodgkin's disease. In *Pathology Annual* **13,** 289–327 (Eds Sommers S.C. & Rosen P.P.). Appleton-Century-Crofts, New York.

Nelson D.F., Cooper S., Weston M.G. & Rubin P. (1981) Second malignant neoplasms in patients treated for Hodgkin's disease with radiotherapy or radiotherapy and chemotherapy. *Cancer* **48,** 2386–93.

Newell G.R. (1970) Age differences in the histology of Hodgkin's disease. *J. Natl. Cancer Inst.* **45,** 311.

Nicholson W.M., Beard M.E.J., Crowther D., Stansfield A.G., Vartan C.P., Malpas J.S., Hamilton Fairley G. & Bodley Scott R. (1970) Combination chemotherapy in advanced Hodgkin's disease. *Brit. Med. J.* **iii,** 7–10.

Olweny C.L.M., Zeigler J.L., Berard C.W. & Templeton A.C. (1971) Adult Hodgkin's disease in Uganda. *Cancer* **27,** 1295–1301.

Order S.E., Bloomer W.D., Jones A.G., Kaplan W.D., Davis M.A., Adelstein S.J. & Hellman S. (1975) Radionuclide immunoglobulin lymphangiography: a case report. *Cancer* **35,** 1487–92.

Order S.E., Chism S.E. & Hellman S. (1972) Studies of antigens associated with Hodgkin's disease. *Blood* **40,** 621–33.

Order S.E. & Hellman S. (1972) Pathogenesis of Hodgkin's disease. *Lancet* **i,** 571–3.

Peckham M.J. (1973) Lung involvement. In *Hodgkin's Disease,* pp. 118–127 (Ed Smithers D.W.). Churchill Livingstone, Edinburgh.

Peckham M.J. & Cooper E.H. (1969) Proliferation characteristics of the various classes of cells in Hodgkin's disease. *Cancer* **24,** 135–45.

Peters M.V. (1950) Study of survivals in Hodgkin's disease treated radiologically. *Amer. J. Roent.* **63,** 299–311.

Pilgrim H.I. (1972) Relationship of the selective metastatic behaviour of tumours of reticular tissues to the migration patterns in their normal cells of origin. *J. Natl. Cancer Inst.* **49,** 3–6.

Plager J. & Stutzman L. (1971) Acute nephrotic syndromes as a manifestation of active Hodgkin's disease. Report of 4 cases and review of the literature. *Amer. J. Med.* **50,** 56–66.

Ranlov P. & Videback A. (1963) Cyclic haemolytic anaemia synchronous with Pel-Ebstein fever in a case of Hodgkin's disease. *Acta Med. Scand.* **174,** 583–8.

Rappaport H. & Strum S.B. (1970) Vascular invasion in Hodgkin's disease; its incidence and relationship to the spread of the disease. *Cancer* **25,** 1302–11.

Rather L.J. (1972) Who discovered the pathognomonic giant cell of Hodgkin's disease? *Bull. N.Y. Acad. Med.* **48,** 943–50.

Razis D.V., Diamond H.D. & Craver L.F. (1959) Familial Hodgkin's disease: its significance and implications. *Ann. Intern. Med.* **51,** 933–71.

Reed D.M. (1902) On the pathological changes in Hodgkin's disease with especial reference to its relation to Tuberculosis. *Johns Hopkins Hosp. Rep.* **10,** 133–96.

Richmond J., Sherman R.S., Diamond H.D. & Craver L.F. (1962) Renal lesions associated with malignant lymphomas. *Amer. J. Med.* **32,** 184–207.

Roberts W.C., Glancy D.L. & DeVita V.T. (1968) The heart in malignant lymphoma (Hodgkin's disease, lymphosarcoma, reticulum cell sarcoma and mycosis fungoides). A study of 196 autopsy cases. *Amer. J. Cardiol.* **22,** 85–107.

Rosenberg S.A. (1966) Report of the Committee on the staging of Hodgkin's disease. *Cancer Res.* **26,** 1310.

Rosenberg S.A. (1971) A critique of the value of laparotomy and splenectomy in the evaluation of patients with Hodgkin's disease. *Cancer Res.* **31,** 1737–40.

Rosenberg S.A. (1972) Updated Hodgkin's disease. Place of splenectomy in evaluation and management. *J. Amer. Med. Ass.* **222,** 1296–8.

Rosenberg S.A. & Kaplan H.S. (1966) Evidence for an orderly progression in the spread of Hodgkin's disease. *Cancer Res.* **26,** 1225–31.

Rosenthal S.R. (1936) Significance of tissue lymphocytes in the prognosis of lymphogranulomatosis. *Arch. Path.* **21,** 628–46.

Ross E.J. (1972–74) Metabolic manifestations of malignancy. *Medicine (Lond.)* **2,** 125–9.

Ruuskanen C. (1971) Tonsillectomy, appendicectomy and Hodgkin's disease. *Lancet* **i,** 1127–8.

Sacks E.L., Donaldson S.S., Gordon J. & Dorfman R.F. (1978) Epithelioid granulomas associated with Hodgkin's disease. *Cancer* **41,** 562–7.

Sahakian G.J., Mondmiry A.I., Lacher M.J. & Connelly C.E. (1974) Acute leukaemia in Hodgkin's disease. *Cancer* **33,** 1369–75.

Schier W.W., Roth A., Ostroff G. & Schrift M.H. (1956) Hodgkin's disease and immunity. *Amer. J. Med.* **20,** 94–9.

Schimpff S., Serpick A., Stoler B., Rumach B., Mellin H., Joseph J.M. & Block J. (1972) Varicella/zoster infection in patients with cancer. *Ann. Intern. Med.* **76**, 241–54.

Shapiro R.F. & Zvaifler N.J. (1973) Concurrent intrathoracic Hodgkin's disease and hypertrophic osteoarthropathy. *Chest* **63**, 912–16.

Sheagren J.N., Block J.B. & Wolff S.M. (1967) Reticulo-endothelial system phagocytic function in patients with Hodgkin's disease. *J. Clin. Invest.* **46**, 855–62.

Simons M.J. & Amiel J.L. (1977) HLA and malignant disease. In *HLA and disease*, pp. 212–132 (Eds Dausset J. & Svejgaard A.). Munksgaard, Copenhagen.

Sinkovics, J.G. & Schullenberger (1975) Hodgkin's disease. *Lancet* **2**, 506.

Smetana H.F. & Cohen B.M. (1956) Mortality in relation to type in Hodgkin's disease. *Blood* **11**, 211–24.

Smithers D.W. (1967) Hodgkin's disease. *Brit. Med. J.* **2**, 263–8 and 337–41.

Smithers D.W. (1970) Malignant lymphomas of the thyroid gland. In *Tumours of the Thyroid Gland*, Chapter 8, pp. 141–154 (Ed Smithers D.W.). E. and S. Livingstone, Edinburgh and London.

Smithers D.W. (ed) (1973a) *Hodgkin's Disease*. Churchill Livingstone, Edinburgh.

Smithers D.W. (1973b) Skin Involvement. In *Hodgkin's Disease*, Chapter 14, pp. 138–142 (Ed Smithers D.W.). Churchill Livingstone, Edinburgh.

Smithers D.W. (1974) Patterns of lymph node involvement in relation to hypothesis about the mode of spread of Hodgkin's disease. *Cancer* **34**, 1779–86.

Sood V.D. & Pasricha J.S. (1974) Pemphigus and Hodgkin's disease. *Brit. J. Derm.* **90**, 575–8.

Sparling H.J. & Adams R.D. (1946) Primary Hodgkin's sarcoma of brain. *Arch. Path.* **42**, 338–44.

Spriggs A.I. (1971) Clonal proliferation in Hodgkin's disease. *Lancet* **1**, 857.

Sternberg C. (1898) Uber erne eigenartige unter dem bilde der pseudoleukamie verlanfende tuberculose des lymphatischen apparates. *Zeitschrift für Heilkunder* **19**, 21.

Stiehm E.R., Ammann A.J., Barnett E.V., Craddock C.G., Fudenberg H.H. & Lawler G.J. (1972) Disease of cellular immunity. *Ann. Intern. Med.* **77**, 101–16.

Strum S.B., Park J.K. & Rappaport H. (1970) Observation of cells resembling Sternberg-Reed cells in conditions other than Hodgkin's disease. *Cancer* **26**, 176–90.

Strum S.B. & Rappaport H. (1971a) Inter-relations of the histologic types of Hodgkin's disease. *Arch. Path.* **91**, 127–34.

Strum S.B. & Rappaport H. (1971b) Persistence of Hodgkin's disease in long term survivors. *Amer. J. Med.* **51**, 222–40.

Sutcliffe S.B.J., Wrigley P.F.M., Smyth J.F., Webb J.A.W., Tucker A.K., Beard M.E., Irving M., Stansfield A.G., Malpas J.S., Crowther D. & Whitehouse J.M.A. (1976) Intensive investigation in the management of Hodgkin's disease. *Brit. Med. J.* **2**, 1343–7.

Swan H.T. & Knowelden J. (1971) Prognosis in Hodgkin's disease related to the lymphocyte count. *Brit. J. Haematol.* **21**, 343–9.

Sybesma J.P.H.B. (1972) Antibody response related to HL-A antigens in Hodgkin's disease and other lymphomas. *Lancet* **2**, 884.

Symmers D. (1944) Clinical significance of deeper anatomic changes in lymphoid diseases. *Arch. Intern. Med.* **74**, 163–71.

Symmers W. St. C. (1968) A survey of the eventual diagnosis in 600 cases referred for a second histological opinion after an initial biopsy diagnosis of Hodgkin's disease. *J. Clin. Path.* **21**, 650–3.

Szur L., Harrison C.V., Levene G.M. & Samman P.D. (1970) Primary cutaneous Hodgkin's disease. *Lancet* **i**, 1016–20.

Taylor C.R. (1974) The nature of Reed-Sternberg cells and other malignant 'reticulum' cells. *Lancet* **ii**, 802–7.

Taylor C.R. & Burns J. (1974) The demonstration of plasma cells and other immunoglobulin-containing cells in formalin-fixed, paraffin-embedded tissues using peroxidase-labelled antibody. *J. Clin. Path.* **27**, 14–20.

Thomas L.B. & Berard C.W. (1973) Hodgkin's disease: relationship of histological type at diagnosis of clinical parameters and to histological progression and anatomical distribution at autopsy. *Gann. Monog. on Cancer Res.* **15**, 253–73.

Todd G.M. & Michaels L. (1974) Hodgkin's disease involving Waldeyer's lymphoid ring. *Cancer* **34**, 1769–78.

Todd I.D.H. (1967) Intracranial lesions in Hodgkin's disease. *Proc. Roy. Soc. Med.* **60**, 734–6.

Tubiana M., Attié E., Flamant R., Gérard-Marchant R. & Hayat M. (1971) Prognostic factors in 454 cases of Hodgkin's disease. *Cancer Res.* **31**, 1801–10.

Ultmann J.E., Cunningham J.K. & Gellhorn A. (1966) The clinical picture of Hodgkin's disease. *Cancer Res.* **26**, 1047–62.

Valagussa P., Santoro A., Kenda R., Fossati Bellani F., Franchi F., Banfi A., Rilke F., Bonadonna G. (1980) Second malignancies in Hodgkin's disease: a complication of certain forms of treatment. *Br. Med. J.* **280**, 216–19.

Verloop M.C. (1955) Anaemia in systemic diseases. *Acta Med. Scand.* **151**, 367–80.

Vianna N.J. (1976) Evidence for infectious component of Hodgkin's disease and related considerations. *Cancer Res.* **36**, 663–6.

Vianna N.J., Greenwald P., Brady J., Polan A.K., Dwork A., Mauro J. & Davies J.N.P. (1972) Hodgkin's disease. Cases with features of a community outbreak. *Ann. Intern. Med.* **77**, 169–80.

Vianna N.J., Greenwald P. & Davies J.N.P. (1971a) The nature of the Hodgkin's disease agent. *Lancet* **1**, 733–6.

Vianna N.J., Greenwald P. & Davies J.N.P. (1971b) Tonsillectomy and Hodgkin's disease: the lymphoid tissue barrier. *Lancet* **1**, 431–2.

Vianna N.J. & Polan A.K. (1973) Epidemiologic evidence for transmission of Hodgkin's disease. *N. Eng. J. Med.* **289**, 499–502.

Wagener D.J.T. & Haanen C. (1975) Incubation period in Hodgkin's disease. *Lancet* **ii**, 747–8.

Walton J.N., Tomlinson B. & Pearce G.W. (1968) Subacute 'poliomyelitis' and Hodgkin's disease. *J. Neurol. Sci.* **6**, 435–45.

Williams H.M., Diamond H.D., Craver L.F. & Parsons H. (1959) *Neurological Complications of Lymphomas and Leukaemias.* Charles C. Thomas, Springfield.

Willis R.A. (1967) *Pathology of Tumours*, 4th ed, pp. 788–9. Butterworth's, London.

Wright C.J.E. (1960) The 'benign' form of Hodgkin's disease (Hodgkin's paragranuloma). *J. Path. Bact.* **80**, 157–71.

Wrigley P.F.M., Hamilton Fairley G. & Matthias J.Q. (1973) Anaemia and Bone Marrow Involvement. In *Hodgkin's Disease*, Chapter 16, pp. 154–62 (Ed. Smithers D.W.). Churchill Livingstone, Edinburgh.

Young R.C., Corder M.P., Haynes H.A. & DeVita V.T. (1972) Delayed hypersensitivity in Hodgkin's disease; a study of 103 untreated patients. *Amer. J. Med.* **52**, 63–72.

Zervas J.D., Delamore I.W. & Israels M.C.G. (1970) Leucocyte phenotypes in Hodgkin's disease. *Lancet*, **2**, 634–5.

After a lymphoma has been diagnosed histologically in a lymph node, the major decision is whether or not it is Hodgkin's disease. If not, the usual inelegant description is 'non-Hodgkin's lymphoma'. In such a lymph node three features usually occur in both nodular and diffuse lymphomas:

1   loss of overall tissue pattern, the usual neat arrangement into follicles, pulp and sinusoids has disappeared

2   loss of the normal reticulin pattern

3   atypical cells are present.

Further subclassification is controversial. The first statement that should be made is whether or not the lesion is follicular (or nodular) or not, and the second is whether or not the component cells are clearly and evidently lymphocytic or not. If it is lymphocytic then it is important to state whether the lymphocytes are small or large. If it is not lymphocytic then the term 'histiocytic' is commonly used (in the past the term 'reticulum' cell was used). Sometimes some of the neoplastic cells are evidently lymphocytic, others not. This can be described by saying that the lesion is mixed lymphocytic-histiocytic. Beyond this simple description lies a morass, and there are hidden snags in even these statements. Nearly all of the non-Hodgkin lymphomas derive anyway from lymphocytes, usually B-lymphocytes; few are of genuinely histiocytic (monocyte-macrophage) origin. Nodular lymphomas and small lymphocytic lymphomas have a better prognosis, and non-nodular (diffuse) lymphomas have a worse prognosis. Fibrosis may be present, and may infer a marginally better prognosis. Good overall reviews are those of Mann *et al.* (1979) and Berard (1981). The classification of non-Hodgkin's lymphoma has a troubled history. Kundrat (1893) pointed out the existence of neoplasms composed of small lymphoid cells, later called lymphosarcoma, and Roulet (1930) recognized a group of neoplasms of rather large cells later called reticulum cell sarcoma. Brill *et al.* (1925) and Symmers (1927) described follicular lesions of good prognosis, some of which were probably reactive and others more malignant. Robb-Smith (1938) classified systematically according to cell of origin. Gall and Mallory (1942) studied

618 cases and correlated histology and prognosis successfully. They described a stem cell lymphoma, a neoplasm of large lymphoid stem cells, and a clasmatocytic lymphoma, a neoplasm of slightly smaller cells resembling histiocytes. Lymphoblastic and lymphocytic lymphomas were lesions of large and small lymphocytes. This classification had reasonable predictive value; stem cell, clasmatocytic and lymphoblastic lymphomas (and Hodgkin's sarcoma) had a poor prognosis with median survival from 0.6 to 1.1 years, lymphocytic lymphoma and Hodgkin's disease rather better with median survival of 2.4 and 3.2 years and follicular lymphoma the best prognosis with median survival of 5.0 years. In general, lesions tended to remain within one subgroup during the course of the disease.

The next major contribution was the view put forward by Rappaport *et al.* (1956), that malignant lymphomas of whatever cellular type may have either a nodular or diffuse pattern. Many of the best available studies are couched in this classification and its subsequent updated form (Nathwani 1979). Lymphomas are classified as nodular or diffuse in pattern, and as lymphocytic or histiocytic in cell type. Small lymphocytes are regarded as well-differentiatied (WD) and large lymphocytes as poorly differentiated (PD). Where a non-lymphocytic lymphoma does not show clear evidence of histiocytic differentiation, it is described as undifferentiated. When it is not clear whether a lesion is lymphocytic or histiocytic, it is described as 'mixed'. This classification has disadvantages. The term 'histiocytic' is inappropriate; most 'histiocytic' tumours derive from B-lymphocytes. It does not distinguish between subgroups of large cell, or 'histiocytic' lesion. And 'mixed' lesions are in fact of B-lymphocytic origin.

Next Lukes and Collins (1975a and b) proposed that lymphoma be classified according to the cell type of origin as defined immunologically. A lesion can therefore be of T-lymphocytic, B-lymphocytic or true histiocytic origin, of uncommited (U) cell (Null) type or frankly unclassifiable. Most NHL is of B cell origin and essentially follicular derivation. These views developed initially from a study of the way in which, *in vitro*, small lymphocytes 'transform' in the presence of antigen, and from parallel histological studies. It is likely that round (B) lymphocytes arrive at the periphery of the follicle and move in; the hitherto round nucleus becomes irregular, indented or cleaved; the 'small cleaved' cell enlarges, retaining the nuclear cleavage (the 'large cleaved cell'); the nucleus, now large, becomes round or oval, once more losing its cleavage (the 'large non-cleaved cell'); nucleoli appear and enlarge. The cytoplasm is now markedly pyroninophilic. The large non-cleaved cell divides and probably moves out into the interfollicular tissue, as a B immunoblast which matures into a plasma cell. If the stimulus disappears it is possible that the immunoblast can regress to a small 'memory' lymphocyte.

Most NHL is of B cell and essentially follicular origin and can be categorized as of:

1   small non-cleaved cell
2   small cleaved cell
3   large cleaved cell
4   large non-cleaved cell origin.

Tumours of the large non-cleaved cell, the dividing cell of the follicle, are very malignant; if more than 25% of cells are large or if there are focal areas where they predominate, prognosis is poor. Tumours with a pronounced nodular (follicular) pattern are usually composed largely of small cleaved cells which tend to form follicles or clusters; these small cleaved cells ('haematogones') may be present in blood and seed, possibly by the usual B cell homing mechanisms to marrow, spleen and liver. Nevertheless the prognosis is good with a median survival of more than 5 years (the classical Brill–Symmers lesion) even in the presence of disseminated disease. Tumours of large cleaved cells have a more diffuse pattern with relatively slow progression and often show fibrosis. Lymphomas of large non-cleaved cells of diffuse pattern are highly malignant. Large foci of these cells in a cleaved cell lymphoma may herald progression to the more malignant large non-cleaved cell form. Tumours evolve from follicular to diffuse becoming more malignant.

The immunoblastic nature of lesions may be particularly evident. Such lesions have been reported to occur in patients with chronic abnormal immune disorders such as rheumatoid arthritis, systemic lupus erythematosus, Sjögren's syndrome, macroglobulinaemia and α-chain disease, and in patients with immune defects or on immunosuppressives. There is often associated production of abnormal immunoglobulin. These are regarded in this terminology as immunoblastic sarcomas of B cell type. A few of these immunoblastic sarcomas originate in angioimmunoblastic adenopathy.

T cell lymphomas as proved by marker studies are rare, and include mycosis fungoides, Sézary syndrome, and lymphoblastic lymphoma, often accompanied by leukaemia. True histiocytic lymphomas, as classified by marker studies and ultrastructure, occur only rarely. The remaining groups are those which are undefined because they have no markers, and those which are unclassifiable for technical reasons. Very similar conclusions have been expressed differently by Lennert *et al.* (1975), using the term centrocyte to describe cleaved cells and centroblast to describe non-cleaved cells.

The use of immunologic markers in the study of the non-Hodgkin's lymphomas has been reviewed by Stein *et al.* (1980). Nodular lymphomas are clearly of B cell origin while diffuse lymphocytic lymphomas are usually B cell, but sometimes T cell (lymphoblastic lymphoma). 95% of diffuse histiocytic lymphomas were classified as B cell, the rest T cell. Some lymphomas do not express surface markers ('null cell' lymphomas). These tend to have a rather poor prognosis. Monoclonal lesions are usually malignant (Stein *et al.* 1980). It does not seem that marker studies are yet of great value in management of individual patients (see also Azar *et al.* 1980; Yamanaka *et al.* 1981). Other classifications based on morphology have been put forward by Bennett *et al.* (1974) leading to that used in a recent British histologic text (Stuart *et al.* 1981).

The six best known classifications have recently been compared by an international group. The classifications all work in the hands of their originators, but there is no agreement as to which is best (National Cancer Institute Sponsored Study 1982). However, agreement was reached on a working formulation by means of which the various classifications may be harmonized. This formulation will probably be widely accepted. A useful result of this work has been the publication of a table of expected clinical results based on large numbers of patients. The various lesions will now be described in terms of the British text (Stuart *et al.* 1981) and the international working formulation (IWF), with cross reference to the Rappaport classification (R) (see Table 5.1).

Follicular lymphoma

Follicular lymphoma is uncommon below the age of 25 and rare in children. The lesion is composed of neoplastic follicles, which contain varying proportions of small and large lymphoid cells. The small cells have irregular, elongated or

British	Rappaport (R)	International working formulation (IWF)
		Low Grade Malignancy
a Diffuse lymphocytic	**a** Diffuse lymphocytic well-differentiated (DLWD)	**a** Small lymphocytic, diffuse Consistent with CLL Plasmacytoid
b Follicular (small cell)	**b** Nodular lymphocytic poorly differentiated (NLPD)	**b** Follicular Predominantly small cleaved cell Diffuse areas Sclerosis
c Follicular (mixed small & large cell)	**c** Nodular mixed lymphocytic—histiocytic (NM)	**c** Follicular Mixed small cleaved and large cell Diffuse areas Sclerosis
		Intermediate Grade Malignancy
d Follicular (large cell)	**d** Nodular histiocytic (NH)	**d** Follicular Predominantly large cell Diffuse areas Sclerosis
e Diffuse intermediate	**e** Diffuse lymphocytic poorly differentiated (DLPD)	**e** Diffuse Small cleaved cell Sclerosis
f Diffuse mixed	**f** Diffuse mixed lymphocytic/histiocytic (DM)	**f** Diffuse Mixed, small and large cell Sclerosis Epithelioid cell component
g Diffuse large cell	**g** Diffuse histiocytic (DH)	**g** Diffuse, large cell Cleaved cell Non-cleaved cell Sclerosis
		High Grade Malignancy
h	**h**	**h** Large cell immunoblastic Plasmacytoid Clear cell Polymorphous Epithelioid cell component
i Lymphoblastic	**i** Lymphoblastic	**i** Lymphoblastic Convoluted cell Non-convoluted cell
		j Small non-cleaved cell Burkitt's Follicular areas
		Miscellaneous Composite Mycosis fungoides Histiocytic Extramedullary plasmacytoma Unclassifiable Other
Diffuse histiocytic		

(After Stuart *et al.* 1981 and The Non-Hodgkin's Lymphoma Pathologic Classification Project 1982.)

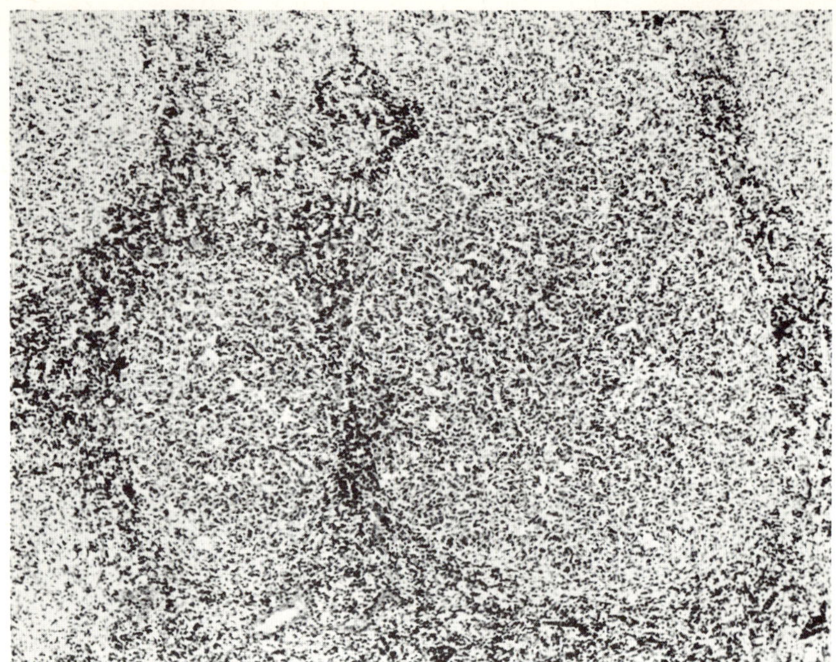

Fig. 5.1 Nodular (follicular) lymphoma showing closely related irregular shaped follicles, devoid of the clearly arranged collar of small lymphocytes and the large tingible body macrophages found in normal follicles. × 45.

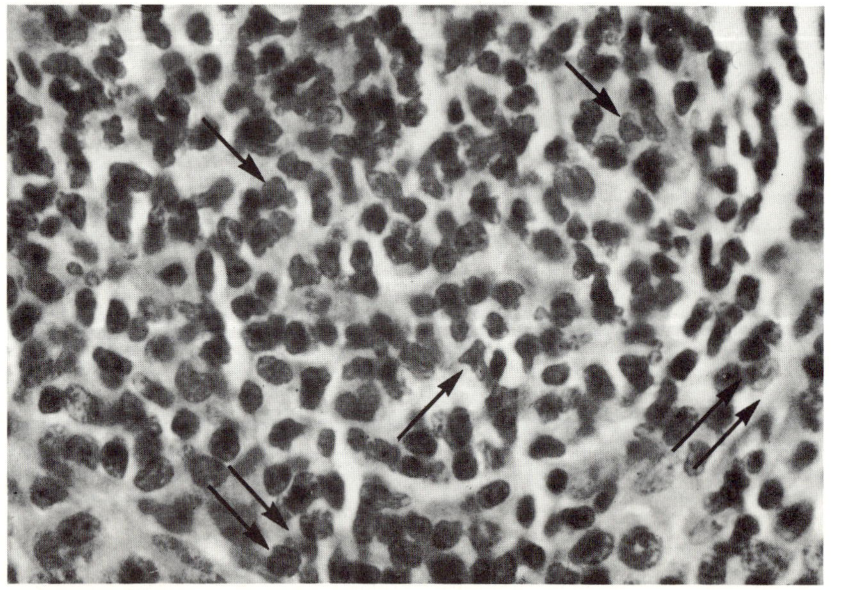

Fig. 5.2 Follicular lymphoma, small cell type: Part of a neoplastic 'follicle' showing a predominance of small follicle cells with characteristic irregularly contoured nuclei (arrows). The 'cleaved' appearance seen in blood preparations is not readily apparent in tissue sections. Note the early interfollicular infiltration with the neoplastic lymphocytes (double arrows). × 840.

indented nuclei, which stain less densely than the nuclei of mature small lymphocytes, and are less round. These are 'cleaved' cells, but the cleavage or very deep indentation usually shows poorly by light microscopy; it is more evident by electron microscopy. The large cells have either nuclei which are ovoid and irregularly outlined with relatively inconspicuous nucleoli, or have a rounded nucleus of smooth regular outline. A large cell is probably best defined as one larger than a non-neoplastic histiocyte as seen in the same sections (see Figs 5.1, 5.2, 5.3).

Since prognosis is generally believed to be related to the proportion of large cells present, the follicular lymphomas have been subdivided as follows (ML = malignant lymphoma and see Table 5.1 to which the small prefixed letters refer):

(b) Predominantly small cell type (less than a third large cells)
(ML—nodular lymphocytic poorly differentiated (R), ML follicular, small cleaved cell (IWF).)

(c) Mixed small and large cell type (between a third and two thirds large cells)
(ML—nodular lymphocytic-histiocytic (R), ML follicular, mixed small cleaved and large cell (IWF).)

(d) Predominantly large cell type (more than two thirds large cells)
(ML—nodular histiocytic (R), ML follicular predominantly large cell (IWF)—the least common type.)

If the pattern is only partly follicular, the lesion is still called a follicular lymphoma; the presence of diffuse areas implies a worse prognosis. If only a trace of nodular appearance is present the lesion should be regarded as diffuse. In general follicular lymphomas are relatively benign but diffuse lymphoma of high grade malignancy may develop at any time. Sclerosis either in the form of bands or a fine compartmentalizing fibrosis is more commonly seen in lymphomas of follicular origin than in other types of lymphoma, and may indicate a marginally better prognosis (Bennet and Millett 1969; Bennett 1975; Rosas-Uribe and Rappaport 1972). The progression of nodular to diffuse lymphomas is particularly evident in postmortem series (Risdall *et al.* 1979).

The differentiation between a nodular lymphoma and a reactive hyperplasia can be very difficult. The important points in favour of lymphoma are:

1   pleomorphism of nuclei
2   spillage of follicles
3   destruction of normal architecture of the node.

In non-neoplastic germinal centres large macrophages containing nuclear debris are prominent; inflamed nodes often show polymorphs.

Diffuse lymphoma

In these lesions either no residue or only a very faint residue of follicular structure remains.

(a) *Diffuse lymphoma, lymphocytic (ML Lymphocytic well-differentiated diffuse (R), ML—Small lymphocytic, consistent with CLL (IWF)).*
These lesions are composed of monotonous sheets of small round lymphocytes with darkly staining nuclei and no obvious cytoplasm similar to those occurring in the cuff of small lymphocytes surrounding germinal centres (Fig. 5.4). Mitosis is infrequent. Most are manifestations of chronic lymphocytic leukaemia; it is essential to be aware of the patient's haematologic status before reporting them. In these lesions there are often small foci of pale staining areas which are composed of larger lymphoid cells—the so-called proliferation centres (Lennert *et al.* 1975). The lesion may progress to a more malignant lymphoma, usually histiocytic lymphoma (so-called Richter's syndrome) (Harousseau *et al.* 1981).

(a) *Diffuse lymphoma, lymphocytic, plasmacytoid*
Some similar tumours may show plasmacytoid differentiation and may be associated with a monoclonal gammopathy, e.g. Waldenström's disease. In a few patients with chronic lymphocytic leukaemia, malignant lymphoma, usually histiocytic lymphoma, but rarely Hodgkin's disease may supervene (reviewed by Harousseau *et al.* 1981).

(e) *Diffuse lymphoma intermediate type (Poorly differentiated lymphocytic—diffuse (R), ML diffuse—small cleaved cell (IWF))*
This tumour is the diffuse counterpart of the predominantly small cell type of follicular lymphoma (Fig. 5.5). In many tumours of this type, in addition to the characteristically irregularly nucleated lymphocytes, there are scattered large lymphoid cells occurring singly, in contrast to the focal aggregates of lymphoid cells seen in the well-differentiated group. Mitosis is frequent.

(i) *Diffuse lymphoma lymphoblastic (ML lymphoblastic (R) (IWF))*
Lymphoblastic lymphoma (reviewed by Nathwani *et al.* 1981) is a distinct lesion, more common in males that females, often but not always accompanied by a mediastinal mass, and often (50%) a manifestation of acute lymphoblastic leukaemia. There is a biphasic age incidence—the second and third

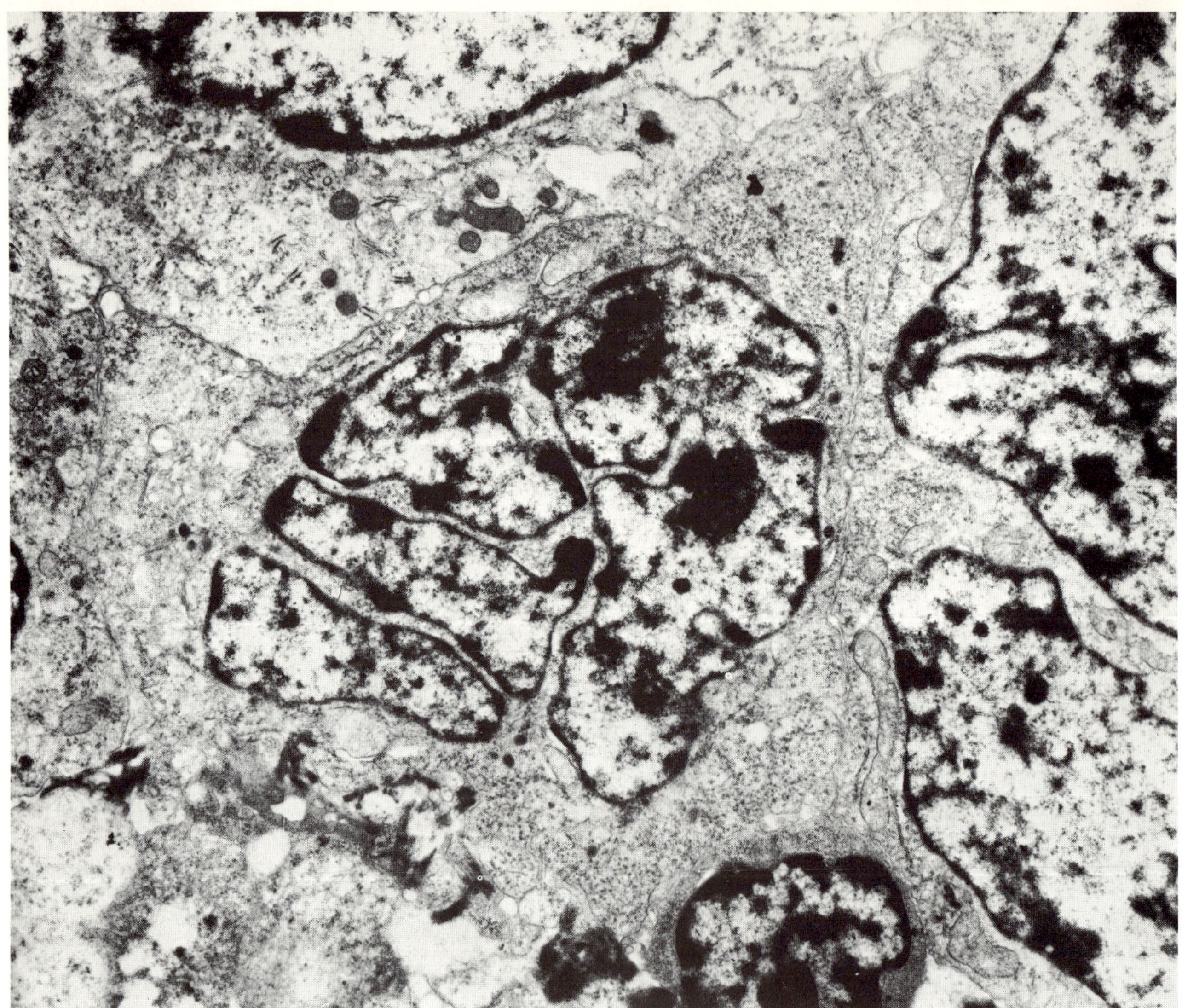

Fig. 5.3. Electron micrograph of lymphocytic lymphoma of nodular or follicular type showing the deeply indented nuclei, indicative of follicular origin. ×8,900.

decade and the seventh decade. The lesion (Fig. 5.6) is a diffuse lymphoma composed of immature large lymphocytes, or lymphoblasts, whose nuclei have delicate chromatin and few nucleoli and sometimes a linear 'chicken's foot' accumulation of chromatin. Clumping of chromatin indicates maturation into prolymphocytes. Crush artefact is common, and the cells often arrange in single files and infiltrate the capsule of the lymph node. The 'starry sky' appearance of scattered macrophages seen against a background of lymphocytes is seen in about 10% of cases. There is a relationship between mitosis and survival—less than 50 mitotic figures per 10 high fields suggesting a better chance of survival. These are T cell lesions, and are the only lymphomas commonly to show TDT transferase.

(j) *Burkitt's lymphoma*, described elsewhere (p. 117) is composed of monomorphous lymphoblasts with fine nuclear chromatin-containing lipid vacuoles and characteristically numerous large macrophages laden with cell debris.

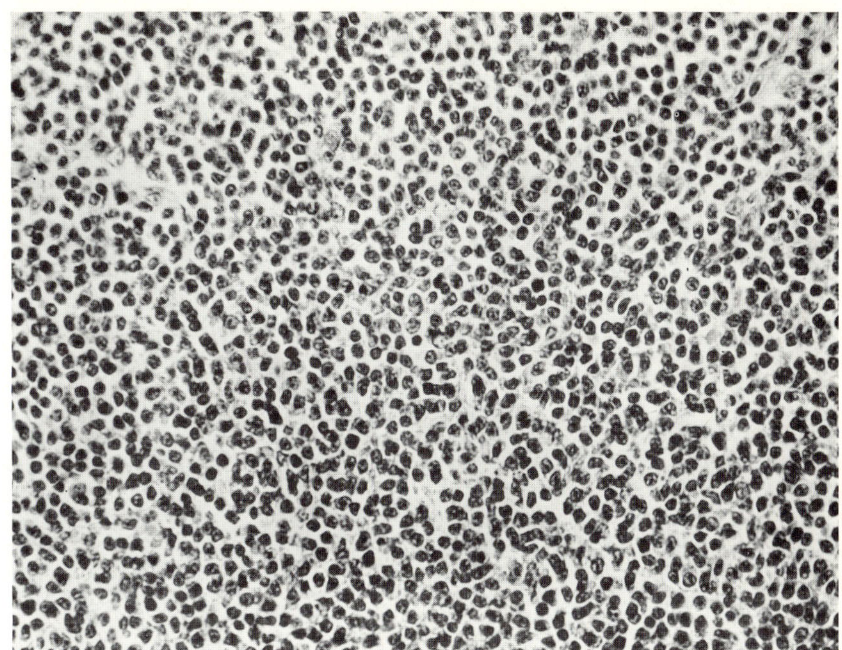

Fig. 5.4. A lymph node diffusely infiltrated with small round lymphocytes from a patient with chronic lymphatic leukaemia. ×108.

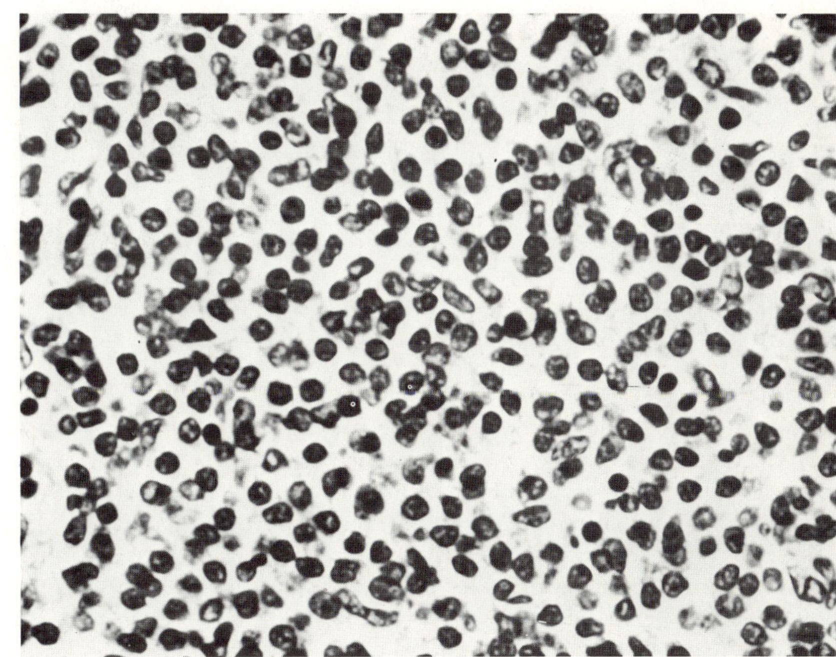

Fig. 5.5. A lymph node diffusely infiltrated by abnormal small follicle lymphocytes, small 'cleaved' cells. The nuclei are irregular in shape. Malignant lymphoma, diffuse, intermediate (diffuse lymphocytic poorly differentiated) ×216.

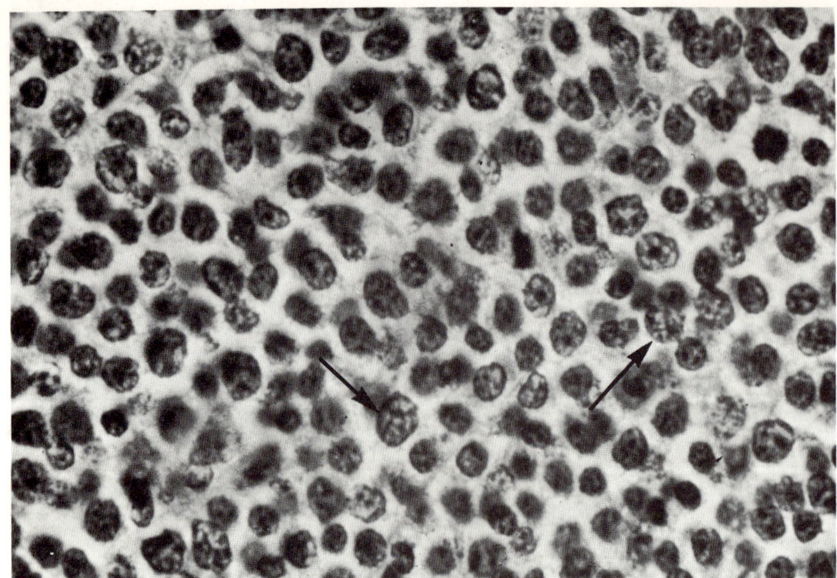

Fig. 5.6. A mediastinal lymph node infiltrated by large lymphocytes (lymphoblasts) whose nuclei have a delicate linear chromatin pattern. Lymphoblastic lymphoma. × 480.

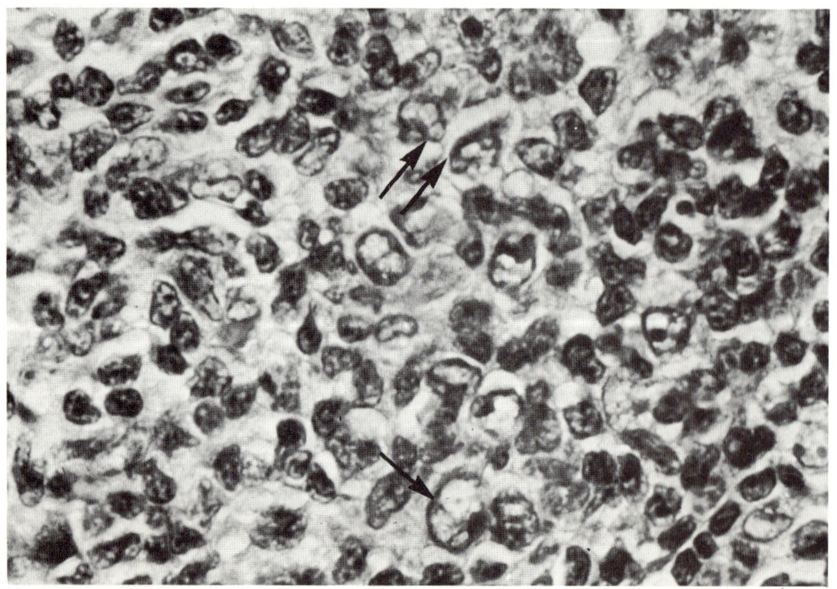

Fig. 5.7. A lymph node diffusely infiltrated with small follicular (cleaved) lymphocytes and large follicular (cleaved) lymphocytes (arrows). Malignant lymphoma diffuse mixed. × 840.

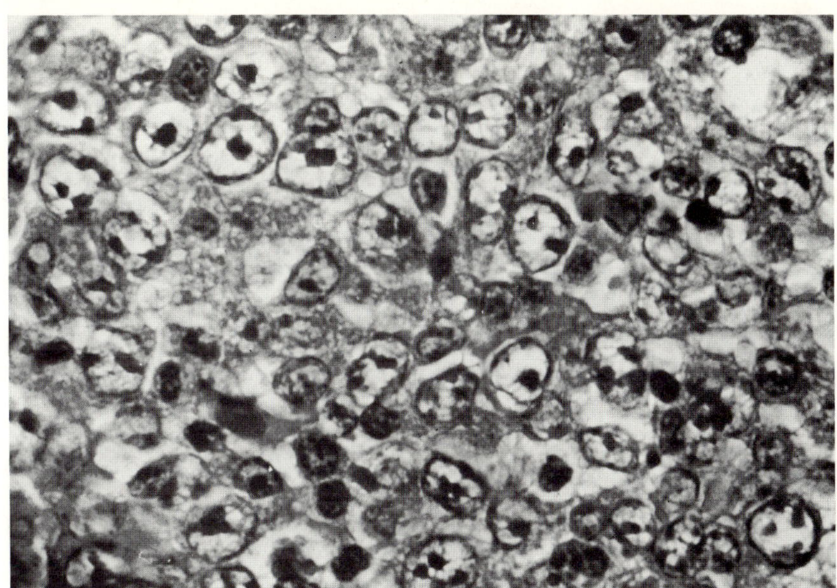

Fig. 5.8. A lymph node diffusely infiltrated with large nucleolated cells with a variable amount of cytoplasm. Malignant lymphoma, large cell type ('histiocytic' diffuse). ×840.

(f) *Diffuse lymphoma, mixed type (Mixed lymphocytic histiocytic diffuse (R), ML diffuse mixed small and large cell (IWF))*
The term 'mixed lymphoma' is restricted to tumours composed of a mixture of small and large lymphoid cells, thought to be the diffuse counterpart of the mixed type of follicular lymphoma (Fig. 5.7). The percentage of larger cells necessary to qualify for this term is variously held between 25 and 60%. The smaller lymphocytic cells are analogous to the follicular centre lymphocytes, therefore show irregular nuclei and may also show plasmacytoid differentiation. In evaluating these lesions, it should be remembered that infiltrating reactive cells may be seen in other lymphomas.

(g and h) *(Diffuse lymphoma large cell type (Histiocytic lymphoma diffuse (R), ML diffuse, large cell (g) and large cell immunoblastic (h) (IWF))*
This group consists mainly of tumours composed of large lymphoid cells with or without plasmacytoid differentiation (Fig. 5.8). Some true histiocytic tumours and possibly other types of lymphomas will be included, unless electron microscopy and immunohistologic techniques are used. The large lymphoid cells have a large round-to-ovoid nucleus and prominent nucleoli, and a variable amount of pyroninophilic cytoplasm. Where pyroninophilic cytoplasm is prominent the lesion is regarded as immunoblastic.

Diffuse lymphoma (histiocytic)—'true histiocytic'

True tumours of histiocytes (macrophages or mononuclear phagocytes) are rare, though commoner in Britain, and best defined by electron microscopy (Henry 1975) (Fig. 5.9 and 5.10) and by the identification of histiocytic cell markers. The neoplastic histiocytes may be quite well-differentiated, approximating closely in appearance to tissue histiocytes with reniform nuclei and cytoplasmic inclusions, or they may be larger and less well-differentiated. They have lumpy or lobulated nuclei, and eosinophilic, often pyroninophilic cytoplasm which may be voluminus with an ill-defined edge. Multinucleate cells may be present.

Diffuse lymphoma—plasma cell type

Plasma cell tumours are rare in lymph nodes and spleen and more common outside the lymph nodes. The term should only be applied to tumours composed largely of recognizable plasma cells with a perinuclear halo, and round nuclei. In less differentiated plasma cell tumours multinucleated cells are common. The lesion shades into large cell (immunoblastic) lymphoma.

Several further rare variants of non-Hodgkin's lymphoma do not fit neatly into the above categories.

The signet-ring variant of lymphocytic lymphoma

Here the neoplastic cells have a signet ring appearance, due to content of immunoglobulin. This lesion may be mistaken for carcinoma and has a rather poor prognosis (Kim *et al.* 1978a).

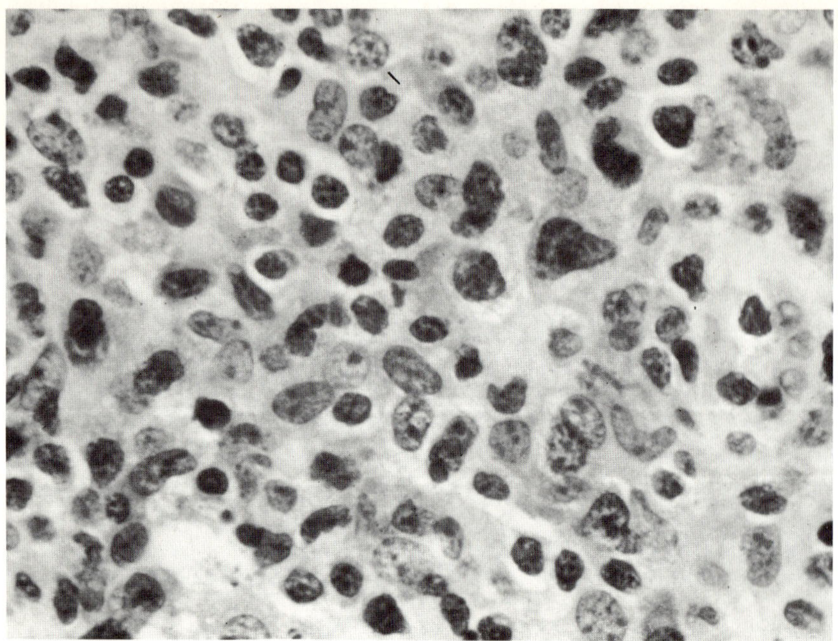

Fig. 5.9. A lymph node diffusely infiltrated with large cells, some of which have indented or reniform nuclei. Malignant lymphoma—true histiocytic. ×434.

Lymphoma with epithelioid histiocytes

In another rare variant of lymphocytic lymphoma, epithelioid histiocytes are prominent, and are seen in patients over the age of 20, often in cervical nodes. The node is diffusely infiltrated by small and large lymphoid cells and by groups of large epithelioid histiocytes. The prognosis is poor. This lesion is distinguished from Hodgkin's disease by the fact that the lymphocytes are atypical, the capsule is infiltrated and true Reed–Sternberg cells are rare or absent (Kim *et al.* 1978b and 1980).

Sinusoidal large cell lymphoma

Here, the lymph node sinusoids are infiltrated by pleomorphic large lymphoma cells, containing immunoglobulin but not lysozyme (Osborne *et al.* 1980). This can be confused with metastatic carcinoma or melanoma.

Mycosis fungoides

The lymph node lesion in mycosis fungoides may range from dermatopathic lymphadenopathy, to a frank lymphoma showing infiltration of the lymph node with pleomorphic lymphoid cells with hyperconvoluted lymphoid cells. It is hard to determine exactly when there is true neoplastic infiltration of the node, and prognosis appears to depend more on the extent of the skin lesion (Colby *et al.* 1981).

A few lymphomas remain unclassified, usually because of insufficient material or technical inadequacy.

In all these new classifications, it is important to realize that whatever the conceptual advances involved, the immediate effects of diagnosis in the hands of the general histopathologist are less clear. Obviously follicular lymphomas have a good prognosis, whereas diffuse lymphomas have a bad one, unless they are of a small lymphocytic type usually found in chronic lymphatic leukaemia; intermediate forms have an intermediate prognosis. It is important to use a classification understood by the relevant clinicians; in most areas, whatever classification is used, it is useful also to define the lesion by the Rappaport classification, which is widely understood, and it is useful to state whether the lesion is of low, intermediate or high grade malignancy.

NON-HODGKIN'S LYMPHOMA—THE CLINICAL ASPECTS

Non-Hodgkin's lymphomas have a maximum incidence between 50 and 70 years of age; most studies show a male preponderance, but in our experience the sex incidence is

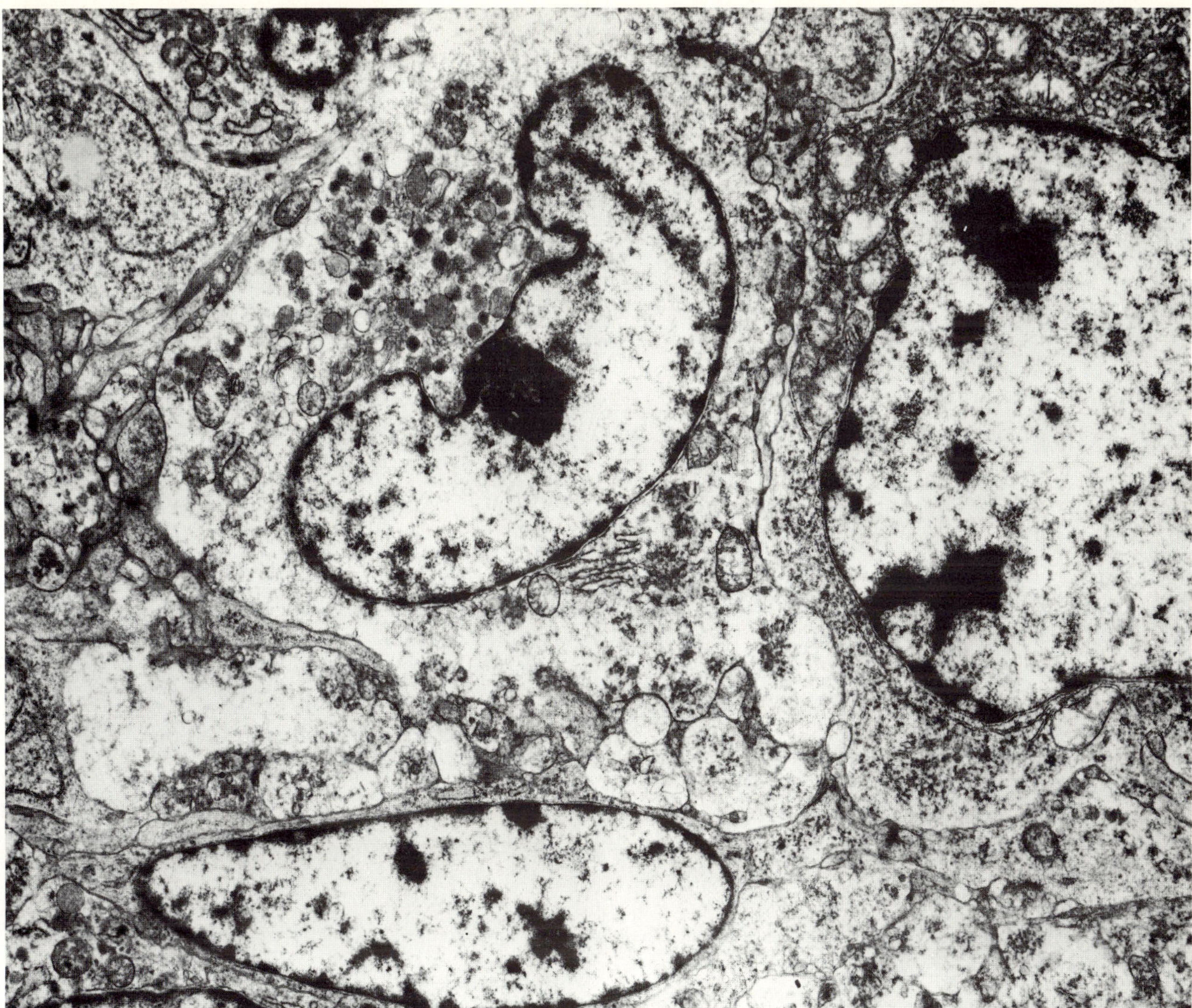

Fig. 5.10. Electron micrograph of lesion seen in Figure 5.9. A cell with a reniform nucleus and prominent nucleolus contains several lysosomes. The appearances in this context suggest that this is a 'true histiocytic' lymphoma.

about equal. In the Sheffield area we see over 40 new cases each year from a population of about $1\frac{1}{2}$ million.

The presenting features of 342 consecutive adult patients are summarized in Table 5.2; the patients have been grouped according to the histological categories described in the Working Formulation (National Cancer Institute Sponsored Study 1982). However, in the text below, unless otherwise stated, the Rappaport terminology is employed, since this has been most widely used in clinical studies.

Diffuse lymphomas tend to occur in young adults and in elderly; nodular lymphomas preponderate in middle age (Jones *et al.* 1973). There is an increased incidence of lymphomas (particularly of the brain) in immunodepressed organ transplant patients (Penn and Starzl 1972; Kinlen *et al.*

Table 5.2 Presenting features of 342 consecutive adult patients presenting to the Sheffield lymphoma group (1971–80).

Age:	<35 years	12%	Sex:	Male	49%
	36–64 years	49%		Female	51%
	>65 years	39%			
Clinical presentation	Neck nodes	25%	Clinical Stage: (Ann Arbor)	I	15%
	Axillary/groin nodes	27%		II	22%
	Other nodes	9%		$I_E II_E$	12%
	Extranodal mass	19%		III	19%
	'symptoms'	20%		IV	32%
Symptom status: (Ann Arbor)	A	70%	Histology: (Working formulation)	Low grade	32%
	B	30%		Intermediate grade	42%
				High grade	18%
				Miscellaneous	8%

1979) in association with congenital immunodeficiency syndromes (Gatti and Good 1971) and with autoimmune disease, e.g. systemic lupus erythematosus, Sjögren's syndrome. Pseudolymphoma development with hydantoin treatment is recognized (Saltzstein and Ackerman 1959), but there may also be an increased coincidence of malignant lymphoma in such patients (Li *et al.* 1975).

The clinical presentation of non-Hodgkin's lymphoma bears some resemblance to that of Hodgkin's disease but there are important distinguishing features. Superficial painless mobile cervical lymphadenopathy is still the commonest form of presentation, but there is often far more widespread disease that in Hodgkin's disease. The latter tends to be centripetal in presentation and the non-Hodgkin's centrifugal, so that the involvement of popliteal, trochlear and mesenteric nodes, Peyer's patches and Waldeyer's ring is much commoner. Widespread disease is more commonly seen with a diffuse than with a nodular histological pattern (Jones *et al.* 1973). particularly with histiocytic lymphoma. Extranodal disease occurs with greater frequency in non-Hodgkin's lymphoma (particularly of diffuse type) than Hodgkin's disease and may account for nearly a quarter of cases (Freeman *et al.* 1972). Extranodal lymphoma is discussed in Chapters 6 and 7, but a degree of overlap is inevitable.

Another important point is that whereas in Hodgkin's disease the involvement at presentation and sites of recurrence can often be predicted from the original disease site, in non-Hodgkin's lymphoma the disease is often not contiguous and may recur in any lymph node or extranodal site.

Obstructive phenomena, related to occlusion of either viscera or vessels, are commoner in nodular lesions. Jaundice is a rare presenting symptom, but up to 10% of patients at some time during their illness are jaundiced; extrahepatic obstruction is the commonest single cause of this.

In our experience patients often present with symptoms occurring from some complication of the lymphoma rather than actual recognition of an abnormal mass.

Childhood non-Hodgkin's lymphoma is generally regarded as being highly malignant; blood, bone marrow and central nervous system involvement are frequent, but one of the most common clinical presentations is with intra-abdominal disease (up to a third of cases).

Waldeyer's ring

Involvement of Waldeyer's ring either as the extranodal primary focus, or as part of more generalized disease, is far more frequent with non-Hodgkin's lymphoma than with Hodgkin's disease (Banfi *et al.* 1972) and occurs in about 5% of cases at presentation (Rosenberg *et al.* 1961). The tumour usually arises in the tonsil or nasopharyngeal space, and the commonest presenting finding is cervical lymph node enlargement.

Alimentary system

Gastrointestinal lesions may be primary (Allen *et al.* 1954) or secondary, and occur in about 15% of cases at presentation

(Jones *et al.* 1973). At autopsy about half of patients have involvement (Rosenberg *et al.* 1961) which is more frequent with diffuse rather than nodular histology (Jones *et al.* 1973) and the sites frequently involved are stomach and small intestine (the large intestine is seldom involved and the oesophagus rarely). Intestinal lesions are particularly common in the Middle East (Gelpi 1970) and in children, where they account for about one third of lymphoma cases. Gastric and colonic lesions may simulate carcinoma, whereas small intestinal lesions, though they may present with obstructive features, are a recognized cause of malabsorption (Sleisenger *et al.* 1953). Patients with initial gastrointestinal disease have a better prognosis if their lymphoma is nodular in type (Jones *et al.* 1973).

Ascites (occasionally chylous) may be seen as a result of obstruction of retroperitoneal lymph nodes

Respiratory system

Pleural involvement with non-Hodgkin's lymphoma is seen at autopsy in 30% of cases and may be associated with pleural effusion. The latter may also arise from lymphatic obstruction by intra-thoracic tumour, and may occasionally be chylous in nature.

Mediastinal and hilar lymphadenopathy at presentation occurs less frequently than Hodgkin's disease, and is seen in only about a quarter of patients (Jones *et al.* 1973). Lung parenchymal involvement may occur, particularly with disseminated disease (in about 20% of cases) and is seen radiologically as infiltration or discrete deposits. Clinically such patients are often asymptomatic but they may present with cough, dyspnoea or local pain. Superior vena caval obstruction is seen in some cases of superior mediastinal gland enlargement. Pulmonary hypertrophic osteoarthropathy is a rare finding with intra-thoracic lymphoma. Over 50% of patients at some stage present some abnormality on a straight chest X-ray.

Haemopoietic system

Anaemia of a non-specific type with a normocytic, normochromic blood film can occur as a presenting feature in non-Hodgkin's lymphoma. Often the anaemia is a feature of generalized disease but it may be exacerbated by blood loss, myelosuppressive therapy, bone marrow infiltration, hypersplenism and uraemia. A macrocytic blood picture can also be encountered; this is sometimes, but not always, accompanied by folate deficiency as seen in other malignant disease.

Serum ferritin levels may be elevated in malignant lymphoma; this may be as a result of reticuloendothelial block of iron release or production of abnormal isoferritins (Hancock *et al.* 1979); the level of elevation correlates with response to treatment, high levels at presentation indicating a potentially poor prognosis (Hancock *et al.* 1980).

A particular feature of non-Hodgkin's lymphoma is the significant incidence of haemolytic anaemia of autoimmune type. This haemolytic anaemia may be due to warm or cold antibodies (Dacie 1967) and surprisingly may occur even in the presence of hypogammaglobulinaemia. The warm antibodies are usually of IgG class and may show a specificity for particular blood group antigens mainly in the Rh system (Worlledge and Blajchman 1972). Cold antibodies are usually of IgM class and have anti-I specificity, though occasionally anti-i activity is seen. In both types of autoimmune haemolytic anaemia the broad spectrum Coombs' antiglobulin test is positive, and the red cell survival time shortened, usually in association with reticulocytosis and depressed haptoglobin levels. The warm antibody type autoimmune haemolytic anaemia may show a gratifying response to corticosteroid therapy; the cold antibody type usually responds only to treatment of the underlying lymphoma and to the avoidance of cold.

Bone marrow involvement occurs in about 15% of cases of non-Hodgkin's lymphoma at presentation, usually in the presence of generalized disease (Jones *et al.* 1973). It is identified more often the harder it is looked for. Positive identification is easier in marrow sections than in smears, and easier the more numerous and larger the biopsies. It is seen much more frequently in lymphocytic lymphomas of nodular and diffuse types than with histiocytic lymphomas. This high incidence of bone marrow involvement may cause confusion with leukaemia. Indeed leukaemic transformation occurs frequently in patients with lymphocytic lymphomas with involvement of the peripheral blood, either as a well-differentiated chronic lymphocytic leukaemia, a 'lymphosarcoma cell' leukaemia, or as acute leukaemia, the latter particularly in children with childhood lymphocytic or undifferentiated lymphoma. Patients with initial bone marrow disease have a better prognosis if their lymphoma is nodular in type (Jones *et al.* 1973).

Rarely marrow infiltration may cause a leuco-erythroblastic blood picture. Leucocytosis (including eosinophilia and monocytosis) and thrombocytosis are occasionally seen in all lymphomas (Gall and Mallory 1942). Neutropenia and thrombocytopenia usually follow intensive myelosuppressive therapy but may occur with hypersplenism. Thrombocytopenic purpura (thought to be due to platelet auto-antibodies) is an occasional finding with non-Hodgkin's lymphoma. Lymphopenia may occur with generalized disease and is exacerbated by cytotoxic chemotherapy. The ESR and haemoglobin level are useful pre- and post-treatment follow-up markers; low haemoglobin and elevated ESR at presentation are unfavourable prognostic indices.

Cardiovascular system

At autopsy cardiovascular involvement, particularly with histiocytic lymphoma, is seen in about 20% of patients. Cardiac involvement is seldom recognized during life and is seen in less than 1% of cases (Rosenberg *et al.* 1961; Roberts *et al.* 1968). The effect of the lymphomatous infiltration is either inflow obstruction, cardiac tamponade or frank restriction of cardiac function.

Bone

Histiocytic lymphoma of bone, especially of long bones, pelvis and scapulae is usually seen in younger age groups (Rosenberg *et al.* 1961). Widespread bone involvement is commoner in non-Hodgkin's lymphoma than in Hodgkin's disease, and occurs in a quarter or more of cases (Gall and Mallory 1942). The patient often presents with bone pain or with local pressure effects, and the lesions on radiological examination are usually osteolytic. Hypercalcaemia may supervene (Moses and Spencer 1963) sometimes in the absence of overt bone disease (Greaves and Hancock 1980).

Genito-urinary system

The genito-urinary tract is involved in about half of the cases at autopsy (Rosenberg *et al.* 1961) but clinical involvement is seen in only 3% of patients.

Infiltration of renal parenchymal tissue occurs most frequently with lymphocytic lymphoma with evidence of bone marrow involvement (Richmond *et al.* 1962). If renal failure develops it is most often due to ureteric obstruction by enlarged retro-peritoneal nodes. Serum uric acid levels are commonly elevated in lymphoma, and urate nephropathy may result in uraemia, particularly after initiation of chemotherapy in a sensitive bulky tumour. Kidney involvement

leading to uraemia is rare (Richmond *et al.* 1962), and nephrocalcinosis and amyloidosis may also occur (Kiely *et al.* 1969).

Involvement of the reproductive tract is seen at autopsy in a quarter of patients, females being twice as commonly affected as males. Clinical involvement, however, is uncommon, even in generalized disease. Chorlton *et al.* (1974) in a clinical study reported 12 patients with non-Hodgkin's lymphoma presenting with lesions of uterus and vagina. A tumour of the testis may rarely be a presenting sign in non-Hodgkin's lymphoma (Tanenbaum *et al.* 1972).

Nervous system (see also Chapter 7)

Primary involvement of the nervous system is rare, except in the young. At autopsy it has been reported in 5–10% of cases. Clinical involvement (Williams *et al.* 1959) may be specific or non-specific. As in Hodgkin's disease primary or secondary lymphomatous deposits may present as intra-cerebral space-occupying lesions or as transverse spinal cord compression syndromes. Peripheral neuropathy is occasionally seen, and involvement of head and neck structures may result in cranial nerve palsies. Non-specific neurological manifestations include *Herpes zoster* infection, vincristine neurotoxicity and malignant cachexia. In the patient with unexplained central nervous system signs the possibility of opportunistic infection must be excluded.

There is an increased incidence of lymphomas involving the brain in immunosuppressed organ transplant patients (Doak *et al.* 1968; Penn and Starzl 1972; Kinlen *et al.* 1979).

Spleen

Splenomegaly is seen in about one third of patients presenting with non-Hodgkin's lymphoma (Rosenberg *et al.* 1961) and at autopsy in over half of cases. It is less common with histiocytic lymphoma, and as an isolated finding at presentation splenic enlargement occurs in less than 1% of patients. The spleen is usually moderately enlarged but occasionally may reach massive proportions. As with Hodgkin's disease, clinical size does not always correlate with pathological involvement.

Liver

About one third of patients have heptomegaly at presentation and in many cases this indicates hepatic involvement with lymphoma. At autopsy 50% of cases have hepatic deposits. Jaundice is seen in some of these patients but cannot be correlated with the extent of hepatic disease. This may also be due to extrahepatic biliary obstruction, drug toxicity or accompanying haemolytic anaemia.

Elevation of serum alkaline phosphate is often seen in patients with lymphoma, but it is sometimes difficult to assess the part played by bone and hepatic disease, the patient often remaining asymptomatic. Iso-enzyme studies may be of help.

Skin

Cutaneous involvement is seen in about 20% of cases (Gall and Mallory 1942). Both histiocytic and lymphocytic lymphoma may involve the skin as the primary extranodal focus. Usually, however, the skin presentation is a marker of more disseminated disease. The cutaneous lesion often takes the form of purplish-red papules of varying number and size. Ulceration may occur. The non-specific effects of lymphoma include pruritus, various skin eruptions, erythroderma, stomatitis and herpes infections. Mycosis fungoides is a unique primary lymphoma of skin described on p. 110. It may show prolonged localization to the skin and indeed, occasionally patients die from infection and toxaemia without apparent dissemination of the disease. The remainder die of a condition difficult to distinguish from histiocytic lymphoma.

Other organs

Lesions in the breast are uncommon. Salivary gland and thyroid lesions are also uncommon, happening more frequently in females. Adrenal and pancreatic infiltration is seen at autopsy in a quarter of cases but clinical involvement is rare. Involvement of pituitary gland, orbital structures and tongue is rare, even at autopsy.

Systemic symptoms

Fever, night sweats, weight loss, general ill health and pruritus occur in up to a quarter of patients. Such symptoms are encountered in histiologically diffuse rather than nodular lymphomas and tend to occur with more generalized disease (Jones *et al.* 1973); however, their presence does not appear to affect prognosis as adversely as in Hodgkin's disease.

Immunological aspects

The classical immune abnormality in non-Hodgkin's lymphoma, particularly of the lymphocytic lymphoma type, is of B-cell (humoral) depression so that, as in chronic lymphocytic leukaemia, hypogammaglobulinaemia may develop. Cellular immunity is not usually affected until the disease is far advanced (Hancock *et al.* 1976) or until the patient undergoes immunosuppressive therapy. Depressed lymphocyte transformation and lymphopenia at presentation are bad prognostic features (Hancock *et al.* 1980).

In some patients polyclonal hypergammaglobulinaemia is seen, and in others a monoclonal immunoglobulin or paraprotein (particularly of IgM class) may lead to a hyperviscosity syndrome causing a haemorrhagic diathesis and cardiac failure (Hamilton Fairley 1974).

As a result of immune deficiency, infections (including those with opportunistic organisms, as in Hodgkin's disease) occur in these patients, particularly when the disease is widespread and during immunosuppressive (particularly chemo-) therapy. *Herpes zoster* is the commonest offender and occurs in up to 10% of patients (Schimpff *et al.* 1972). The incidence of this infection and also of tuberculosis is less than with Hodgkin's disease.

Autoimmune disease and co-existent cancer may occur with increased incidence in non-Hodgkin's lymphoma, as with Hodgkin's disease (Chapter 4); autoimmune haemolytic anaemia, collagen-vascular disorders (particularly systemic lupus erythematosus) and nephrotic syndrome are all recognized associations.

Second malignancies

Moertel and Hagedorn (1957) reported an incidence during life of 3.6% of co-existent cancer in 1,514 patients with lymphosarcoma. 7.3% of 109 cases had second malignancies at autopsy. Similar incidences were seen in the clinical and autopsy series of Rosenberg *et al.* (1961) and in our own study 3 second neoplasms were seen in 50 autopsies.

Cause of death

As in Hodgkin's disease the usual patterns of death are of severe infection and disseminated lymphoma, e.g. in 50 Sheffield autopsies (Table 5.3) infection, usually bronchopneumonia, was seen in 50% and cardiorespiratory failure in 16% of cases, both in association with disseminated lymphoma. Five patients without active lymphoma died of infection, presumably partly associated with the effects of immunosuppressive therapy.

Table 5.3 Autopsy findings in Sheffield patients

Non-Hodgkin's lymphoma	+pneumonia	50%
	+other infections	4%
	+cardiorespiratory failure	16%
	+other neoplasm	2%
	+other complications	12%
Second neoplasm,	no active lymphoma	4%
Bronchopneumonia,	no active lymphoma	8%
Septicaemia,	no active lymphoma	2%
Other disease,	no active lymphoma	2%

MANAGEMENT AND PROGNOSIS

After biopsy diagnosis, usually from an enlarged lymph node but occasionally from an extranodal site, the disease is investigated and staged in a similar way to Hodgkin's disease (see Chapters 4 and 13). This is often complicated, however, because lesions are not contiguous. Since non-Hodgkin's lymphoma is acknowledged in many cases to be a disseminated disease requiring systemic therapy, and since staging laparotomy often discloses no more disease than would be found with standard closed investigations, this operation is not at present routinely indicated, except in the case of primary abdominal disease.

The survival figures quoted in Gall and Mallory's (1942) paper are, as clearly indicated by the authors, inaccurate in that many of the patients were still alive at the time of writing, but are more closely related to the natural history of the disease than more modern figures. Large lymphocytic lymphoma had a median survival time of 0.6 years, histiocytic lymphoma 1.1 years, lymphocytic lymphoma 2.4 years and follicular lymphoma 5 years (in the same series Hodgkin's disease for comparison has a median survival time of 3.2 years and Hodgkin's sarcoma 0.9 years.) Primary extranodal presentation was associated with a rather better prognosis. Actuarial survival data indicate that patients with nodular lymphomas survive longer than patients with diffuse lymphomas. Patients with well-differentiated lymphocytic lymphoma have a good prognosis; those with undifferentiated lymphomas a poor one. The differences between the other groups are not striking, except that nodular histiocytic lymphomas have a distinctly worse prognosis than other nodular lymphomas (Jones *et al.* 1973).

Young patients with diffuse lymphocytic and mixed cell lymphomas have a worse prognosis than older patients with similar histology. Conversely, older patients with nodular lymphocytic and mixed cell lymphoma have a relatively poorer prognosis.

The survival figures from a recent international study (NCI 1982) are shown in Table 5.4. Application of the Working Formulation to the series of 342 patients seen in Sheffield emphasises the vital role of accurate pathological assessment—a clear cut survival pattern was seen for the different histology grades; the 5-year figures for low grade (a, b, c) lesions was 53%, for intermediate grade (d, e, f, g) 27%, and for high grade (h, i, j) 20% (Hancock *et al.* 1983).

It is obviously important to distinguish between extranodal, local nodal, regional nodal and generalized disease from the point of view of treatment and prognosis. However, conventional staging classifications (e.g. Ann Arbor) are less useful than in Hodgkin's disease, since the disease is more often widespread than clinically suspected. In our experience stage IV disease carries a significantly poorer outlook than other stages, whereas localised extranodal lesions without B symptoms have a relatively good prognosis (20% and 56% 5-year survival figures respectively).

Details of treatment are given more fully in Chapter 13. In general, in patients with more favourable histology types, local irradiation, single agent chemotherapy or whole body irradiation may be appropriate. These disorders are acknowledged to be indolent in their behaviour and it is doubtful whether they are ever actually cured (with the exception of truly localised lesions)—the median survival is above 50% at 5 years. Progression to more malignant histology types is common after a period of time.

With the more malignant histology types the best hope of complete remission and cure, particularly where the disease is widespread, is aggressive combination chemotherapy. Complete remission rates of above 50% are possible (Lewis and DeVita 1978; Canellos and Lister 1978). Bulky disease (particularly abdominal) and bone marrow or CNS involvement are poor prognostic features (Canellos and Lister 1978). Maintained remission is possible for over one third of such patients (DeVita *et al.* 1975). However, radical radiotherapy is undoubtedly successful in a proportion of truly localised nodal and extranodal tumours; 5-year survival figures of up to 50% are commonly reported (reviewed by Hellman *et al.* 1977).

Childhood lymphomas, with the possible exception of those presenting with localised neck node disease, are best treated with aggressive and combined protocols similar to those in acute lymphoblastic leukaemia (Murphy 1978).

Table 5.4 Clinical features of patients in the non-Hodgkin's Lymphoma Pathologic Classification Project 1982

Pathologic subtype	(%)	Age range	Median age	Survival median (years)	Survival 5 yr (%)	Complete response rate (%)	Median time to relapse of complete responders (years)
(a)	3.6	26–79	60.5	5.8	59.0	61	>5.4
(b)	22.5	3–87	54.3	7.2	70.0	73	5.0
(c)	7.7	26–99	56.1	5.1	50.0	65	5.2
(d)	3.8	16–82	55.4	3.0	45.0	61	>8.0
(e)	6.9	10–91	57.9	3.4	33.0	56	2.1
(f)	6.7	22–90	58.0	2.7	38.0	69	4.3
(g)	19.7	10–88	56.8	1.5	35.0	59	>8.4
(h)	7.9	10–81	51.3	1.3	32.0	53	3.5
(i)	4.2	11–90	16.9	2.0	26.0	69	1.1
(j)	5.0	3–90	29.8	0.7	23.0	48	>7.7

In Sheffield, the overall 5-year survival for the 342 patients treated between 1971 and 1980 was 34%—a disappointingly low figure. However, with recent improvements in staging and therapy, our complete response rates are improving. With generalised disease of unfavourable histology type the complete remission rate (using CHOP, see Chapter 13) is now over 50% and, as might be expected from the now well-recognised fact that one of the most important indices of successful outcome is good response to intial therapy, the survival figures are starting to improve—a reassuring prospect for those who have seen the outlook in non-Hodgkin's lymphoma lagging far behind that in Hodgkin's disease with all its recent impressive advances.

REFERENCES

ALLEN A.W., DONALDSON G., SNIFFEN R.C. & GOODALE F. (1954) Primary malignant lymphoma of the gastrointestinal tract. *Ann. Surg.* **140**, 428–38.

AZAR H.A., JAFFE E.S., BERARD C.W., CALLIHAN T.R., BRAYLAN R.R., COSSMAN J. & TRICHE T.S. (1980) Diffuse large cell lymphomas (histiocytic cell sarcomas, histiocytic lymphomas). Correlation of morphologic features with functional markers. *Cancer* **46**, 1428–41.

BANFI A., BONADONNA G., RICCI S.B., MILANI F., MOLINARI R., MOFARDINI S. & ZUCALI R. (1972). Malignant lymphomas of Waldeyer's ring—natural history and survival after radiotherapy. *Brit. Med. J.* **3**, 140–3.

BENNETT M.H. (1975) Sclerosis in non-Hodgkin's lymphomata. *Brit. J. Cancer*, **31**, Suppl II, 44–52.

BENNETT M.H., FARRER-BROWN G., HENRY K. & JELLIFFE A.M. (1974) Classification of non-Hodgkin's lymphomas. *Lancet* ii, 405–6.

BENNETT M.H. & MILLETT Y.L. (1969) Nodular sclerotic lymphosarcoma—a possible new clinico-pathological entity. *Clin. Radiol.* **20**, 339–43.

BERARD C.W. (Moderator) (1981) A multidisciplinary approach to non-Hodgkin's lymphomas. *Ann. Int. Med.* **94**, 218–35.

BRILL M.E., BAEHR G. & ROSENTHAL N. (1925) Generalized giant lymph follicle hyperplasia of the lymph nodes and spleen. A hitherto undescribed type. *J. Amer. Med. Ass.* **84**, 665–71.

CANELLOS G.P. & LISTER T.A. (1978) The staging and treatment of non-Hodgkin's lymphoma. *Brit. J. Haem.* **39**, 477–82.

CHORLTON I., KARNEI R.F., KING F.M. & NORRIS H.J. (1974) Primary malignant reticulo-endothelial disease involving the vagina, cervix and corpus uteri. *Obstet. Gyn.* **44**, 735–48.

COLBY T.V., BURKE J.S. & HOPPE R.T. (1981) Lymph node biopsy in mycosis fungoides. *Cancer* **47**, 351–9.

DACIE J.V. (1967) Secondary or symptomatic haemolytic anaemias. In *The Haemolytic Anaemias*, Part III, Chapter 13, pp. 719–809. J.A. Churchill, London.

DEVITA V.T., CANELLOS G.P., CHABNER B., SCHEIN P., HUBBARD S.P. & YOUNG R.C. (1975) Advanced diffuse histiocytic lymphoma, a potentially curable disease. Results with combination chemotherapy. *Lancet* i, 248–50.

DOAK P.B., MONTGOMERIE J.Z., NORTH J.D.K. & SMITH F. (1968) Reticulum cell sarcoma after renal homotransplantation and azathioprine and prednisone therapy. *Brit. Med. J.* **4**, 746–8.

FREEMAN C., BERG J.W. & CULTER S.F. (1972) Occurrence and prognosis of extranodal lymphomas. *Cancer* **29**, 252–60.

GALL E.A. & MALLORY T.B. (1942) Malignant lymphoma. A

clinico-pathological survey of 618 cases. *Amer. J. Path.* **18**, 381–429.

GATTI R.A. & GOOD R.A. (1971) Occurrence of malignancy in immunodeficiency disease—a literature review. *Cancer* **28**, 89–98.

GELPI A.P. (1970) Malignant lymphoma in the Saudi Arab. *Cancer* **25**, 892–5.

GREAVES M. & HANCOCK B.W. (1980) Hypercalcaemia in malignant lymphoma, case descriptions and discussion of underlying mechanisms. *Postgrad. Med. J.* **56**, 34–7.

HAMILTON FAIRLEY G. (1972–74) Lympho-proliferative diseases. *Medicine (Lond.)* **24**, 1412–20.

HANCOCK B.W., AITKEN M., ROSS C.M.D. & DUNSMORE I.R. (1983) Non-Hodgkin's lymphoma in Sheffield 1971–80. *Clin. Oncol.* **9**, 109–19.

HANCOCK B.W., BRUCE L., SUGDEN P., WARD A.M. & RICHMOND J. (1976) Immune status in untreated patients with lymphoreticular malignancy—a multifactorial study. *Clin. Oncol.* **3**, 57–63.

HANCOCK B.W., MAY K., BRUCE L. & RICHMOND J. (1979) Ferritin; a sensitising substance in the leucocyte migration test in patients with malignant lymphoma. *Brit. J. Haem.* **43**, 223–33.

HANCOCK B.W., MAY K., BRUCE L., DUNSMORE I.R., CLARK A. & WARD A.M. (1980) Haematological and immunological markers in malignant lymphoma. *Tumour Diagnostik* **3**, 140–4.

HAROUSSEAU J.V., FLANDRIN G., TRICOT G., BROUET J.C., SELIGMAN M. & BERNARD J. (1981) Malignant lymphoma supervening in chronic lymphocytic leukemia and related disorders. *Cancer* **48**, 1302–8.

HELLMAN S., CHAFFEY J.T., ROSENTHAL D.S., MOLONEY W.C., CANELLOS G.P. & SKARIN A.T. (1977) The place of radiation therapy in the treatment of non-Hodgkin's lymphomas. *Cancer* **39**, 843–51.

HENRY K. (1975) Electron microscopy in the non-Hodgkin's lymphoma. *Brit. J. Cancer* **31**, Supple II, 73–93.

JONES S.E., FUKS Z., BULL M., KADIN M.E., DORFMAM R.F., KAPLAN H.S., ROSENBERG S.A. & KIM H. (1973) Non-Hodgkin's lymphomas. IV. Clinico-pathological correlation in 405 cases. *Cancer* **31**, 806–23.

KIELY J.M., WAGONER L.D. & HOLLEY K.E. (1969) Renal complications of lymphoma. *Ann. Intern. Med.* **71**, 1159–75.

KIM H., DORFMAN R.F. & RAPPAPORT H. (1978a) Signet ring cell lymphoma: a rare morphologic and functional expression of nodular (follicular) lymphoma. *Amer. J. Surg. Path.* **2**, 119–32.

KIM H., JACOBS C., WARNKE R.A. & DORFMAN R.F. (1978b) Malignant lymphoma with a high content of epithelioid histiocytes. *Cancer* **41**, 620–35.

KIM H., NATHWANI B.N. & RAPPAPORT H. (1980) So-called 'Lennert's lymphoma'. Is it a clinicopathologic entity? *Cancer* **45**, 1379–99.

KINLEN L.J., SHEIL A.G.R., PETO J. & DOLL R. (1979) Collaborative United Kingdom–Australasian study of cancer in patients treated with immunosuppressive drugs. *Brit. Med. J.* **2**, 1461–6.

KUNDRAT H. (1893) Ueber Lymphogranulomatose. *Wien. klin. Wschr.* **6**, 211–34.

LENNERT K., STEIN H. & KAISERLING E. (1975) Cytological and functional criteria for the classification of malignant lymphomata. *Brit. J. Cancer*, **31**, Suppl. II, 29–43.

LEWIS B.J. & DEVITA V.T. (1978) Combination therapy of the lymphomas. *Seminar Haem.* **15**, 431–57.

LI F.P., WILLARD D.R. & GOODMAN VAWTER G. (1975) Malignant lymphoma after diphenylhydantoin (Dilantin) therapy. *Cancer* **36**, 1359–62.

LUKES R.J. & COLLINS R.D. (1975a) A functional classification of malignant lymphomas. In *The Reticuloendothelial System* (Eds) Rebuck J.W., Berard C.W. & Abell M.R. Williams and Wilkins, Baltimore.

LUKES R.J. & COLLINS R.D. (1975b) New approaches to the classification of the lymphomata. *Brit. J. Cancer* **31**, Suppl. II, 1–28.

MANN R.B., JAFFE E.S. & BERARD C.W. (1979) Malignant lymphomas—a conceptual understanding of morphologic diversity. *Am. J. Path.* **94**, 105–92.

MOERTEL C.G. & HAGEDORN A.B. (1957) Leukaemia or lymphoma and co-existent primary malignant lesions. A review of the literature and study of 120 cases. *Blood* **12**, 788–803.

MOSES A.M. & SPENCER H. (1963) Hypercalcaemia in patients with malignant lymphoma. *Ann. Intern. Med* **59**, 531–7.

MURPHY S.B. (1978) Current concepts in cancer: childhood non-Hodgkin's lymphoma. *New. Engl. J. Med.* **299**, 1446–8.

NATHWANI B.N. (1979) A critical analysis of the classification of non-Hodgkin's lymphoma. *Cancer* **44**, 347–84.

NATHWANI B.N., DIAMOND L.W., WINBERG C.D., KIM H., BEARMAN R.M., GLICK J.H., JONES S.E., GAMS R.A., NISSEN N.I. & RAPPAPORT H. (1981) Lymphoblastic Lymphoma: A clinicopathologic study of 95 patients. *Cancer* **48**, 2347–57.

NATIONAL CANCER INSTITUTE SPONSORED STUDY OF CLASSIFICATIONS OF NON-HODGKIN'S LYMPHOMAS. (1982) Summary and description of a working formulation for clinical usage. *Cancer* **49**, 2112–35.

OSBORNE B.M., BUTLER J.J. & MACKAY B. (1980) Sinusoidal large cell ('Histiocytic') Lymphoma. *Cancer* **46**, 2484–91.

PENN I. & STARZL T.E. (1972) Malignant tumours arising de novo in immunosuppressed organ transplant recipients. *Transplantation* **14**, 407–17.

PROSNITZ L.R., HELLMAN S., VON ESSEN C.F. & KLIGERMAN M.M. (1969) The clinical course of Hodgkin's disease and other malignant lymphomas treated with radical radiation therapy. *Amer. J. Roentgenol.* **105**, 618–28.

RAPPAPORT H., WINTER W. & HICKS E.B. (1956) Follicular lymphoma. A re-evaluation of its position in the scheme of malignant lymphomas, based on a survey of 253 cases. *Cancer* **9**, 792–821.

RICHMOND J., SHERMAN R.S., DIAMOND H.D. & CRAVER L.F. (1962) Renal lesions associated with malignant lymphomas. *Amer. J. Med.* **32**, 184–207.

RISDALL R., HOPPE R.T. & WARNKE R. (1979) Non-Hodgkin's lymphoma. A study of the evolution of the disease based upon 92 autopsied cases. *Cancer.* **44**, 529–42.

ROBB-SMITH A.H.T. (1938) Reticulosis and reticulosarcoma: a histological classification. *J. Path. Bact.* **47**, 457–80.

Roberts W.C., Glancy D.L. & DeVita V.T. (1968) The heart in malignant lymphoma (Hodgkin's disease, lymphosarcoma, reticulum cell sarcoma and mycosis fungoides). *Amer. J. Cardiol.* **22**, 85–107.

Rosas-Uribe A. & Rappaport H. (1972) Malignant lymphoma, histiocytic type with sclerosis (Sclerosing reticulum cell sarcoma). *Cancer* **29**, 946–53.

Rosenberg S.A., Diamond H.D., Jaslowitz B. & Craver L.F. (1961) Lymphosarcoma. A review of 1269 cases. *Medicine (Balt.)* **40**, 31–84.

Roulet F. (1930) Das primare Retothelsarkom des Lymphknoten. *Virchows Arch. Path. Anat.* **277**, 15–47.

Saltzstein S.L. & Ackerman L.V. (1959) Lymphadenopathy induced by anti-convulsant drugs and mimicking clinically and pathologically malignant lymphomas. *Cancer* **12**, 164–82.

Schimpff S., Serpick A., Stoler B., Rumach B., Melin H., Joseph J.M. & Block J. (1972) Varicella/zoster infections in patients with cancer. *Ann. Intern. Med.* **76**, 241–54.

Sleisenger M.H., Almy T.P. & Barr D.P. (1953). The sprue syndrome secondary to lymphoma of the small bowel. *Amer. J. Med.* **15**, 666–74.

Stein R.J., Cousar J., Flexner J.M. & Collins R.D. (1980) Correlations between immunologic markers and histopathologic classifications: Clinical implications. *Semin. Oncol.* **7**, 244–54.

Stuart A.E., Stansfeld A.G. & Lauder I. (1981) *Lymphomas Other Than Hodgkin's Disease.* Oxford University Press, New York.

Symmers D. (1927) Follicular lymphadenopathy with splenomegaly. *Arch. Path.* **3**, 816–20.

Tanenbaum B., Sandford R.S., Elquezabal A. & Klinger M.E. (1972) Testicular tumour, presenting signs of lymphoma. *Cancer* **29**, 1223–8.

Williams H.M., Diamond H.D., Craver L.F. & Parsons H. (1959) *Neurological Complications of Lymphomas and Leukaemias.* Charles C. Thomas, Springfield, Illinois.

Worlledge S.M. & Blajchman M.A. (1972) The autoimmune anaemias. *Brit. J. Haematol* **23**, (Suppl), 61–9.

Yamanaka N., Ishii Y., Koshiba H., Mikuni C., Ogasawara M. & Kikuchi K. (1981) A study of surface markers in non-Hodgkin's lymphoma by using anti-T and anti-B lymphocyte sera. *Cancer* **47**, 311–18.

Chapter 6

Extranodal lymphomas and lymphoreticular hyperplasias

Extranodal lymphomas are lymphomas arising in tissue outside the lymphoreticular system—that is, in tissue other than lymph node, spleen, liver and bone marrow (Salzstein 1969). Tonsillar lesions will be included in the present chapter. Lymphomatous infiltration is found in many organs in advanced lymphoma originating within the lymphoreticular system; to fall within the category extranodal lymphoma, only one organ and its draining lymph notes should be involved, the peripheral blood must be normal and there must be no evidence of dissemination for some time after diagnosis, arbitrarily 3 months to 1 year. True lymphomas must be distinguished from pseudolymphomas; these are lymphoreticular infiltrates which do not show progressive neoplastic growth. The term lymphoreticular infiltrate, or lymphoreticular hyperplasia, is preferable.

Extranodal lymphomas and lymphoreticular infiltrates may occur in any organ. They are found most commonly in the alimentary tract, in the respiratory tract, in the skin and in the reproductive tract. Lesions in other sites will be mentioned briefly; lymphoma of the CNS is described in Chapter 7 (The Rappaport pathologic classification is used throughout the chapter).

In general up to one quarter of malignant lymphomas arise in extranodal sites (Freeman *et al.* 1972). Such a presentation appears to be particularly common in Italy (Banfi *et al.* 1970) and Israel (Modan *et al.* 1969). Extranodal histiocytic lymphomas are more common than extranodal lymphocytic lymphomas; the histology is diffuse in most cases, and subclassification may be particularly difficult.

Localized radiation (with local surgery where necessary) may be curative and good 5-year disease-free survival is possible particularly if the lesion is localized (without evidence of regional spread).

Lymphocytic extranodal lymphomas fare better as a whole than histiocytic lesions. Lymphomas of stomach, tonsil and lung have a far better prognosis than the corresponding carcinomas of these sites. Only lymphomas of the breast and testis appear to do worse than corresponding carcinomas. Nodular lesions in general have a better prognosis than diffuse lesions. In general prognosis varies with histological subtype as in nodal lesions.

A typical spectrum of localized extranodal disease is illustrated in Table 6.1 which shows the Sheffield incidence by site over the 10-year period (1971–1980).

LYMPHORETICULAR LESIONS OF THE BUCCAL CAVITY

THE BENIGN LYMPHOEPITHELIAL LESION OF SALIVARY GLANDS

This is a lesion which appears usually unilaterally, but in about 10% of cases bilaterally, as a swelling of a salivary gland, usually the parotid. Grossly it may be a single or multilobular mass. Histologically it consists of reactive lymphoreticular tissue, often with germinal centres among which lie ductal and acinar epithelial elements in varying quantities, either well-preserved or degenerate.

The epithelium may occasionally show metaplastic change. There is much disagreement in the earlier literature on the best name for this lesion—the term used here (Godwin 1952; Cruikshank 1965) seems to be the best one. Similar lesions are found elsewhere in the oral cavity—notably in the buccal mucosa, tongue and floor of mouth, and often evidently from minor salivary glands (Tomich and Schafer 1975) (Fig. 6.1).

A similar lesion is seen in salivary glands in Sjögren's syndrome, accompanied by such features as inflammation of the cornea and conjunctiva, nose, pharynx and larynx, by polyarthritis, and is seen rarely in rheumatoid disease. Therefore, this diagnosis should be followed by immunological investigation for autoantibodies and rheumatoid factor.

Malignant lymphoma in salivary glands is uncommon and usually of lymphocytic type; as usual nodular lesions have a better prognosis (Patey *et al.* 1965; Freedman 1971). Occasionally, a lesion initially reported as a benign lymphoepithelial lesion recurs and proves to be true malignant lymphoma (Seligman *et al.* 1974).

Table 6.1 Site of presentation in 83 consecutive cases of extranodal malignant lymphoma

Waldeyer's ring	Tonsil	15
	Other	3
Gastrointestinal	Stomach	7
	Intestine	7
Skin	Mycosis fungoides	5
	Other	5
Thyroid		10
Bone		6
Respiratory tract (excluding	Upper	6
Waldeyer's ring)	Lung	2
Spinal cord		5
Salivary gland		3
Orbit		3
Breast		2
Testis		2
Cervix uteri		1
Ovary		1

Lymphoproliferative lesions in the hard palate have a rather worse prognosis than those elsewhere in the mouth. Of 21 cases described by Tomich and Shafer (1975) in patients with an average age of 70 years, all were described as lymphocytic lymphomas. When 14 of these patients were followed-up, 8 had died of disseminated lymphoma, and 3 had disease persistent after therapy.

STOMACH

Gastric lymphomas are among the most common of the extranodal lymphomas, forming up to 5% of gastric malignant neoplasms. The mean age incidence ranges from 48 to 57 years and the incidence in the male is slightly higher. The usual presentation is similar to that of gastric cancer—abdominal pain, weight loss and anorexia, less frequent bleeding, nausea and vomiting, and occasionally an epigastric mass. Radiologically, the lesion may present as a large superficial ulcer on the posterior wall or lesser curvature; as thickened gastric rugae; as a thick non-pliable wall, or as multiple polypoid masses or ulcers. These things favour a diagnosis of lymphoma rather than carcinoma, but are of course not diagnostic.

The gross specimen may be very similar to a carcinoma; there may be a polypoid mass or masses, the lesion may be ulcerated, or spread within the wall producing gross mural thickening. The gastric rugae may occasionally be thickened and brain-like.

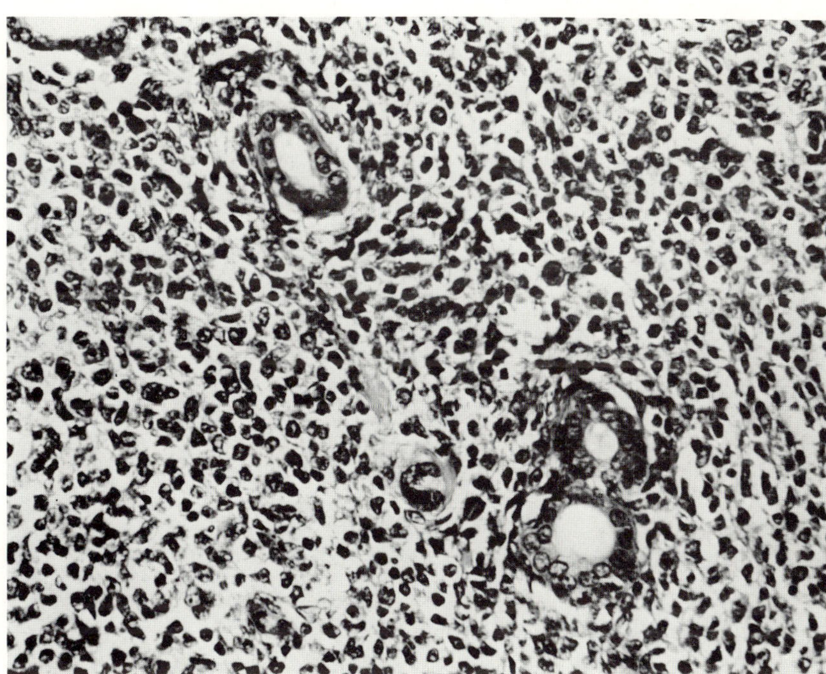

Fig. 6.1. A section of the benign lympho-epithelial lesion of salivary gland showing diffuse infiltration of salivary tissue with lymphoreticular cells, mostly mature small lymphocytes and a few residual glandular epithelial structures. ×216.

Histologically the usual range of patterns of lymphoma is found. The prognosis is rather better in patients with lymphocytic lymphomas, and in those where the lesion is very superficial. The 5-year survival rate is about 34%, though this varies from series to series. Lymphocytic lymphomas have a better prognosis as do those with a nodular pattern. Increased size, deep invasion and nodal involvement materially worsen the prognosis. Good accounts of gastric lymphomas are to be found in articles by Thorbjarnson *et al.* (1956); Azzopardi and Menzies (1960); Dawson *et al.* (1961); Joseph and Lattes (1966); Saltzstein (1969).

Easily confused with gastric lymphoma is gastric lymphoid hyperplasia, sometimes called gastric pseudo-lymphoma (Faris and Saltzstein 1964). This is found in a similar age group to true lymphoma but usually in people with a prior history of peptic ulceration. The gross appearances may be similar to those of a true lymphoma though a large tumour mass does not form. Histologically, the cellular infiltrate may penetrate through all coats of the stomach, but it is likely to be a mixed infiltrate in which many inflammatory cells are clearly recognizable. Individual cells do not show enlarged hyper-chromatic nuclei and mature lymphoid germinal centres may be present; the draining lymph nodes will show merely reactive changes. Nevertheless it may be very hard indeed to differentiate the reactive from the neoplastic. Only one of 21 patients (Faris and Saltzstein 1964) later developed lymphoma.

SMALL INTESTINE

Malignant lymphoma of the small intestine, while a fairly uncommon lesion, forms a significant proportion—up to one-third—of neoplasms arising in the small intestine. These neoplasms usually present with abdominal pain, symptoms of intestinal obstruction and changes of bowel habit. Malabsorption, as will be discussed below, is relatively common. Radiologically there may be discrete tumour masses, ulceration or merely thickening of mucosal folds. The gross lesions may be plaque-like, annular, protuberant or polypoid, and may be single or, less often, multiple, sometimes very numerous (Sheahan *et al.* 1961). As in the stomach, any of the histological types of lymphoma may be found (Isaacson *et al.* 1979). Hodgkin's disease is uncommon and a plasmacytoid variant of histiocytic cell lymphoma fairly common (Azzopardi and Menzies 1960; Dawson *et al.* 1961; Weaver and Batsakis 1964; Saltzstein 1969). The prognosis of small intestinal lymphoma is probably rather worse than that for the

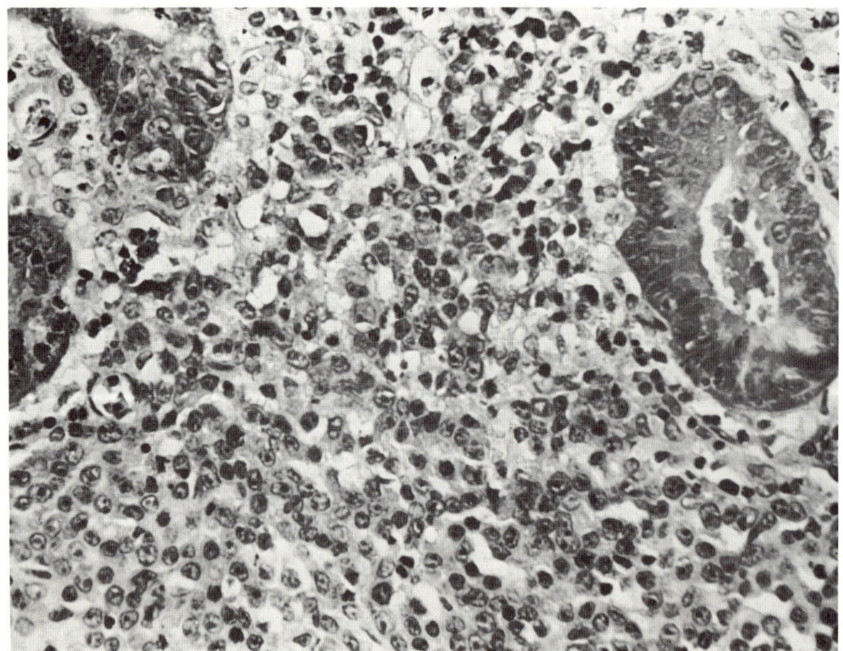

Fig. 6.2. Malignant lymphoma of small intestine showing diffuse lymphomatous infiltrate of pleomorphic histiocytic cells and some residual epithelial structures. ×216.

stomach; the 5-year survival is about 33%. As is usual the prognosis of nodular lymphomas is better than this (50% 5-year survival), and that of diffuse lymphocytic and histiocytic lymphomas worse (25% and 10% 5-year survival respectively). Hodgkin's disease in this site seems to have a particularly bad prognosis. One view (Isaacson and Wright 1978), based on immunohistochemical as well as morphological evidence, is that many of these lesions are in fact variants of malignant histiocytosis.

As in the stomach a lymphoid hyperplasia (pseudo-lymphoma) occurs with an entirely benign prognosis. This is again a mixed lymphoreticular hyperplasia. It may be predisposed to by chronic gastritis, sprue and regional enteritis and may cause intestinal obstruction.

LARGE INTESTINE

Lymphoma occurs less commonly in the colon than elsewhere in the gut, and is very much less common than carcinoma in this site. As in carcinoma, the patient presents with abdominal pain, weight loss, rectal bleeding and often has an abdominal mass or tenderness. Radiologically a filling defect or mass may be visible. The gross lesion is usually caecal, less often recto-sigmoid, and is usually a circumscribed mass projecting into the lumen or into the peritoneal cavity. It is sometimes multiple, much less often diffuse or annular. It may complicate ulcerative colitis (Cornes *et al.* 1961a). The usual histological types of lymphoma are found (Fig. 6.3). The 5-year survival rate for localized disease is 55%, and is rather better for histiocytic than lymphocytic lymphomas. Hodgkin's disease is uncommon (Azzopardi and Menzies 1960; Dawson *et al.* 1961).

Pseudo-lymphomas or benign lymphoid polyps of the large intestine, and in particular of the rectum and anal canal, are very common (Cornes *et al.* 1961b; Saltzstein 1969). These usually present with bleeding but sometimes with prolapse or abdominal pain. The lesions are commonly sessile or pedunculated polyps and may be very numerous. They are characteristically composed of well-differentiated areas of lymphoreticular tissue with germinal centres intersected by broad bands of collagen. The germinal centres characteristically contain mitotic figures and large tingible body macrophages. The overlying mucosa is usually intact.

MANAGEMENT OF GASTROINTESTINAL LYMPHOMA

In extranodal gastrointestinal lymphoma, which accounts for

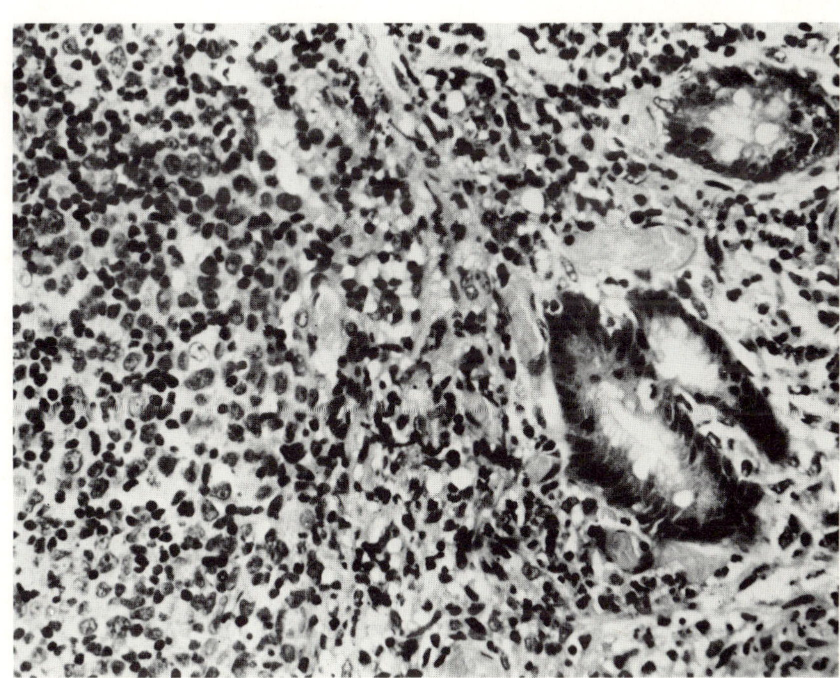

Fig. 6.3. Malignant lymphoma of rectum showing a mixture of lymphocytes and histiocytes invading lamina propria of rectal wall. ×216.

only 2% of all GI malignancy, isolated gut involvement is found in only about half of the cases; regional nodal involvement or extra-abdominal disease are found in others. For isolated involvement surgery followed by radiotherapy may be adequate; in other cases combination chemotherapy (perhaps together with irradiation and debulking surgery) is needed for improved survival.

THE ASSOCIATIONS OF INTESTINAL LYMPHOMA

The most important association is with malabsorption. It is clear that lymph nodes in malabsorption syndromes show marked histological changes, notably prominence of germinal centres and hyperplasia of interstitial histiocytes (Whitehead 1968; Isaacson & Wright 1978). It is also clear that the malabsorption syndrome occurs as a result of intestinal lymphoma (Kent 1964; Gough *et al.* 1962; Eakins *et al.* 1964; Dutz *et al.* 1971). It seems likely, as suggested by several of these authors, that the lesion of coeliac disease, villous atrophy and lymphoreticular infiltration may result in intestinal lymphoma. Many such cases may be examples of malignant histiocytosis of the intestine (Isaacson and Wright 1978).

Malbsorption and abdominal lymphoma are particularly common in the Mediterranean region in Persians and Ashkenazi Jews, forming as many as 2% of lymphomas in some areas (Dutz *et al.* 1971), and are well reviewed by Haghighi and Nasr (1973). Their patients were in the main young, male and poor from the rural areas in southern Iran; similar patients have been described from Israel and South Africa. They present with abdominal pain, weight loss, diarrhoea, nausea, vomiting, and occasionally perforation and obstruction. There may be clubbing of the fingers and osteoarthropathy. Radiologically the pattern after a barium meal suggests only malabsorption, and diagnosis depends on peroral biopsy or if necessary laparotomy. Grossly the upper small intestine shows either diffuse infiltration, focal ulceration or focal nodularity. The lesion is histologically usually lymphocytic, often large lymphocytic, sometimes histiocytic, but never, in the series studied, Hodgkin's disease. Rappaport *et al.* (1972) describe 22 patients with malabsorption; all had a diffuse plasma cell infiltrate of the mesenteric mucosa; 14 had gut lymphomas and two had intestinal nodal lymphomas. Other conditions less commonly associated with intestinal lymphoma are ulcerative colitis and carcinoma (Cornes *et al.* 1961a).

This lymphoma may be associated with abnormal circulating immunoglobulins, notably α-chain disease (Isaacson 1979.)

HEPATIC LYMPHOMA

Proved primary lymphoma of the liver probably is very rare, despite the fact that a significant fraction of the liver is made up of macrophages. In occasional cases at necropsy the major lesion present is in the liver. The hepatic sarcomas, variously reported in haemangiosarcoma and Kupffer cell sarcoma occurring many years after administration of thorotrast, may or may not be of true lymphoreticular origin. Three cases of haemangioendothelial sarcoma of the liver were reported by MacSween *et al.* (1973). These were rapidly progressive lesions and, in one case, there was suggestive evidence of Kupffer cell origin. The same may be postulated of the hepatic lesions reported as occurring in patients exposed to vinyl chloride (Lee and Harry 1974).

RESPIRATORY TRACT

This will be considered as upper respiratory and pulmonary.

UPPER RESPIRATORY TRACT

Malignant lymphoma of Waldeyer's ring is a fairly common lesion, usually in elderly people. Tonsillar lymphomas form some 5% of all lymphomas, and lymphomas in the nasopharynx are a little less common. Common presentations are persistent sore throat, local mass or bleeding and less often pain referred to the ear. In a large series 14% presented with a local lesion only, 42% had distant adenopathy and 26% were multifocal (Banfi *et al.* 1970). The ratio of histiocytic to lymphocytic lymphoma is 8:1. The lesion may spread to other parts of the gastrointestinal tract; the 5-year survival of patients with localized tonsillar lesions is 55%, though this falls to about 30% when there is regional spread (Catlin 1948; Terz and Farr 1969; McNelis and Pai 1969; Freeman *et al.* 1972).

Histologically, in this site, it can be very difficult to distinguish inflamed lymphoreticular tissue from neoplasm. The most important histological point in diagnosis is disappearance of the normal reticulin pattern and infiltration of adjacent tissues by neoplastic cells; it is therefore important to

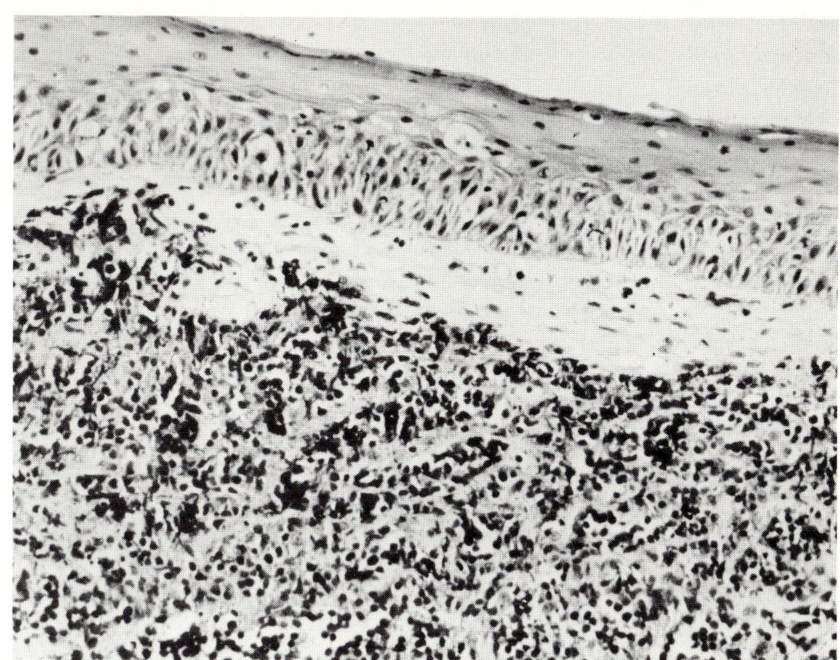

Fig. 6.4. Tonsil showing anaplastic small cell neoplasm. It is often very difficult to decide whether such lesions are carcinoma or lymphoma. At necropsy the pattern of spread of disease is usually that of lymphoma. ×108.

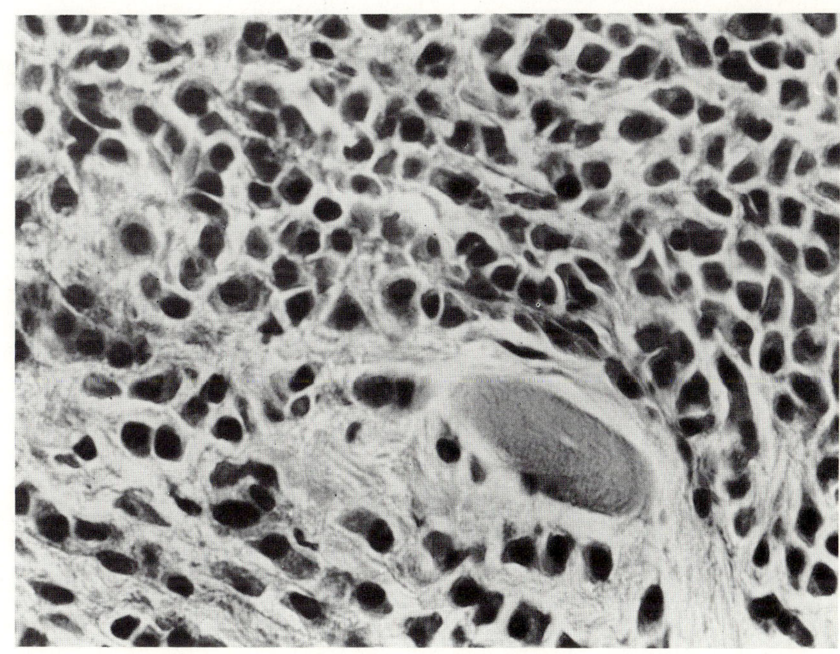

Fig. 6.5. A plasmacytoma of larynx composed of predominantly well differentiated plasmacytes with some residual striated muscle. Such lesions usually terminate in multiple myeloma, often after many years. ×450.

obtain a biopsy with some adjacent normal pharyngeal mucosa. The lesion may be lymphocytic, in which case diagnosis can be very hard or it may be a large cell lesion. Where the reticulin pattern is box-like and pericellular the lesion may be described as histiocytic lymphoma, but often in the absence of this pattern it is impossible to decide whether the lesion is lymphoid or epithelial, and it is best described as a large cell anaplastic neoplasm. Ultrastructural examination may be helpful in distinguishing carcinoma from lymphoma. Tonsillar neoplasms, with the exception of the uncommon well-differentiated squamous carcinoma, often show early and distant metastasis (Fig. 6.4).

Lymphomas may uncommonly be found elsewhere in the upper respiratory tract presenting with hoarseness, haemoptysis or upper respiratory obstruction according to site, e.g. in the larynx (Babbitt *et al.* 1973). Perhaps the least rare of these lesions is solitary plasmacytoma (Webb *et al.* 1962). These are well-circumscribed aggregates composed of differentiated plasma cells; they may be entirely benign, but should be regarded with caution. Many are followed, sometimes after many years, by the development of fatal multiple myeloma. It is therefore necessary always to carry out skeletal X-ray survey and investigation of plasma immunoglobulins (Fig. 6.5).

Truly localised lymphomas of Waldeyer's ring are usually

treated by irradiation; 5-year survivals of at least 50% are possible, particularly if the cervical lymph nodes are not involved.

LUNG

Lymphomas of the lung are rare (Sternberg *et al.* 1959; Saltzstein 1963 and 1969). They commonly present as a radiological abnormality ranging from large masses to small coin lesions. Less commonly they present with local symptoms—pain or cough—or systemic manifestations—chills, fatigues, weakness, and weight loss. Grossly the lesions form masses of varying size, sometimes occupying a whole lobe and usually penetrating to the pleural surface. The lesions may be solid or cystic (Saltzstein 1969). The usual histological variations are found. The lymphocytic type tends to spread within alveolar septa; the histiocytic and Hodgkin's type lesions tend to have a more circumscribed periphery (Fig. 6.6).

Lymphocytic lymphoma is easily confused with pseudolymphoma. The prognosis varies with histological type. The combined 5-year survival of the two types is 70%. The prognosis of histiocytic lymphoma in this site is a little worse—about 50% 5-year survival. Primary Hodgkin's

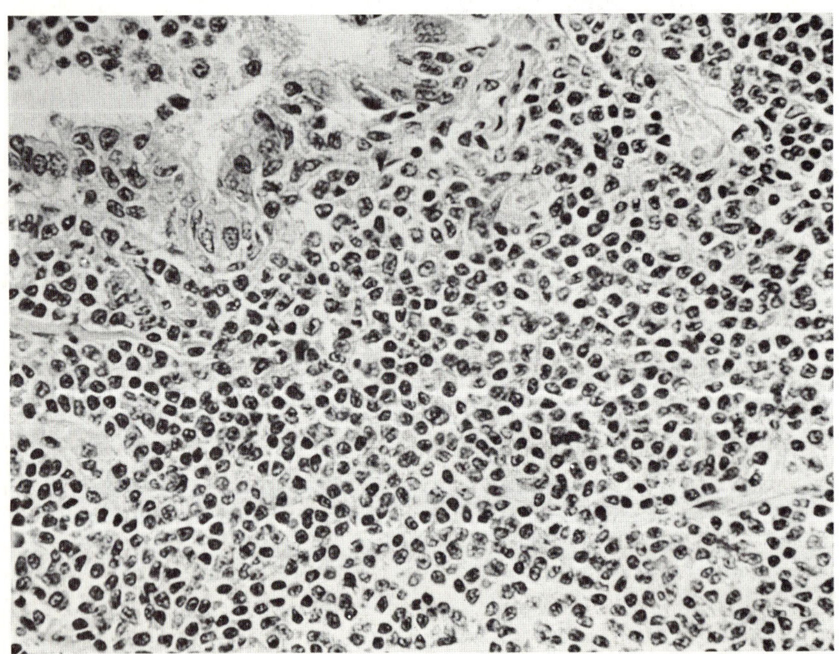

Fig. 6.6. Malignant lymphoma of lung showing massive peritracheal infiltrate of lymphocytes. ×216.

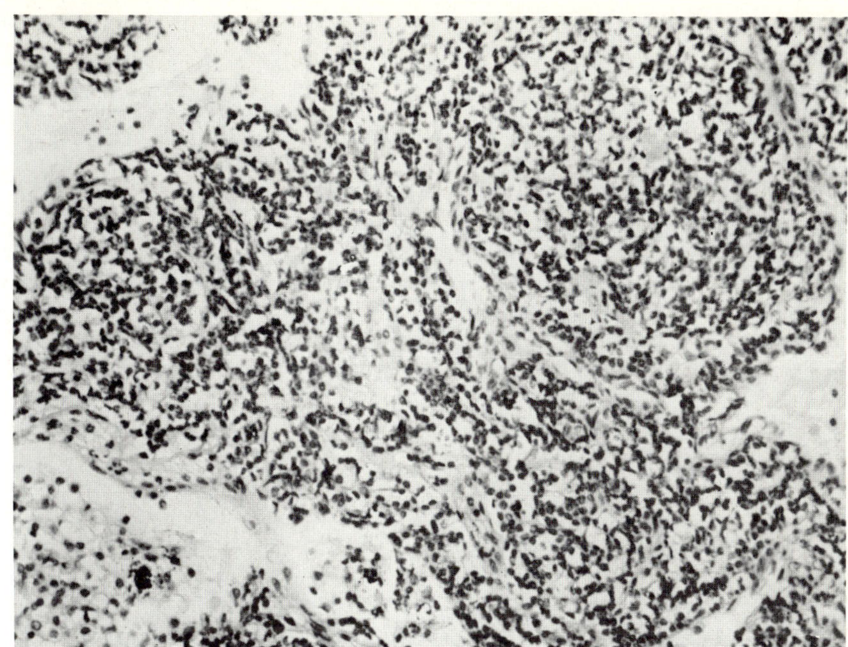

Fig. 6.7. Lymphoreticular hyperplasia or pseudolymphoma in lung showing arrangement of lymphoreticular tissue into follicular aggregates. × 108.

disease of the lung is rare and prognosis therefore hard to predict; Kern *et al.* (1961) described a case with a radiological history lasting over 12 years.

Pseudo-lymphomas or lymphoreticular proliferations in the lung may be difficult to distinguish from lymphomas, and may similarly present as a radiological shadow. The inflammatory infiltrate tends to be poorly demarcated at the edge, to be composed of mixed inflammatory cells including plasma cells and mature macrophages, and to contain lymphoid germinal centres (Titus *et al.* 1962; Saltzstein 1963 and 1969) (Fig. 6.7). Pulmonary lymphomas must also be distinguished from Wegener's granulomatosis in which there is vasculitis and necrosis, the former readily demonstrable by elastic stains, and from mediastinal angiofollicular hyperplasia of lymph nodes (Castleman *et al.* 1956) (see Chapter 3).

CUTANEOUS LYMPHOMAS AND LYMPHORETICULAR HYPERPLASIA

Benign lymphoreticular infiltrates of the skin are common and lymphomas not uncommon; diagnosis may be difficult (reviewed by Lever and Schaumberg-Lever 1975; Mihm *et al.* 1974). The specimen presents as a skin biopsy very often with little clinical information; the first thing that must be done is to establish whether the patient has a generalized skin eruption (Fig. 6.9), of what sort, whether there is a generalized adenopathy and splenomegaly, and whether the patient is systemically ill; if there is any suspicion of a malignant lymphoreticular lesion, haematological examination should be carried out to exclude leukaemia.

The next stage is to examine several sections from the biopsy to allow sufficient sampling. The nature and the site of cellular infiltration should be noted. The present text is concerned only with lymphoreticular infiltrates, and the much commoner mixed inflammatory infiltrates will not be discussed. The cellular infiltrates may be of the following types:

1 Lymphocytic.
2 Macrophagic, i.e. composed of mature macrophages.
3 Histiocytic, i.e. composed of pleomorphic hyperchromatic histiocytes often with mitotic figures.
4 Mixed cells.
5 Hodgkin's disease, i.e. the typical mixed infiltrate of Hodgkin's disease.

On examination of a skin biopsy containing a lymphoreticular lesion, the following histopathological diagnosis may be made:

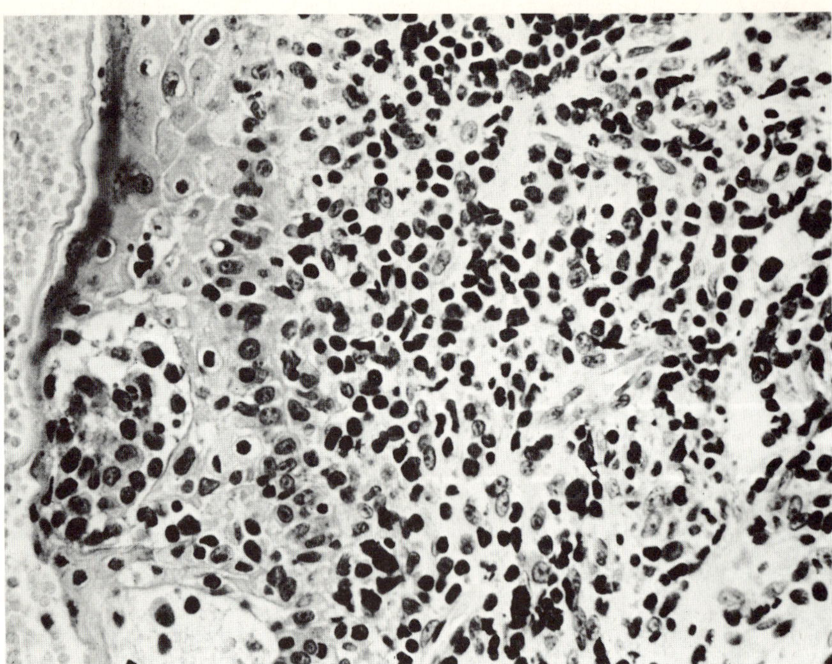

Fig. 6.8. Malignant lymphoma of skin. There is a pleomorphic infiltrate of lymphoma cells in the dermis invading the epidermis. ×216.

1 Benign lymphoreticular infiltration of skin

In these lesions the aggregates may be pure lymphocytic, often with germinal centres, or may have an admixture of histiocytes and plasma cells. There are usually few atypical cells and few mitotic figures. The infiltrate does not usually invade the epidermis and normally occupies only half or less of the dermis.

Within this class of lesion fall 'lymphocytic' infiltration of skin (Jessner and Kanof 1953) and cutaneous lymphocytoma, or lymphoplasia (Mach and Wilgram 1966)—where there are benign papular lesions, erythema annulare centrifugum—where the infiltrate lies in the superficial part of the dermis, palpable migratory arciform erythema and discoid palpable erythema (Clark *et al.* 1974). There are within this group two basic clinical patterns—patients with erythema and patients with one or several skin nodules (reviewed by Clark *et al.* 1974). Three clinical and histological patterns were distinguished in the former group:

(a) Erythema annulare centrifugum presents as complex annulare bizarre erythemas of trunk and extremities. Histologically there is an exudate, predominantly of lymphocytes but with some histiocytes and eosinophils, affecting the superficial part of the dermis. The venules may show endothelial swelling. The disorder may be chronic, lasting up to several years, and may be associated with neoplasia, e.g. of breast and lung.

(b) Palpable migratory arciform erythema appears as elevated dull reddish erythematous plaques, usually on the trunk. The lesions appear to migrate, i.e. to move several inches over a period of several months, though it is not clear whether this represents the appearance of a new lesion. Histologically there is dense perivascular infiltration of the vessels and appendages of the deeper part of the dermis, with lymphocytes. The appearances mimic those of lymphocytic leukaemia closely.

(c) Discoid palpable erythema (Jessner–Kanoff) is an erythematous disc on the face. Histologically there is perivascular infiltration in the area of the subpapillary venous plexus and, to a lesser extent, deeper in the dermis. The cellular infiltrate is predominantly lymphocytic but some histiocytes also may be present.

Cutaneous lymphoplasia (lymphocytoma cutis or Spiegler–Fendt pseudo-lymphoma) is a solitary elevated nodule up to 5 cm in diameter (though usually smaller) most often found in the face. It is characterized by lymphoid aggregates often with germinal centres and displacing rather than infiltrating the

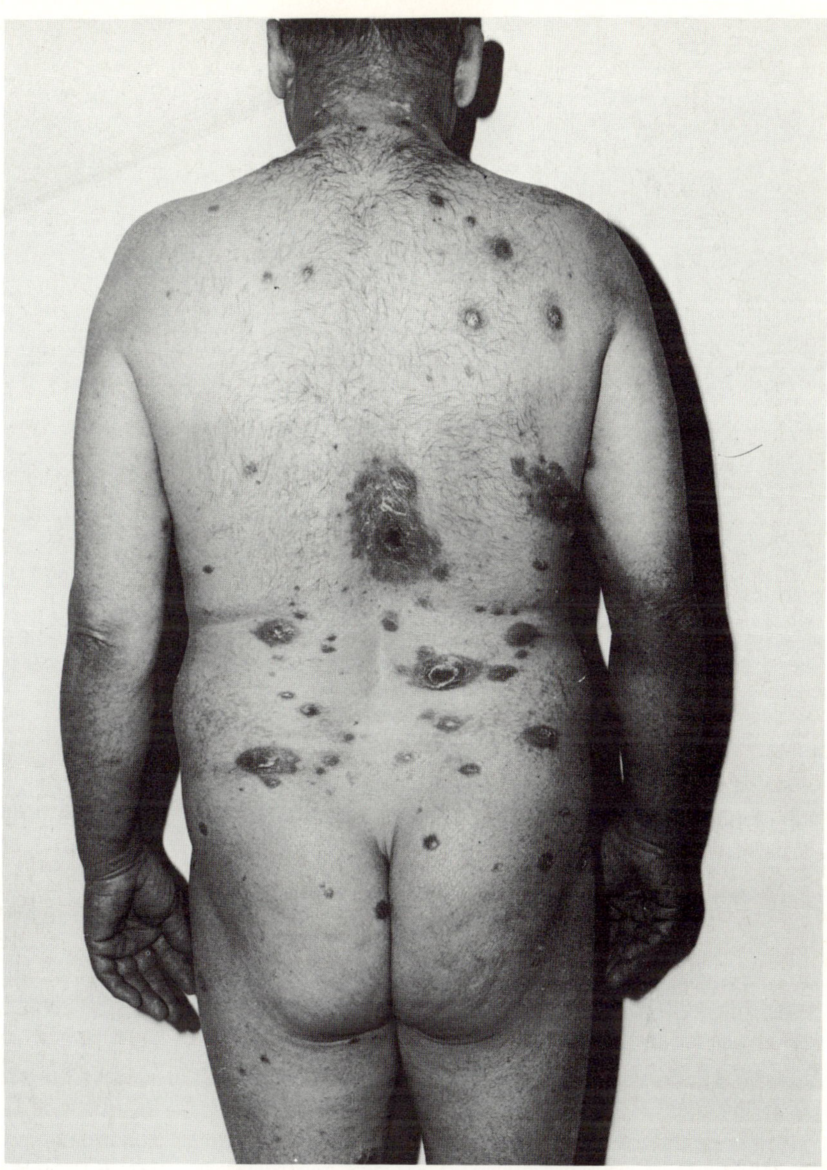

Fig. 6.9. Extensive macular and nodular skin eruption in a patient with mycosis fungoides.

surrounding collagen. Eosinophils may be prominent and the centres of the germinal centres may show numerous mitotic figures. The lesion is usually solitary but may be multiple (Fig. 6.10).

A variant of this lesion is lymphomatoid papulosis (Macaulay 1968; Feuerman and Sandbank 1972) where the patient presents with a crop of small papules which suddenly disappear. The histological picture is confusing, however, because the lesions contain many pleomorphic mononuclear cells. Similarly in actinic reticuloid (Ive *et al.* 1969), a chronic dermatitis associated with severe photosensitivity, there may be considerable cellular atypia in the infiltrate.

Another benign lesion which may mimic lymphoma is a persistent insect bite where there may be a pleomorphic mixed cellular infiltrate with considerable squamous epithelial hyperplasia; eosinophils are notable in the infiltrates. A search should be made in serial sections for insect mouth parts; these appear as sharply defined objects whose chitin is

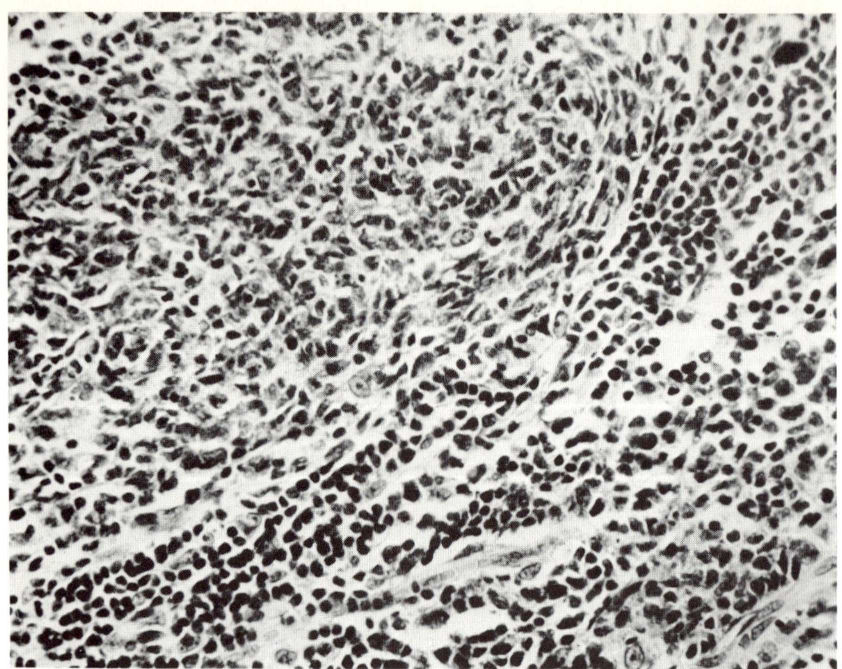

Fig. 6.10. A mass of lymphoreticular cells in the dermis. Benign lymphocytoma cutis. The patient is well and devoid of lesions five years after biopsy. ×216.

PAS-positive. So-called angiolymphoid hyperplasia is characterized by an inflammatory infiltrate containing many small blood vessels. It is probably an atypical pyogenic granuloma.

2 True cutaneous lymphoma

Hodgkin's disease is rare, but the full spectrum of non-Hodgkin's lymphomas may be seen, the most common being diffuse histiocytic lymphoma. The usual features of cellular atypia and pleomorphism are present (Burke *et al.* 1981). Where the lesion shows a mixed infiltrate with atypical cells it can be regarded as a true lymphoma (see Fig. 6.8). Lymphocytic lesions on the other hand, if single, may be truly benign. Multiple pure lymphocytic lesions are best regarded as malignant, but may be very indolent indeed in their behaviour. The characteristic skin lesion is a reddish-purple papular infiltration, single or multiple, and of widely varying size.

It can be difficult to determine malignancy (Evans *et al.* 1979). The malignant lesion typically does not preferentially involve the upper dermis, is composed predominantly of medium to large lymphocytes or histiocytes, and is devoid of well-developed germinal centres. It is peculiarly difficult to distinguish benign from malignant lymphoreticular infiltra-

tion in the conjunctiva. Here small lymphocytic lesions commonly occur. Because of the risks to the eye involved in radiotherapy in this site these should, in the presence of normal haematological findings, be accepted as malignant only on very convincing evidence.

3 Sézary's syndrome and mycosis fungoides

These are now considered to be closely related and to be cutaneous T cell lymphomas (reviewed by Zackheim 1981). The term Sézary's syndrome is used to describe a syndrome in which erythroderma is combined with the presence of abnormal circulating lymphocytes (Sézary and Bouvrain 1938; reviewed by Winkelmann and Linman 1973). The patients are usually over 40 years of age and have, in addition to erythroderma, severe pruritus, alopecia and nail dystrophy. Skin biopsies show a monomorphous band-like cellular infiltrate around the rete pegs. Abnormal lymphocytes, 10–20 μm in diameter, occur in the blood; they have folded or notched nuclei like a 'thumbprint swirl in wet paint'. They contain no peroxidase or acid phosphatase, have no surface Ig receptors, respond to PHA stimulation and are not phagocytic. Ultrastructurally they have deeply cleft nuclei and contain many cytoplasmic microfilaments (Lutzner and Jordan 1968;

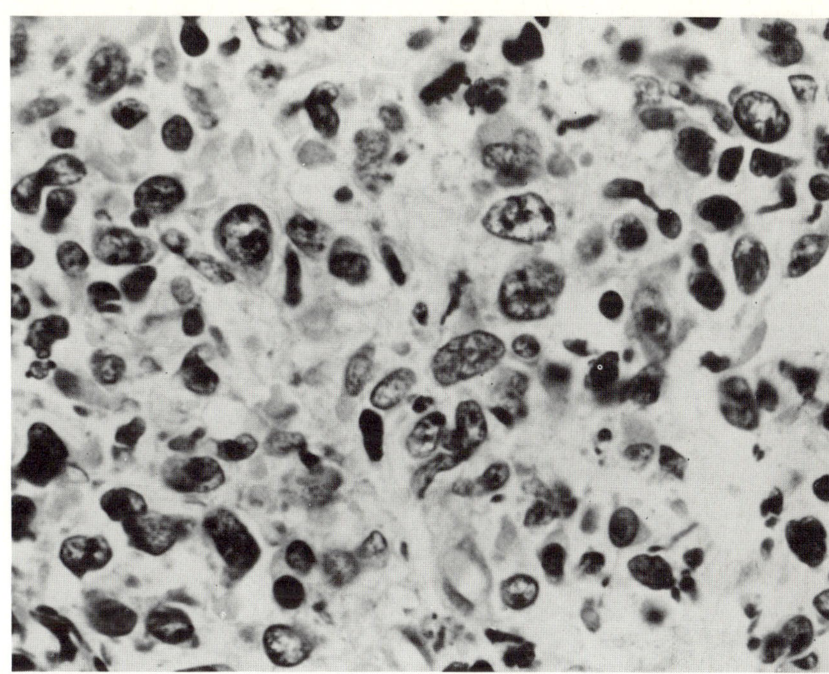

Fig. 6.11. Skin showing cutaneous malignant lymphoma-mycosis fungoides. The nuclei of the malignant lymphoma cells are elongated often indented with large nucleoli. ×450.

Lutzner *et al.* 1973; Winkelmann and Linman 1973; Zucker-Franklin *et al.* 1974); some of the cells seen in the skin biopsies are similar. These patients may have hepatosplenomegaly at the time of presentation; 5 of 34 cases developed lymphoma or leukaemia (Winkelmann and Linman 1973). Sézary cells have been described in the terminal disseminated lymphomatous lesions (Paradinas and Harrison 1974).

The term mycosis fungoides is used to describe a cutaneous lymphoma which characteristically progresses from a non-specific 'premycotic' erythroderma in which there is non-specific lymphoreticular infiltration of skin, via a stage where indurated neoplastic plaques are present in the skin, to the situation where large nodules are present. The term was used to describe a clinical entity (Clendenning *et al.* 1964); it is now widely believed to be a specific pathologic entity. Curiously, widespread dissemination and early death are much commoner in the U.S.A. than in Britain.

Rappaport and Thomas (1974) have analysed a series of 45 cases of mycosis fungoides; the criterion for initial diagnosis was the presence of a band-like cellular infiltrate of atypical lymphoid cells, with irregular, indented, folded, or convoluted nuclei. Some of these infiltrate the epidermis, producing the so-called Pautrier microabscesses; also seen are very large atypical hyperchromatic cells—'mycosis cells' some with a deeply indented cerebriform nucleus. Visceral infiltrates occurred in 32 of these patients. Twenty four of them showed lymph node infiltration; lesions were also found in lung, spleen, liver, kidney, thyroid, pancreas, marrow and heart. The infiltrates characteristically caused rather less tissue destruction than might have been expected (see Fig. 6.11). The infiltrating cells showed chromosomal abnormalities (Erkman-Balis & Rappaport 1974) and at the EM level varying degrees of nuclear indentation (Brownlee and Murad 1970; Lutzner *et al.* 1973; Rosas-Uribe *et al.* 1974). The specificity of these cells has been questioned (Fisher *et al.* 1972). The presence of considerable numbers of such cells indicates mycosis fungoides. Cell marker studies have shown that they are T cells (Edelson *et al.* 1974). The lymph node changes in mycosis fungoides range from dermatopathic lymphadenopathy with florid paracortical expansion, to frank lymphoma (Colby *et al.* 1981). These are difficult to distinguish. There is disagreement as to whether prognosis relates more to the extent of the skin lesion than to the presence of frank malignancy in the draining lymph nodes (Colby *et al.* 1981; Scheffer *et al.* 1980).

MANAGEMENT OF SKIN LYMPHOMAS

In the early stages of mycosis fungoides, local symptomatic

therapy, e.g. steroid application, is all that is needed. For more severe skin disease photochemotherapy (PUVA—psoralen and ultraviolet light) and radiotherapy (local field or whole body superficial electrons) may be required. Visceral spread and Sézary's syndrome are notoriously resistant to treatment, though some responses to combination chemotherapy are seen.

For skin lymphomas other than mycosis fungoides it is very important to exclude extracutaneous disease at presentation. Truly localized lesions are cured by radiotherapy; for disseminated disease the outlook is poor but chemotherapy may be effective.

HISTIOCYTOMA

The commonest lesion alleged to be a neoplasm of histiocytes is the histiocytoma or fibrous histiocytoma. This is a firm, slowly growing cutaneous nodule found characteristically on the extremities of adults. It is composed of numerous macrophage-like cells with large oval nuclei vacuolated and giving positive staining reactions for iron and fat. Some multinucleated giant cells may be present (Fig. 6.12). This lesion was first described as a histiocytoma by Woringer and Kwiatowski (1938). Intermediate stages between this and a fibroma occur; the lesion is benign. Malignant tumours of similar origin occur (Soule and Enriquez 1972; Kempson and Kyriakos 1972; Mackenzie 1974, for review). These tumours occur in the subcutaneous tissues and in connective tissues elsewhere in the body. They are composed of pleomorphic histiocytes with foci of foamy histiocytes and sometimes giant cells. The growth rate, and the tendency to local recurrence and metastasis are widely variable, and do not appear to be predictable from histological appearances. Where there is extensive collagen deposition the lesion is known as malignant fibrous histiocytoma, and where giant cells are numerous as giant cell tumour. There appears to be little doubt (Merkow *et al.* 1971; Guccion and Enzinger 1972) of the histiocytic nature of these lesions.

At least some examples appear to contain unequivocally malignant fibroblasts and macrophages, a few intermediate cells and some undifferentiated ones, raising the possibility that both the principal cell types, at least in a neoplasm, arise from the same undifferentiated stem cell (Fu *et al.* 1975). There is no good evidence that 'Epithelioid Sarcoma' is a histiocytic tumour, despite its name (Mackenzie 1974).

Kyriakos and Kempson (1976) described 7 patients with a variant which they labelled as inflammatory fibrous histiocytoma, characterized by the histological appearance of malignant histiocytes and an inflammatory reaction; this is an

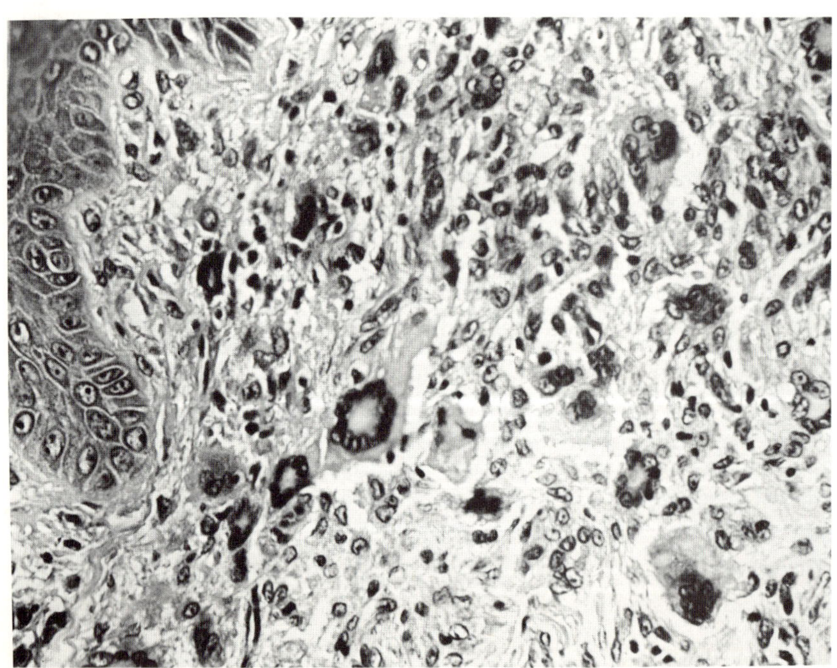

Fig. 6.12. Skin showing benign histiocytoma. The dermis is infiltrated with benign mesenchymal cells, some fibroblasts and some histiocytes and multinucleate giant cells. ×216.

aggressive and lethal condition characterized by local recurrence followed later by metastasis, the mean survival being approximately 4 years. Radiotherapy and chemotherapy are only occasionally successful in treating this condition; extensive surgery is sometimes required (Hancock and Crawford 1982).

OVARY AND UTERUS

Primary lymphoma of the ovary is rare. Patients may present with menstrual abnormality or abdominal discomfort. The gross lesion is firm in texture, sometimes cystic or necrotic and is histiologically lymphocytic, less often histiocytic, more often diffuse than nodular (Cooper *et al.* 1974; Paladugu *et al.* 1980.)

Primary lymphoma of the uterus is a little less rare; Fox and More (1965) refer to 14 cases, 9 in the corpus uteri and 5 in the cervix. Chorlton *et al.* (1974b) described 6 cases in the cervix, 3 in the corpus uteri and 4 in the vagina, usually presenting with abdominal menstrual bleeding, perineal discomfort, or discharge. Stransky *et al.* (1973) described one case and referred to 7 others less often histiocytic, usually of diffuse rather than nodular pattern. Hodgkin's disease in this site is very rare. The number of published cases is so small that prognosis is difficult. Chorlton *et al.* (1974b) indicate a 5-year survival rate with treatment of 22% for ovarian lesions and 60% for uterine lesions. Of two cases of histiocytic lymphoma, primary in cervix uteri, described by us (Carr *et al.* 1976), both patients are alive and well after treatment, one 7 years after primary radiotherapy, the other 5 years after primary radiotherapy, followed by chemotherapy for recurrence (Fig. 6.13).

BREAST

Malignant lymphoma of the breast is a rare disease of middle-aged to elderly women; histiocytic lymphoma occurs at a mean age of 57 years and lymphosarcoma about ten years younger (De Cosse *et al.* 1962; Lawler and Richie 1967; Oberman 1966; Yoshida 1970; Bushkin *et al.* 1973) (Fig. 6.14). Hodgkin's disease is rare in this site.

The lesion is characteristically a rapidly growing lump in a well woman; the best treatment is as yet uncertain but Bushkin *et al.* (1973) suggest that if the diagnosis is made on a frozen section it is best to excise the lump, not the breast and await a definite paraffin section report. The best reported survival rate after radical surgery and irradiation is 64% at 5 years and 54% at 10 years (De Cosse *et al.* 1962). Freeman *et*

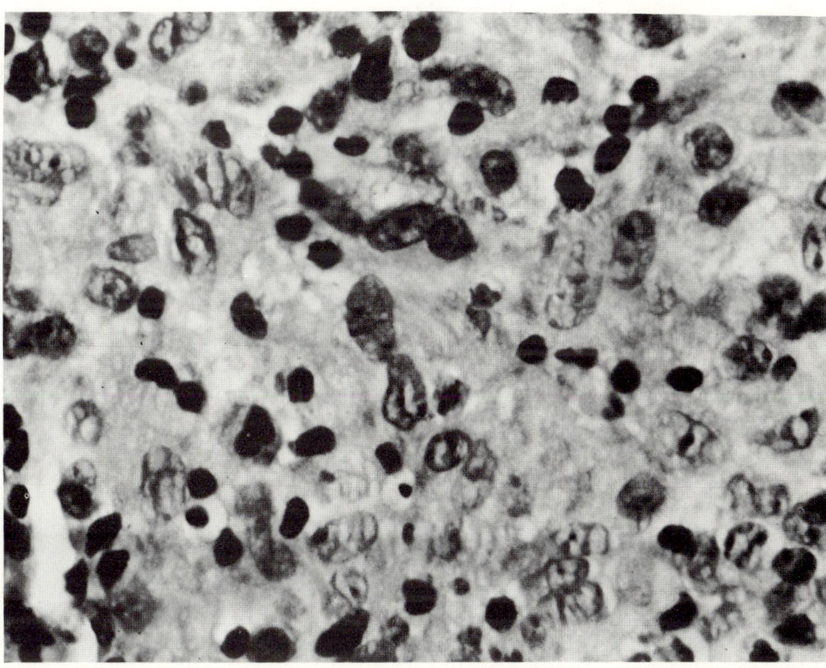

Fig. 6.13. Uterine cervix showing a pleomorphic cellular infiltrate composed of lymphocytes and malignant histiocytic cells. The appearances are those of malignant lymphoma of histiocytic type. ×450.

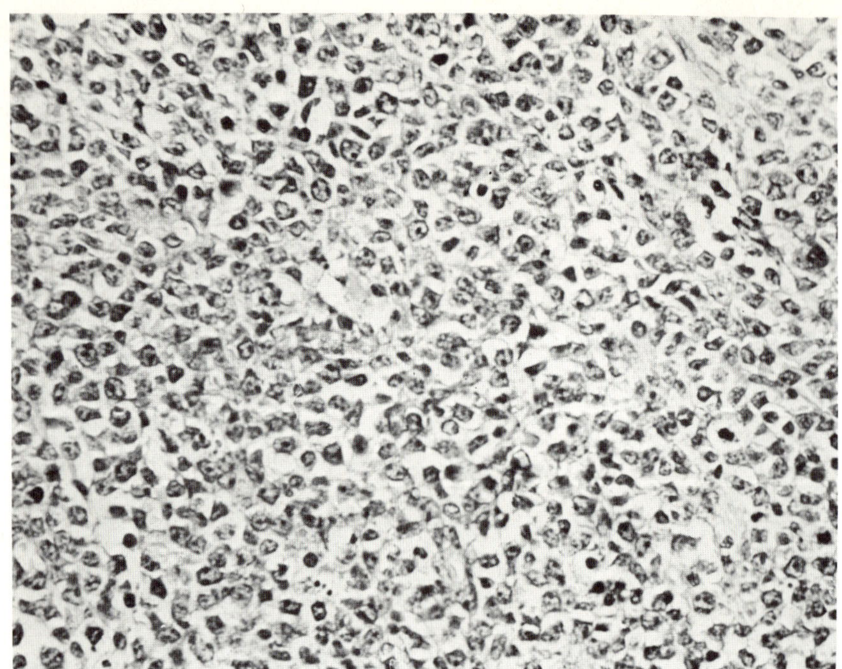

Fig. 6.14. Breast showing diffuse infiltration by monomorphous histiocytic lymphoma. ×216.

al. (1972) in their review of cancer registry patients quote a 5-year survival of 44% for localized disease. Many patients show disseminated relapse after primary surgery and radiotherapy and it may be that early systemic chemotherapy is advisable.

True lymphoma must be distinguished from pseudo-lymphoma (Fisher *et al.* 1979; Lin *et al.* 1980) by the usual criteria; the benign lesion shows small well-differentiated lymphocytes and germinal centres.

TESTIS

Lymphomas of the testis (Gowing 1964; Collins and Pugh 1964; Hamlin *et al.* 1972; Gowing 1976) have a similar presentation to other testicular tumours usually in middle-aged or elderly males. Of 9 cases (Hamlin *et al.* 1972) 2 were Hodgkin's disease, 3 histiocytic lesions and the rest lymphocytic lymphomas. They are occasionally bilateral.

In the large series described by Gowing (1976) all were poorly differentiated, 41% lymphocytic, and 59% histiocytic. None were follicular and there were no examples of Hodgkin's disease (Fig. 6.15). The more recent experience of Paladugu *et al.* (1980) and Turner *et al.* (1981) was similar. These lesions have a marked propensity for invasion of veins. Spread occurs

early and wide, particularly to the nasal and nasopharyngeal regions and skin; in our own experience one patient presented with a mass on the gum. The prognosis was poor; 62% of Gowing's (1976) series were dead within 2 years and the 5-year survival (Freeman *et al.* 1972) was only 21%. This has improved with developments in chemotherapy. Plasmacytomas hardly ever occur in the testis, and rarely a chronic non-specific inflammatory lesion may mimic lymphoma, but should be distinguishable by the mixed and mature nature of the cellular infiltrate, and the presence of fibrosis and lymphoid germinal centres (Gowing 1976).

BONE

Primary malignant lymphoma of bone was described by Parker and Jackson (1939) and has been well reviewed by Boston *et al.* (1974). It presents over a wide age range (mean 44 years) with local pain and swelling and a local mass. Radiologically there is an osteolytic lesion with periosteal reaction—most commonly in pelvis or femur, less often in humerus, ribs or tibia. Histologically most of the lesions show numerous histiocytic cells with a varying number of lymphocytes (Fig. 6.16); less often they are purely lymphocytic and occasionally Reed–Sternberg cells may be seen. It seems

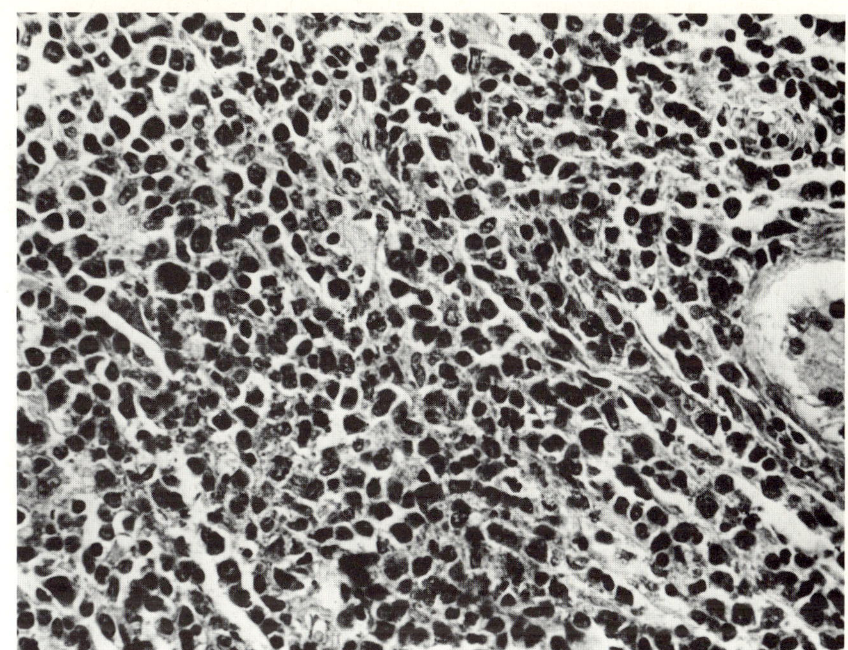

Fig. 6.15. Testis showing diffuse infiltration by pleomorphic malignant histiocytic cells; the residue of a seminiferous tubule is present. It is often difficult to subtype testicular lymphomas. Most as in this instance can be described as histiocytic. ×216.

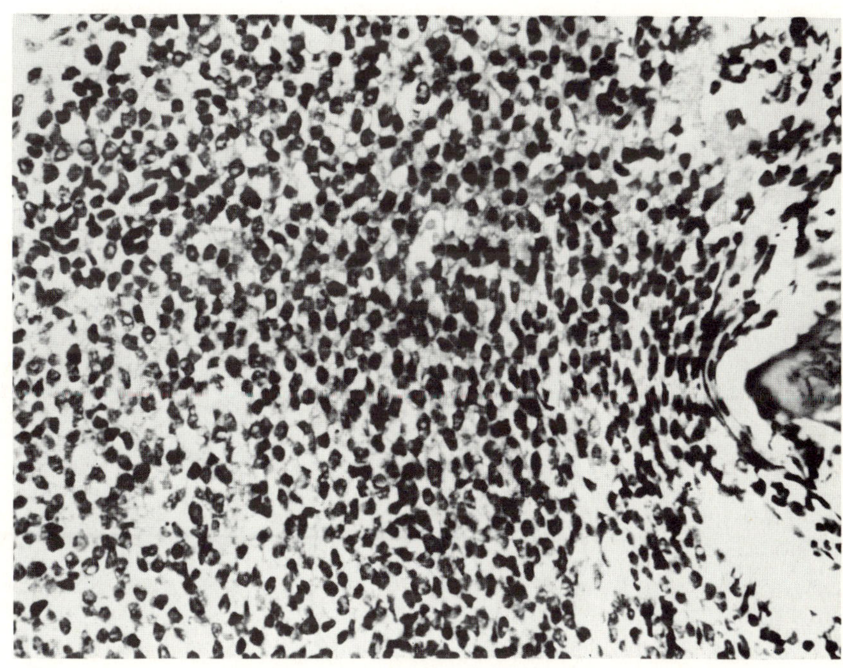

Fig. 6.16. Bone showing diffuse infiltration by malignant lymphoma histiocytic type. It is important but not always easy to distinguish this from Ewing's tumour. The latter contains much intracellular glycogen and little intercellular reticulin. ×216.

(Boston *et al.* 1974) that the histological pattern does not materially affect prognosis. Differential diagnosis from the rather similar Ewing's tumour of bone may be of some importance in that the prognosis of histiocytic lymphoma of bone, after appropriate treatment, is better. The 5-year survival rate is 44% where the lesion has not disseminated from the primary bone site, and 23% where dissemination has taken place. Diagnosis from Ewing's tumour is not always possible; the presence of a dense reticulin network points to malignant lymphoma, while the presence of large amounts of intracellular glycogen suggests Ewing's tumour. Ultrastructural examination may be of value (Friedman and Gold 1968).

Radical radiation therapy remains the treatment of choice for solitary lesions; chemotherapy must be added for disseminated disease.

THYROID

Primary lymphoma of the thyroid is an uncommon tumour of the thyroid occurring usually in middle-aged or elderly women who present with a lump in the neck. On section the mass is homogeneous and pinkish-grey or cream coloured sometimes, with yellowish areas of necrosis, but without the

areas of calcification and cyst formation often found in thyroid carcinomas. Histologically (Fig. 6.17) the neoplasms present the usual variety of lymphocytic lymphoma, histiocytic lymphoma and, least commonly, Hodgkin's disease (Cox 1964; Walt 1957, reviewed by Smithers 1970; Rayfield *et al.* 1971) (Fig. 6.17). In Smithers' own series there were 19 cases of lymphosarcoma, 6 of histiocytic sarcoma and 2 of Hodgkin's disease. In a recent large series (Compagno and Oertel 1980) poor prognosis was indicated by a histologically diffuse lesion, a plasmacytic lesion and the presence of vascular invasion, necrosis and metastasis. Until recently, the outlook for patients with thyroid lymphomas, as for those with anaplastic thyroid carcinomas was bleak; most were dead within a year. It may be hard to predict prognosis from histology; in a group of cases described by Brewer and Orr (1953) as 'struma lymphomatosa', there were some who survived for a long time.

With high dose radiotherapy for local disease and systemic chemotherapy for more advanced cases survivals of about 50% at 5 years are possible (Burke *et al.* 1977), though abdominal relapse is especially common.

It seems likely that there is an increased incidence of thyroid neoplasms in Hashimoto's disease. These are usually carcinomas but lymphomas may occur (Smithers 1970). In a small number of cases it may be difficult to be sure whether a

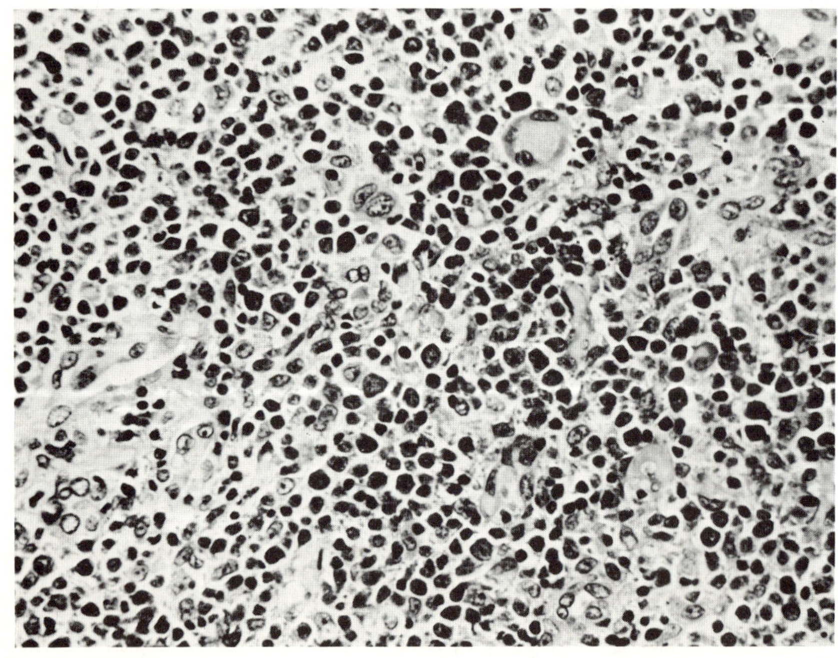

Fig. 6.17. A section of thyroid with a few residual degenerate thyroid epithelial elements, diffusely infiltrated by pleomorphic malignant histiocytic cells and lymphocytes. ×216.

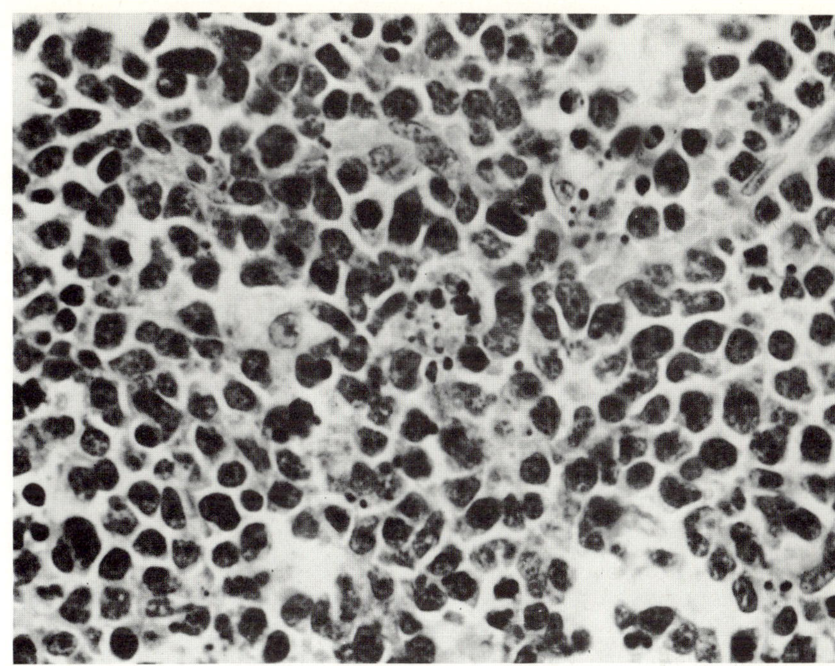

Fig. 6.18. Burkitt's lymphoma. The component neoplastic cells are large lymphocytes (lymphoblasts). Scattered large macrophages containing cellular debris produce a 'starry sky' appearance. ×840.

thyroid shows merely a non-neoplastic lymphoreticular infiltrate, or true lymphoid neoplasm. As in other sites, the criteria for neoplasia are gross cellular and nuclear pleomorphism; true germinal centres are found only in reactive lesions. The absence of thyroid auto-antibodies in the serum is a clear indication that the lesion is neoplastic rather than autoimmune.

ADRENAL

Primary adrenal lymphoma is very rare. Hayes and Christensen (1961) reported a single case of bilateral histiocytic sarcoma and refer to another.

MARROW

Isolated lymphoma of marrow is rare and presents as pancytopenia (Barton *et al.* 1980).

KIDNEY

Primary lymphoma of the kidney is very rare. Silber and

Chang (1973) reported a single case in a 57-year old female who presented with a mass in the loin. She had been treated for many years with steroids for rheumatoid disease. The histological appearances were not clearly presented but the lesion was probably either a large lymphocytic or a histiocytic lymphoma. Primary lymphoma of the bladder is similarly rare (Wang *et al.* 1969).

ORBIT

Orbital lymphoreticular lesions have been described as a distinct group (Tewfik *et al.* 1979; Knowles and Jacobiec 1980; Brisbane *et al.* 1981). As usual they fall into reactive lymphoreticular proliferations and true lymphomas, and the diagnosis in borderline cases can be difficult; recurrence occurs in the first 5 years after treatment if it is going to happen.

BURKITT'S LYMPHOMA

This lymphoma (Burkitt 1958) is found in a belt of tropical Africa where the rainfall is 20″ or more and where the mean temperature of the coldest month is not below 15°C; even at the equator it is not found above an altitude of 5000 feet, leading to the speculation that it is an infectious disease of viral aetiology carried by an insect. Time–space clustering and epidemic drift also suggest an infectious aetiology. The Epstein–Barr virus (EBV) is the strongest contender (Epstein *et al.* 1964) possibly in association with falciparum malaria. The virus, which causes glandular fever in previously healthy people, may act synergistically with the immunosuppression produced by chronic malarial infection, to produce lymphoma. It occurs usually in children, rarely below the age of 2 years and usually in the age range 5–8 years. It has been reported also epidemically in Papua-New Guinea and sporadically, for instance, in the USA, Northern Manitoba and Italy, as reviewed in a *British Medical Journal* leading article (1978).

The classical presentation is of single or multiple tumours of the jaw or with diffuse spread to salivary glands, thyroid, heart, breast, testes and ovaries. In over half the cases where the lesions are disseminated the central nervous system is involved. The spinal cord may be compressed or show ischaemic degeneration and demyelination; there may be meningeal infiltration and cranial nerve palsies. The lesion is very rapidly growing.

Histologically the pattern is that of an expanding nodular mass of undifferentiated lymphoreticular cells, best identified as large lymphocytes, 20 μm or more in diameter. The nuclei are best seen in smears as having finely stippled chromatin. There is marked cytoplasmic basophilia and pyroninophilia; Sudanophilic inclusions are seen in appropriately stained smears. The tissue contains numerous large non-neoplastic macrophages, variously loaded with cytoplasmic debris, producing the 'starry sky' appearance (Fig. 6.18).

The histological diagnosis of Burkitt's lymphoma is easy in the classical case, where it presents as a solid nodal or extranodal tumour. Acute lymphoblastic and myeloblastic leukaemia should be excluded. In malignant lymphoma histiocytic type the cells tend to be larger with large eosinophilic nucleoli, coarse nuclear chromatin, and any Sudanophilic vacuoles present are larger than those in Burkitt's lymphoma. In malignant lymphoma large lymphocytic type the nuclei are smaller than those of histiocytes, and cleaved or indented with coarse chromatin. Pyroninophilia is variable or not marked. For further information on what can be a difficult diagnostic problem, reference should be made to the World Health Organisation Bulletin handbook (1969).

The appropriate treatment in communities without specialized radiotherapy centres is chemotherapy. Dramatic long-term remissions occur with one and two dose treatments of cyclophosphamide vincristine and methotroxate (Burkitt 1967). However relapses are seen even after long-term remissions and the importance of maintenance after combination chemotherapy is now recognized.

The prognosis for localized disease is good with long-term remissions of several years duration and some patients appear to have been completely cured. With generalized disease the prognosis is similar to that encountered in the other non-Hodgkin's lymphomas; overall 5-year survival is 30–40%. Bad prognostic features are older age, bulky disease, and CNS relapse.

A full account of the condition is given by Burkitt and Wright (1970) and more recently by Davies (1975) and Ziegler (1981).

GENERAL ASPECTS OF
MANAGEMENT AND PROGNOSIS
IN EXTRANODAL LYMPHOMA

Although lymphoma (particularly of non-Hodgkin's type) often presents as apparently localized extranodal disease, extensive staging investigations (see Chapter 13) will detect the presence of other regional or more disseminated disease in up to half of these patients. If the lymphoma is localized, i.e. stage I_E, and the patient is clinically well, local irradiation is currently regarded as the treatment of choice though chemotherapy, even at this early stage, has its advocates. For widespread disease systemic chemotherapy is appropriate, but the older age and debilated condition of some patients must be taken into consideration. 5-year survivals of above 50% are possible for many extranodal lymphomas; the best results are seen with skin, salivary gland and Waldeyer's ring tumours and worst with testis, bone and small bowel. Thyroid, stomach and breast occupy intermediate positions (Van der Werf-Messing 1978). In our series of localised (IA_E IIA_E) extranodal lymphomas treated radically by radiotherapy the 5-year survival is 55%.

REFERENCES

AZZOPARDI J.G. & MENZIES T. (1960) Primary malignant lymphoma of the alimentary tract. *Brit. J. Surg.* **47**, 358–66.
BABBITT D.E., YARINGTON C.T. & YONKERS A.J. (1973) Malignant lymphoma of the larynx. *J. Larynx.* **87**, 807–10.
BANFI A., BONADONNA G., CARNEVALI G., MOLINARI R., MONFAR-

DINI S. & SALVINI E. (1970) Lymphoreticular sarcomas with primary involvement of Waldeyer's ring. *Cancer* **26**, 341–51.

BARTON J.C., CONRAD M.E., VOGLER L.B. & PARMLEY R.T. (1980) Isolated marrow lymphoma. An entity of possible T-cell derivation. *Cancer* **46**, 1767–74.

BOSTON H.C., DAHLIN D.C., IVINS J.C. & CUPPS R.E. (1974) Malignant lymphoma (so called reticulum cell sarcoma) of bone. *Cancer* **34**, 1131–7.

BREWER D.B. & ORR J.W. (1953) Struma reticulosa: a reconsideration of the undifferentiated tumours of the thyroid. *J. Path.* **65**, 193–208.

BRISBANE J.V., LESSEL S., FINKEL H.E. & NEIMAN R.S. (1981) Malignant lymphoma presenting in the orbit. *Cancer* **47**, 548–53.

BROWNLEE T.R. & MURAD T.M. (1970) Ultrastructure of mycosis fungoides. *Cancer* **26**, 686–98.

BURKE J.S., BUTLER J.J. & FULLER L.M. (1977) Malignant lymphomas of the thyroid. *Cancer* **39**, 1587–1602.

BURKE J.S., HOPPE R.T., CIBULL M.L. & DORFMAN R.F. (1981) Cutaneous malignant lymphoma. A pathologic study of 50 cases with clinical analysis of 37. *Cancer* **47**, 300–10.

BURKITT D.P. (1958) Sarcoma involving the jaws in African children. *Brit. J. Surg.* **46**, 218–331.

BURKITT D.P. (1967) Long-term remissions following one and two-dose chemotherapy for African lymphoma. *Cancer* **20**, 756–9.

BURKITT D.P. & WRIGHT D.H. (1970) *Burkitt's Lymphoma.* E. and S. Livingstone, Edinburgh and London.

BUSHKIN F.L., DEMIAN S.D.E. & PIERSON K.K. (1973) Primary reticulum cell sarcoma of the breast *Amer. J. Surg.* **126**, 63–6.

CARR I., HILL A.S., HANCOCK B.W. & NEAL F.E. (1976) Malignant lymphoma in the cervix uteri: histology and ultrastructure. *J. Clin. Path.* **29**, 680–6.

CASTLEMAN B., IVERSON L. & PARDO MENENDEZ V. (1956) Localized mediastinal lymph node hyperplasia resembling thymoma. *Cancer* **9**, 822–30.

CATLIN D. (1948) Lymphosarcoma of the head and neck. *Amer. J. Roentgenol.* **59**, 354–8.

CHORLTON I., KARNEI R.F., KING F.M. & NORRIS H.J. (1974b) Primary malignant reticulendothelial disease involving the vagina, cervix and corpus uteri. *Obstet. Gynaecol.* **44**, 735–48.

CLARK W.H., MIHM M.C., REED R.J. & AINSWORTH A.M. (1974) The lymphocytic infiltrates of the skin. *Hum. Path.* **5**, 25–43.

CLENDENNING W.E., BRECHER G. & VAN SCOTT E.J. (1964) Mycosis fungoides. Relationship to malignant cutaneous reticuloses and the Sézary syndrome. *Arch. Derm. (Chicago)* **89**, 785–92.

COLBY T.V., BURKE J.S. & HOPPE R.T. (1981) Lymph node biopsy in mycosis fungoides. *Cancer* **47**, 351–9.

COLLINS D.H. & PUGH R.C.B. (1964) Classification and frequency of testicular tumours. *Brit. J. Urol.* **36**, 1–11.

COMPAGNO J. & OERTEL J.E. (1980) Malignant lymphoma and other lymphoproliferative disorders of the thyroid gland. A clinicopathological study of 245 cases. *Am. J. Clin. Path.* **74**, 1–11.

COOPER J.A., BROAD A.F. & SALM R. (1974) Primary ovarian lymphoma. *J. Obstet. Gynaecol. Brit. Commonw.* **81**, 571–4.

CORNES J.S., SMITH J.C. & SOUTHWOOD W.F.W. (1961a) Lymphosarcoma in chronic ulcerative colitis. *Brit. J. Surg.* **49**, 50–3.

CORNES J.S., WALLACE M.H. & MORSON B.C. (1961b) Benign lymphomas of the rectum and anal canal: a study of 100 cases. *J. Path. Bact.* **82**, 371–82.

COX M.T. (1964) Malignant lymphoma of the thyroid. *J. Clin. Path.* **17**, 591–601.

CRUIKSHANK A.H. (1965) Benign lymphoepithelial salivary lesion to be distinguished from adenolymphoma. *J. Clin. Path.* **18**, 391–400.

DAVIES J.N.P. (1975) Burkitt's lymphoma. In *Lymphoproliferative disease* (Ed Molander D.W.). Thomas, Springfield.

DAWSON I.M.P., CORNES J.S. & MORSON B.C. (1961) Primary malignant lymphoid tumours of the intestinal tract. Report of 37 cases with a study of factors influencing prognosis. *Brit. J. Surg.* **49**, 80–9.

DE COSSE J.J., BERG J.W., FRACCHIA A.A. & FARROW J.M. (1962) Primary lymphosarcoma of the breast. *Cancer* **15**, 1264–8.

DUTZ W., ASVADI S., DADRI S. & KOHOUT E. (1971) Intestinal lymphoma and sprue: a systematic approach. *Gut* **12**, 804–10.

EAKINS D., FULTON T. & HADDEN D.R. (1964) Reticulum cell sarcoma of the small bowel and steatorrhoea. *Gut* **5**, 315–23.

EDELSON R.C., KIRKPATRICK C.H., SCHEVACH E.M., SCHEM P.S., SMITH R.W., GREEN I. & LUTZNER M. (1974) Preferential cutaneous infiltration by neoplastic thymus derived lymphocytes. Morphologic and functional studies. *Ann. Intern. Med.* **80**, 685–92.

EPSTEIN M.A., ACHONG B.G. & BARR Y.M. (1964) Virus particles in cultured lymphoblasts from Burkitt's lymphoma. *Lancet* **1**, 702–3.

ERKMAN-BALIS B. & RAPPAPORT H. (1974) Cytogenetic studies in mycosis fungoides. *Cancer* **34**, 626–33.

EVANS H.L., WINKELMANN R.K. & BANKS P.M. (1979) Differential diagnosis of malignant and benign cutaneous lymphoid infiltrates. A study of 57 cases in which malignant lymphoma had been diagnosed or suspected in the skin. *Cancer* **44**, 699–717.

FARIS T.D. & SALTZSTEIN S.L. (1964) Gastric lymphoid hyperplasia: a lesion confused with lymphosarcoma. *Cancer* **17**, 207–12.

FEUERMAN E.J. & SANDBANK M. (1972) Lymphomatoid papulosis: an additional case of a new disease. *Arch. Derm.* **105**, 233–5.

FISHER E.R., HORVAT B.L. & WECHSLER H.L. (1972) Ultrastructural features of mycosis fungoides. *Amer. J. Clin. Path.* **58**, 99–110.

FISHER E.R., PALEKAR A.S., PAULSON I.D., GOLINGER R. (1979) Pseudolymphoma of breast. *Cancer* **44**, 258–63.

FOX H. & MORE J.R.S. (1965) Primary malignant lymphoma of the uterus. *J. Clin. Path.* **18**, 723–28.

FREEDMAN S.I. (1971) Malignant lymphomas of the major salivary glands. *Arch. Otolaryngol.* **93**, 123–7.

FREEMAN C., BERG J.W. & CUTLER S.J. (1972) Occurrence and prognosis of extranodal lymphomas. *Cancer* **29**, 252–60.

FRIEDMAN B. & GOLD H. (1968) Ultrastructure of Ewing's sarcoma of bone. *Cancer* **22**, 307–22.

FU Y.S., GABBIANI G., KAYE G.I. & LATTES R. (1975) Malignant soft tissue tumours of probably histiocytic origin (malignant fibrous histiocytomas): general considerations and electron microscopic and tissue culture studies. *Cancer* **35**, 176–98.

GODWIN J.T. (1952) Benign lymphoepithelial lesion of the parotid gland (adenolymphoma, chronic inflammation, lymphoepithelioma, lymphocytic tumour, Mikulicz disease). Report of 11 cases. *Cancer* **5**, 1089–1103.

Gough K.R., Read A.E. & Naish J.M. (1962) Intestinal reticulosis as a complication of idiopathic steatorrhoea. *Gut* **3**, 232–9.

Gowing N.F.C. (1964) Malignant lymphoma of the testis. *Brit. J. Urol.* **36**, 85–94.

Gowing N.F.C. (1976) Malignant lymphoma of the testis. In *Pathology of the Testis*, pp. 334–55 (Ed Pugh R.C.B.). Blackwell Scientific Publications, Oxford.

Guccion J.G. & Enzinger F.M. (1972) Malignant giant cell tumour of soft parts: an analysis of 32 cases. *Cancer* **29**, 1518–29.

Haghighi P. & Nasr K. (1973) Primary upper small intestine lymphoma. (So called Mediterranean lymphoma.) *Pathology Ann.* **8**, 231–55.

Hamlin J.A., Kagan A.R. & Friedman N.B. (1972) Lymphomas of the testicle. *Cancer* **29**, 1352–6.

Hancock B.W. & Crawford B.S. (1982) Inflammatory fibrous histiocytoma. *Brit. J. Plastic Surg.* **35**, 471–3.

Hayes J.A. & Christensen O.E. (1961) Primary adrenal lymphoma. *J. Path. Bact.* **82**, 193–4.

Isaacson P. (1979) Middle East lymphoma and α-chain disease. An immunohistochemical study. *Am. J. Surg. Path.* **3**, 432–41.

Isaacson P. & Wright D.H. (1978) Malignant histiocytosis of the intestine: its relationship to malabsorption and ulcerative jejunitis. *Hum. Path.* **9**, 661–7.

Isaacson P., Wright D.H., Judd M.A. & Mepham B.L. (1979) Primary gastrointestinal lymphomas. A classification of 66 cases. *Cancer* **43**, 1805–19.

Ive F.A., Magnus I.A., Warin R.P. & Wilson Jones R. (1969) Actinic reticuloid: a chronic dermatosis associated with severe photosensitivity and the histological resemblance to lymphoma. *Brit. J. Derm.* **81**, 469–85.

Jessner M. & Kanof N.B. (1953) Lymphocytic infiltration of skin. *Arch. Derm.* **68**, 447–9.

Joseph J.I. & Lattes R. (1966) Gastric lymphosarcoma. Clinicopathologic analysis of 71 cases and its relation to disseminated lymphosarcoma. *Amer. J. Clin. Path.* **45**, 653–69.

Kempson R.L. & Kyriakos M. (1972) Fibroxanthosarcoma of the soft tissues. *Cancer* **29**, 961–76.

Kent T.H. (1964) Malabsorption syndrome with malignant lymphoma. *Arch. Path.* **78**, 97–103.

Kern W.H., Crepeau A.G. & Jones J.C. (1961) Primary Hodgkin's disease of the lung. Report of 4 cases and review of the literature. *Cancer* **14**, 1151–65.

Knowles D.M. & Jakobiec F.A. (1980) Orbital lymphoid neoplasms. A clinicopathologic stydy of 60 patients. *Cancer* **46**, 576–89.

Kyriakos M. & Kempson R.L. (1976) Inflammatory fibrous histiocytoma. *Cancer* **37**, 1584–1606.

Lawler M.R. & Richie R.F. (1967) Reticulum cell sarcoma of the breast. *Cancer* **20**, 1438–46.

Leading Article (1978) Non-endemic Burkitt's lymphoma. *Brit. Med. J.* **1**, 1508.

Lee F.I. & Harry D.S. (1974) Angiosarcoma of the liver in a vinyl chloride worker. *Lancet* **i**, 1316–18.

Lever W.F. & Schaumberg-Lever G. (1975) *Histopathology of the skin*, 5th edn. Lippincott, Philadelphia.

Lin J.J., Farha G.J. & Taylor R.J. (1980) Pseudolymphoma of the breast. *Cancer* **45**, 973–8.

Lutzner M.A., Emerit I., Durepaire R., Flanorin G., Grupper C. & Prunieras N. (1973) Cytogenic, cytophotometric and ultrastructural study of large cerebriform cells of the Sézary syndrome and description of a small-cell variant. *J. Natl. Cancer Inst.* **50**, 1145–62.

Lutzner M.A. & Jordan H.W. (1968) The ultrastructure of an abnormal cell in Sézary's syndrome. *Blood* **31**, 719–26.

Macaulay W.L. (1968) Lymphomatoid papulosis. A continuing self-healing eruption clinically benign, histologically malignant. *Arch. Derm.* **97**, 23–30.

Mach K.W. & Wilgram G.F. (1966) Characteristic histopathology of cutaneous lymphoplasia. (Lymphocytoma.) *Arch. Derm. (Chicago)* **94**, 26–32.

Mackenzie D.M. (1975) Miscellaneous soft tissue sarcomas. In *Recent Advances in Pathology* (ed. Hanson C.V.). Churchill Livingstone, Edinburgh.

MacSween R.N.M., Vetters J.M., Ross S.K., Ferguson J., Johnstone J.M. & Sandison A.T. (1973) Haemangio-endothelial sarcoma of the liver. *J. Path.* **109**, 39–44.

McNelis F. & Pai U.T. (1969) Malignant lymphoma of head and neck. *Laryngoscope* **79**, 1076–87.

Merkow L.P., Frich J.C., Slifkin M., Kyreages C.G. & Pardo M. (1971) Ultrastructure of a fibroxanthosarcoma (malignant fibroxanthoma). *Cancer* **28**, 372–83.

Mihm M.C., Clark W.H. & Reed R.J. (1974) The histiocytic infiltrates of the skin. *Hum. Path.* **5**, 45–54.

Modan B., Shani M., Goldman B. & Modan M. (1969) Nodal and extranodal malignant lymphoma in Israel—an epidemiological study. *Brit. J. Haematol.* **16**, 53–9.

Oberman M.A. (1966) Primary lymphoreticular neoplasms of the breast. *Surg. Gynec. Obstet.* **123**, 1047–51.

Paladugu R.R., Bearman R.M. & Rappaport H. (1980) Malignant lymphoma with primary manifestation in the gonad. *Cancer* **45**, 561–71.

Paradinas F.J. & Harrison K.M. (1974) Visceral lesions in an unusual case of Sézary's syndrome. *Cancer* **33**, 1068–74.

Parker F. & Jackson H. (1939) Primary reticulum cell sarcoma of bone. *Surg. Gyn. Obstet.* **68**, 45–53.

Patey D.H., Thackray A.C. & Keeling D.H. (1965) Malignant disease of the parotid. *Brit. J. Cancer* **19**, 712–37.

Rappaport H., Ramot B., Hulu N. & Park J.K. (1972) The pathology of so-called Mediterranean abdominal lymphoma with malabsorption. *Cancer* **29**, 1502–11.

Rappaport H. & Thomas L.B. (1974) Mycosis fungoides: the pathology of extracutaneous involvement. *Cancer* **34**, 1198–1229.

Rayfield E.J., Nishiyama R.H. & Sisson J.C. (1971) Small cell tumours of the thyroid: a clinicopathological study. *Cancer* **28**, 1023–30.

Rosas-Uribe A., Variakojis D., Molnar Z. & Rappaport H. (1974) Mycosis fungoides: an ultrastructural study. *Cancer* **34**, 634–45.

Saltzstein S.L. (1963) Pulmonary malignant lymphomas and pseudolymphomas: classification, therapy and prognosis. *Cancer* **16**, 928–55.

Saltzstein S.L. (1969) Extranodal malignant lymphomas and pseudolymphomas. *Path. Ann.* **4**, 159–84.

Scheffer E., Meijer C.J.L.M. & Van Vloten W.A. (1980) Dermatopathic lymphadenopathy and lymph node involvement in mycosis fungoides. *Cancer* **45**, 137–48.

Seligman B.R., Rosner F. & Davenport J. (1974) Primary lymphosarcoma of the parotid gland. *Cancer* **33**, 239–43.

Sézary A. & Bouvrain Y. (1938) Erythrodermie avec presence de cellules monstrueuses dans le derme et le sang circulant. *Bull. Soc. Franc. Derm. Syph.* **45**, 254–60.

Sheahan D.G., Martin F., Baginsky S., Mallory G.K. & Zamcher N. (1961) Multiple lymphomatous polyposis of the gastrointestinal tract. *Cancer* **28**, 408–25.

Silber J.S. & Chang C.Y. (1973) Primary lymphoma of kidney. *J. Urol.* **110**, 282–4.

Smithers D.W. (1970) Malignant lymphomas of the thyroid gland. In *Tumours of the Thyroid Gland*, pp. 141–54, (Ed D.W. Smithers). Livingstone, Edinburgh and London.

Soule E.M. & Enriquez P. (1972) Atypical fibrous histiocytoma, malignant fibrous histiocytoma, malignant histiocytoma and epithelioid carcinoma. *Cancer* **30**, 128–43.

Sternberg W.H., Sidransky H. & Ochsner S. (1959) Primary malignant lymphomas of the lung. *Cancer* **12**, 806–19.

Stransky G.C., Acosta A.A., Kaplan A.L. & Friedman J.A. (1973) Reticulum cell sarcoma of the cervix. *Obstet. Gynecol.* **41**, 183–7.

Terz J.J. & Farr M.W. (1969) Primary lymphosarcoma of the tonsil. *Surgery* **65**, 772–6.

Tewfik H.H., Platz C.E., Corder M.P., Panther S.K. & Blodi F.C. (1979) A clinicopathologic study of orbital and adnexal non-Hodgkin's lymphoma. *Cancer* **44**, 1022–28.

Thorbjarnson B., Beal J.M. & Peace J.M. (1956) Primary malignant lymphoid tumours of the stomach. *Cancer* **9**, 712–17.

Titus J.L., Harrison E.G., Clagett O.T., Anderson M.W. & Knaff L.J. (1962) Xanthomatous and inflammatory pseudotumours of the lung. *Cancer* **15**, 522–38.

Tomich C.E. & Schafer W.G. (1975) Lymphoproliferative disease of the hard palate: a clinicopathologic entity. *Oral Surg.* **39**, 754–68.

Turner R.R., Colby T.V. & Mackintosh F.R. (1981) Testicular lymphomas: a clinicopathologic study of 35 cases. *Cancer* **48**, 2095–102.

van der Werf-Messing B. (1978) Radiotherapy of extranodal non-Hodgkin's lymphoma: In "Recent results in cancer research: Lymphoid neoplasia II," pp. 111–28 (Ed. Mathe G., Seligmann M. & Tubiana M.). Springer-Verlag, Berlin.

Walt A.J., Woolner L.B. & Black B.N. (1957) Primary malignant lymphoma of the thyroid. *Cancer* **10**, 663–77.

Wang C.C., Scully R.E. & Leadbetter W.F. (1969) Primary malignant lymphoma of the urinary bladder. *Cancer* **24**, 772–6.

Weaver D.K. & Batsakis J.G. (1964) Primary lymphomas of the small intestine. *Amer. J. Gastroent.* **42**, 620–5.

Webb H.E., Harrison E.G., Masson J.K. & Remin W.H. (1962) Solitary extramedullary myeloma (plasmacytoma) of the upper part of the respiratory tract and oropharynx. *Cancer* **15**, 1142–55.

World Health Organisation Bulletin (1969) Histopathological definition of Burkitt's tumour. **40**, 601–7.

Whitehead R. (1968) Primary lymphadenopathy complicating idiopathic steatorrhoea. *Gut* **9**, 569–75.

Winkelmann R.K. & Linman J.W. (1973) Erythroderma with atypical lymphocytes (Sézary syndrome). *Amer. J. Med.* **55**, 192–8.

Woringer F. & Kwiatowski S.L. (1938) L'histiocytome de la peau. *Ann. Derm. Syph.* **3**, 998.

Yoshida Y. (1970) Reticulum cell sarcoma of the breast. Case report and review of the Japanese literature. *Cancer* **26**, 94–9.

Zackheim H.S. (1981) Cutaneous T-cell lymphomas. *Arch. Dermatol.* **117**, 295–304.

Ziegler J.L. (1981) Burkitt's lymphoma. *N. Eng. J. Med.* **305**, 735–44.

Zucker-Franklin D., Melton J.W. & Quagliata F. (1974) Ultrastructural, immunologic and functional studies on Sézary cells: a neoplastic variant of thymus-derived (T) lymphocytes. *Proc. Natl. Acad. Sci. USA*, **71**, 1877–81.

Chapter 7

Central nervous involvement in lymphoma and leukaemia

PRIMARY LYMPHOMA OF THE BRAIN

The macrophages of the brain are known as microglial cells, and tumours arising from these cells are known as microgliomata, cerebral reticulum cell sarcomas (Schaumberg *et al.* 1972; Russell and Rubinstein 1976) or more recently as primary intracranial malignant lymphomas. These tumours account for between 0.3 and 1.5% of all intracranial neoplasms (Zimmerman 1975; Jellinger and Radaszkiewicz 1976) and they represent about 0.8% of all lymphomas from all sites (Henry *et al.* 1974).

Characteristically these tumours are often widely disseminated in the brain with multiple small foci, often microscopic in size, and the tumour cells form dense perivascular cuffs and infiltrate the adjacent cerebral tissues (Figs 7.1 and 7.2).

The histological pattern of primary lymphoma of the nervous system is similar to that seen in lymphomas arising in other sites, and a variety of histological patterns have been described. For instance, in a series of 83 cases studied by Henry *et al.* (1974) 60% were classified as lymphocytic, 28% as Hodgkin's disease, and 13% as histiocytic; whereas Jellinger *et al.* (1975) divided them into three types, the immunoblastoma (59%), lymphoplasmacytoid immunocytoma (28%) and lymphoblastic lymphoma (13%). Nodular or follicular lymphomatous patterns are not seen.

Primary lymphomas of the nervous system resemble extracerebral lymphomas ultrastructurally (Horvath *et al.* 1969; Johnson 1975) and immunologically (Taylor *et al.* 1978). The latter authors showed that most of these tumours are derived from B-lymphocytes. Histologically they may contain predominantly argyrophilic cells with variable numbers of non-argyrophilic cells; the latter resemble cells seen in histiocytic lymphomas, found outside the nervous system. Ultrastructural studies show morphological changes representing various stages in the transformation of one single cell population, showing neither the cytochemical nor the ultrastructural features of monocytes or histiocytes, but resembling transformed lymphocytes or immunoblasts (Henry 1975) (Figs 7.3 and 7.4). All tumours show some

evidence of transformation towards cells with rough endoplasmic reticulum. Immunological studies also show some evidence of intracellular immunoglobulin production—monoclonal in the majority of cases (Taylor *et al.* 1978). Two out of six cases described by Jellinger *et al.* (1979) consisted mainly of lymphocytic blast cells rich in polyribosomes and poor in rough endoplasmic reticulum, and the others showed larger proportions of cells with prominent rough endoplasmic reticulum suggesting some plasmablastic differentiation.

There has been a marked increase in the number of cases of primary lymphoma of the nervous system since the widespread use of immunosuppressive therapy, particularly in the case of the recipients of renal transplants (Schneck and Penn 1971), about 5% of whom develop some form of malignant tumour. The risk of developing malignant lymphoma is approximately 350 times greater than expected in these patients (Hoover and Fraumeni 1973), and out of a series of 25 transplant patients with lymphoma, 52% had disease localised in the brain, as compared with an incidence of 1% in lymphoma patients in general.

There is also an increased incidence of primary lymphomas of the nervous system in patients suffering from other forms of disturbed immunological mechanisms such as Wiscott–Aldrich syndrome (Brand and Marinkovich 1969), the various forms of hyperglobulinaemia, including Waldenström's macroglobulinaemia (Gundersson *et al.* 1971) and those with a complete lack of IgA (Gregory and Hughes 1973); Ulrich and Wuthrich (1974) reported a case of multifocal malignant lymphoma of the central nervous system, also involving the lungs, liver, kidneys and lymph nodes in a patient who had multiple sclerosis treated with azathioprine for fifteen months.

Primary lymphoma of the nervous system may present at any age but usually appears in the sixth decade and affects both sexes equally. Onset is usually fairly rapid and patients may present with focal neurological deficits, seizures, signs of increased intracranial pressure, dementia, psychiatric disturbances, uveitis, or peripheral neuropathy. Uveitis may antedate the neurological symptoms by up to eight years (Neault *et al.* 1972), and peripheral neuropathy may appear in

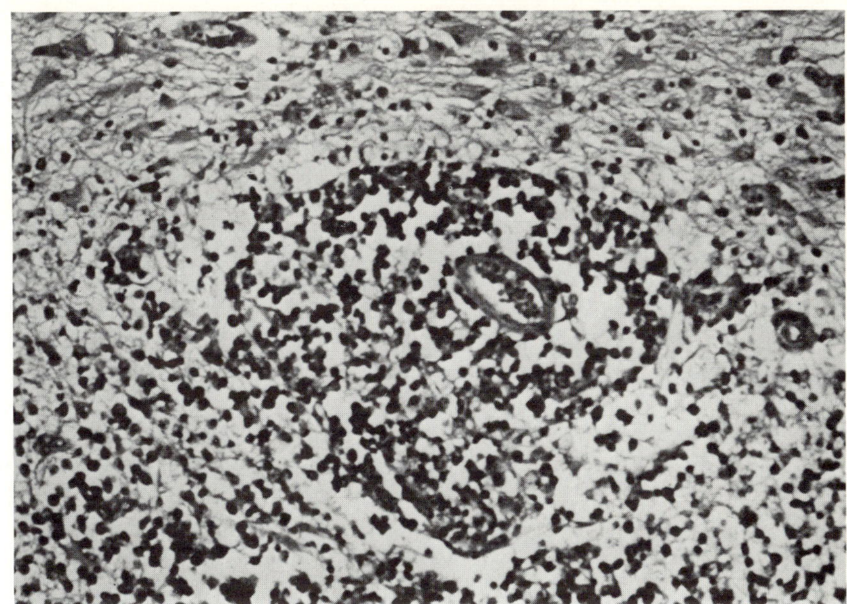

Fig. 7.1. Primary cerebral malignant lymphoma showing a perivascular cuff of tumour cells infiltrating in the adjacent cerebral tissues. × 180.

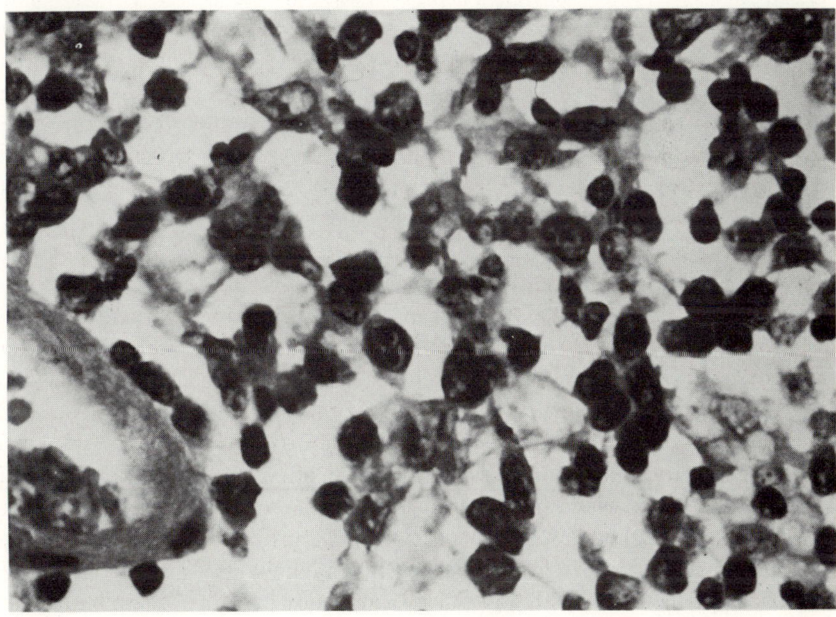

Fig. 7.2. Primary cerebral malignant lymphoma showing cuff of tumour cells around a small intracerebral blood vessel. × 840.

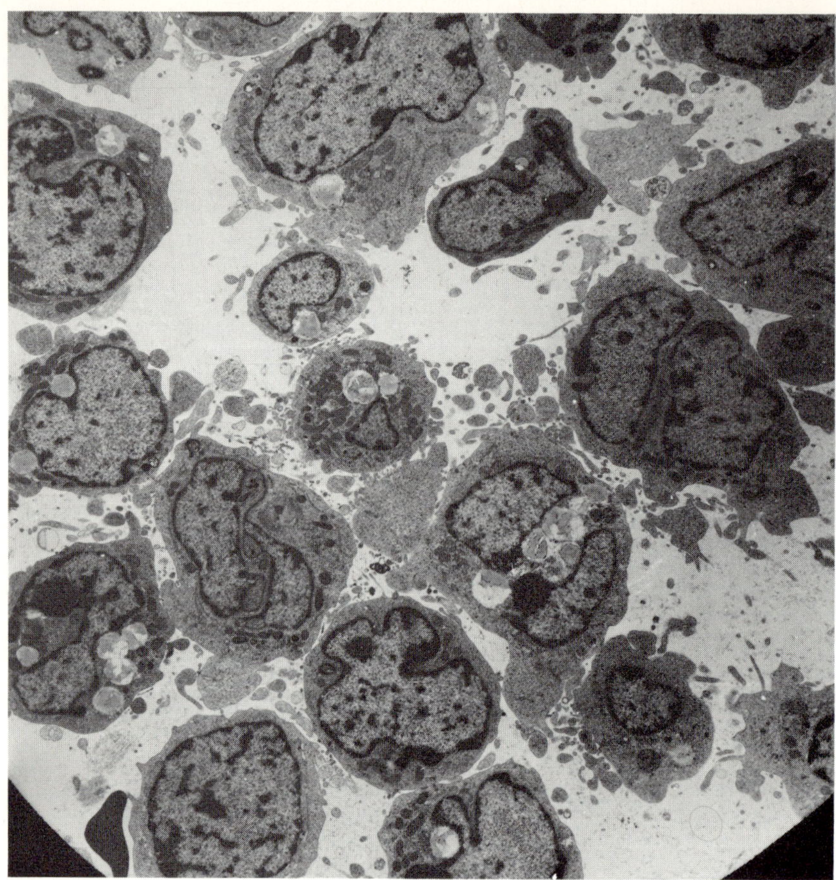

Fig. 7.3. Electronmicrograph of primary cerebral malignant lymphoma. These cells resemble transformed lymphocytes with small amounts of rough endoplasmic reticulum. ×4800.

the absence of direct nerve invasion; this may closely simulate acute infectious polyneuritis (Blanchard 1962; Allison and Gordon 1955).

Multifocal lesions occur in up to almost half of the cases and most lesions are found within the cerebral hemispheres, but other areas of the brain, including the brainstem and cerebellum, may be involved; the spinal cord is rarely affected.

None of the usual routine investigative procedures such as arteriograms, brain scans, electroencephalograms, or compu-terised axial tomography, are diagnostic, but may be helpful in localising lesions. In the presence of multifocal abnormali-ties, particularly with homogeneous contrast enhancement on CAT scanning, the possibility of primary lymphoma of the nervous system should always be considered (Fig. 7.5). Cytological examination of the cerebrospinal fluid can also be helpful and may show the presence of neoplastic cells in up to 30% of cases; the cerebrospinal fluid may also show increased protein, increased cell content and sometimes a reduced glucose concentration.

NON-PRIMARY LYMPHOMAS OF THE CNS

Lymphomas may involve the nervous system in a number of ways. Neurological complications may be a result of either compression or direct invasion, or of remote effects such as progressive multifocal leuco-encephalopathy, peripheral neuropathy, polymyositis, encephalomyelopathy, cerebellar cortical degeneration, or as a result of opportunistic infec-tions. The incidence of malignant lymphoma in tumours of the central nervous system appears to be about 3% and slightly under half of these are primary within the brain (Zimmerman 1975).

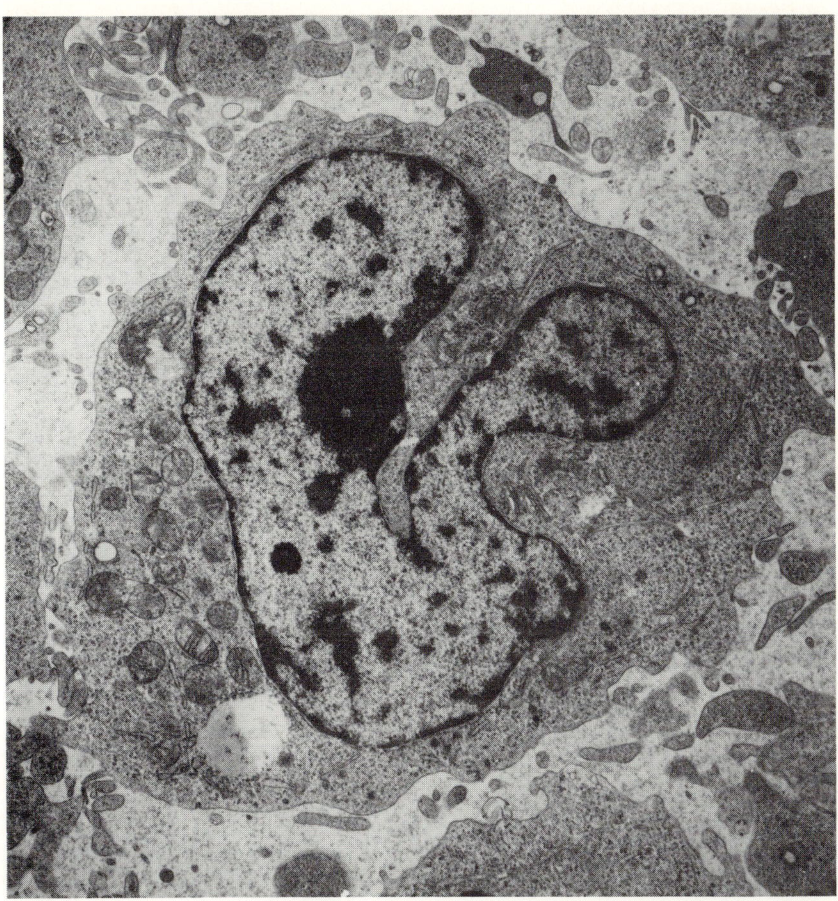

Fig. 7.4. Electronmicrograph of a single cell from a primary cerebral lymphoma. The nucleus has a deep cleft and the cytoplasm contains small amounts of rough endoplasmic reticulum. × 12 000.

Neurological syndromes complicating lymphoma fall into three main groups:

1   acute or subacute spinal cord compression
2   cranial nerve involvement
3   meningeal invasion.

Intracerebral deposits are rare.

Spinal cord involvement is the commonest neurological abnormality associated with the reticuloses (Hutchinson *et al.* 1958) and compression of the cord occurs mostly in the thoracic and lumbar regions (Friedman *et al.* 1976). Epidural lymphoma is rarely a manifestation of localised extranodal disease and usually represents a generalised and progressive disease. Neurological problems usually result from direct compression of the spinal cord or its nerve roots, but vertebral destruction and collapse or interruption of the blood supply to the cord may also be involved. Lymphomatous tissue may either spread through the intervertebral foramina from paraspinal masses, or may extend directly from diseased vertebrae. The tumour may extend around the outside of the cord and even encircle it completely, but the dura mater usually prevents invasion of the cord itself. Usually, vertebral X-rays are normal and abnormal lymphograms are only seen in some cases (Friedman *et al.* 1976).

The usual presenting symptoms include pain, which may or may not be radicular in type, paraesthesiae, sensory abnormalities, weakness or paralysis of the legs, or of all four limbs in some cases, and at a later stage there may be involvement of bowel and bladder function. Motor symptoms usually precede sensory symptoms and paraplegia may be flaccid or spastic; the paraplegia is always associated with extensor plantar responses. Back pain associated with localised tenderness precedes the onset of spinal cord symptoms in most patients, by a few months in most cases. The average interval between the onset of back pain and diagnosis of

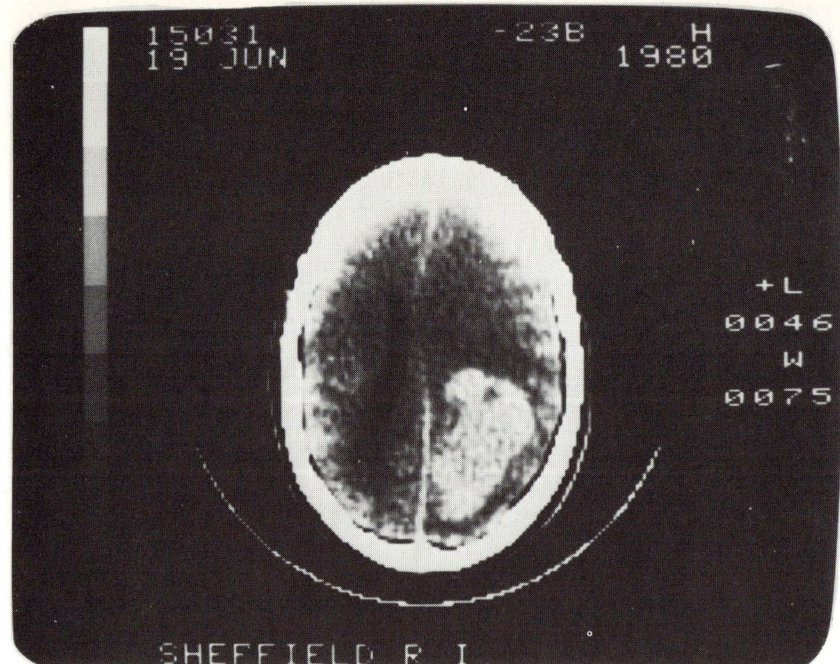

Fig. 7.5. Primary cerebral malignant lymphoma—CAT scan showing homogenous contrast enhancement in a lesion in the right parietal lobe.

epidural disease was just over seven months in a series reported by Mullins *et al.* (1971). It is, however, important to remember that cord compression may be the first manifestation of the disease in some cases, and that the development of a cord lesion indicates a poor prognosis. Myelography is needed to detect the presence of an extradural mass and the cerebrospinal fluid should be examined cytologically.

Intracranial lymphoma appears to be rare (Currie and Henson 1971; John and Nabarro 1955) and usually signifies a poor prognosis (Gendelman *et al.* 1969; Skarin *et al.* 1977). Survival following the development of meningeal lymphoma is usually less than eight months from the time of diagnosis. Intracranial deposits are commoner in association with histiocytic lymphoma, and orbital deposits appear to be more commonly associated with lymphocytic lymphoma. Intracranial deposits are rarely seen in lymphocytic lymphoma unless leukaemia has supervened (John and Nabarro 1955). There appears to have been some increase in the incidence of meningeal infiltration in recent years; for instance Sparling *et al.* (1947) reported one case of meningeal lymphoma in 118 autopsies, whereas more recently Law *et al.* (1975) reported an incidence of approximately 11%. Similarly, Bunn *et al.* (1976) reported an incidence of 25–30% of meningeal involvement following chemotherapy in patients with Stage 3

or 4 diffuse histiocytic and diffuse undifferentitated lymphoma. This may partly be due to the prolonged survival associated with chemotherapy.

Intracranial involvement in Hodgkin's disease usually occurs as a result of direct extension through the base of the skull from involved cervical lymph nodes and tumour may be found extradurally, within the dura, invading the underlying brain, or intracerebrally (Buckley and Warwick 1968). On rare occasions Hodgkin's disease of the skull bones has been known to spread to form an intracranial mass.

Three cases of primary cerebral Hodgkin's disease with no evidence of Hodgkin's disease elsewhere were reported by Kinney and Adams (1943) and by Sparling *et al.* (1947).

Intracranial Hodgkin's disease is much rarer than spinal extradural deposits; before 1955 only twelve cases had been reported in the literature (John and Nabarro 1955) and only eight of these had been confirmed at postmortem. Out of a series of 125 cases of Hodgkin's disease from their own records, they found only one patient with unequivocal evidence of intracranial deposits.

Non-Hodgkin's lymphoma may diffusely infiltrate the meninges (Figs 7.6 and 7.7) and cranial nerve roots, there may be disseminated foci of cellular infiltration, the tumour may extend from adjacent skull bones, or there may be widespread

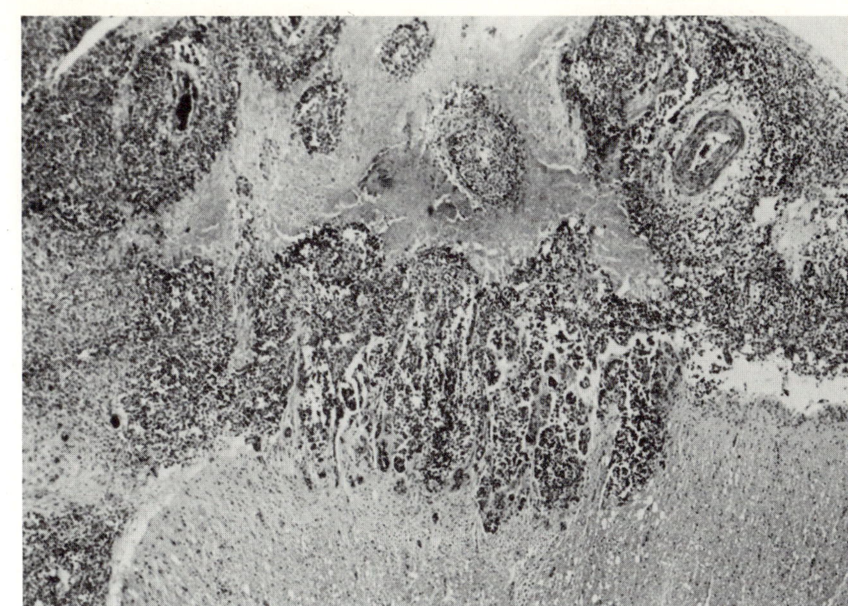

Fig. 7.6. Malignant lymphoma—lymphocytic. Section of spinal cord showing a thick cuff of tumour cells within the meninges. Note columns of tumour cells infiltrating the superficial aspect of the spinal cord. In this particular case the lymphoma appeared to be confined to the region of the cauda equina and lower lumbar region, and no evidence of lymphoma was found elsewhere in the body at post mortem. ×80.

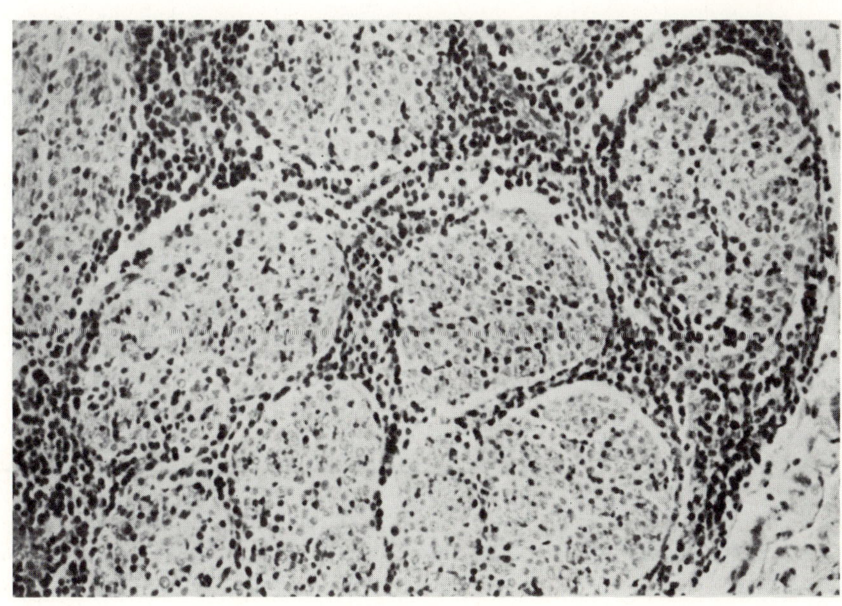

Fig. 7.7. Malignant lymphoma—lymphocytic. Section of spinal nerve root showing diffuse infiltration by lymphoma cells. ×180.

intracerebral deposits. Almost all cases of lymphomatous meningitis are found in patients with diffuse non-Hodgkin's lymphoma (Griffin *et al.* 1971; Skarin *et al.* 1977). Lymphoblastic lymphoma, diffuse histiocytic lymphoma, diffuse undifferentiated lymphoma, and diffuse lymphocytic poorly-differentiated lymphoma have a high incidence of meningeal disease (Nathwani *et al.* 1976). There appears to be a very high correlation between the presence of bone marrow disease and leptomeningeal lymphoma.

A wide variety of neurological abnormalities is encountered, including headaches, papilloedema, cranial nerve palsies, neck stiffness, seizures, paraesthesiae, radicular pain, weakness and mental abnormalities. Mental changes vary from a moderate degree of depression to a rapidly developing dementia (which is usually profound). In the late stages the patient may sink into coma. Mental changes are often not associated with localising neurological signs, particularly in the early stages.

A variety of changes have been described in the retina including papilloedema, optic atrophy and retinal haemorrhages, and it is important to emphasise that retinal haemorrhages and papilloedema can be found in association with Hodgkin's disease in the absence of intracranial deposits and even in the absence of raised intracranial pressure (Hutchinson *et al.* 1958).

Abnormalities may be found in the cerebrospinal fluid, including an increased protein content, increased white cell count, and decreased glucose concentration. The absence of neoplastic cells in the cerebrospinal fluid does not exclude the diagnosis; eight out of thirteen patients with lymphomatous meningitis reported by Billingham *et al.* (1975) were undetected by routine CSF cytological examination.

The incidence of non-metastatic neurological abnormalities in the reticuloses is about 2% (Currie *et al.* 1970). Patients with lymphomas often have reduced immunological function due to the disease itself, or due to treatment by cytotoxic drugs, corticosteroids and radiotherapy. Patients may have lymphopenia, neutropenia, monocytopenia, abnormalities of leucocyte function, abnormalities of chemotaxis, opsonisation, and reduced cell-mediated immune mechanisms. A variety of paraneoplastic syndromes have been described including progressive multifocal leuco-encephalopathy, peripheral neuropathy (Fig. 7.8) and polymyositis. As in the case of other malignancies, myasthenia gravis may occasionally complicate lymphoma. Walton *et al.* (1968) described a case of subacute poliomyelitis associated with Hodgkin's disease and in this case electronmicroscopical examination of tissues taken at postmortem showed virus-like particles.

Any virus which can cause a meningoencephalitis may result in infection in lymphoma, but herpes and measles are the most common. An interesting feature is that a patient who recovers from a severe virus complication in the course of lymphoma may go into remission (Bluming and Ziegler 1971; Gross 1971) and this has led to a number of attempts to treat

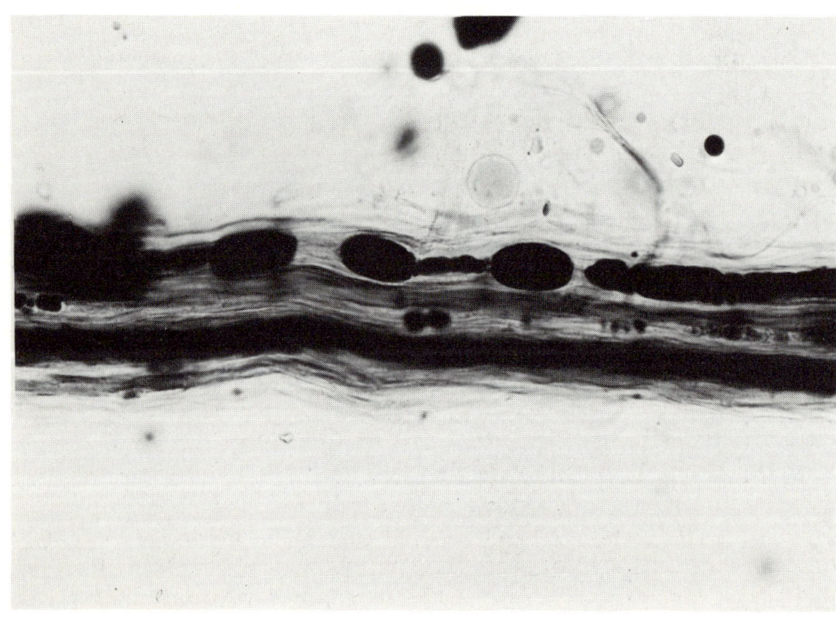

Fig. 7.8. Hodgkin's disease. Longitudinal section of sural nerve showing active demyelination of nerve fibres. Teased nerve fibre preparations stained with osmium tetroxide. ×450.

malignant disease with viruses (Webb *et al.* 1975). Polyneuritis, in association with lymphomas, is usually predominantly sensory (Denny-Brown 1948); histologically there is infiltration of the dorsal root ganglia with lymphocytes and histiocytes with variable degrees of neuronal loss and atrophy. There may be some hyperplasia of Schwann cells and in chronic cases areas of fibrosis are seen. Peripheral neuropathy may occur in the presence of encephalopathy or myelopathy.

Infections of the nervous system may be due to organisms other than viruses. Patients with lymphoma, leukaemia or tumours of the head and spine account for about 80% of all CNS infections in neoplastic disease (Chernick *et al.* 1973 and 1977); in their series the incidence of CNS infection in lymphoma admissions was 0.97%, in leukaemic admissions 1.3%, in patients with tumours of the head and spine 0.53%, and in patients with other tumours 0.03%. In many cases the diagnosis is not made until after death; this is especially true of fungal infections. Bacterial infections account for about 57% (*Listeria monocytogenes*, *Staphylococcus aureus*, *Pseudomonas aeruginosa*, *Streptococcus pneumoniae*, *Streptococcus pyogenes*, *Escherichia coli*, *Klebsiella* species, *Nocardia* species), fungi account for 34% (*Aspergillus* species, *Candida* species, *Cryptococcus neoformans*, *Mucor* species), viruses account for 6% (*Herpes zoster* and *Herpes simplex*), and parasites account for about 3% (*Toxoplasma gondii*) (Gaya 1979). Organisms causing cerebral abscesses are also different from those seen in the general population; Gram-negative bacilli, *Aspergillus* species and *Phycomycetes* species are common (Chernick *et al.* 1973), whereas staphylococci, streptococci, and anaerobic organisms are rarely encountered.

Haemorrhage may of course occur in any of the reticuloses and this is usually due to thrombocytopenia.

Damage may occur to the nervous system as a result of cytotoxic drugs or irradiation. The most common abnormalities are radiation myelitis, neuropathy induced by vincristine, and methotrexate leuco-encephalopathy.

TREATMENT OF CNS LYMPHOMA

Few cytotoxic drugs have the capacity to cross the blood–brain barrier but fortunately localised lymphoma deposits in the CNS respond well to radiotherapy. Co-existent systemic disease must be treated with appropriate chemotherapy (see Chapter 13). More diffuse CNS involvement, e.g. meningeal infiltration, can be treated by irradiation but this is best combined with intrathecal and probably systemic chemotherapy.

The problem of CNS prophylaxis in malignant lymphoma is controversial. CNS lymphoma usually co-exists with non-controlled systemic disease; prophylaxis would therefore only be successful in patients in systemic remission. Nevertheless there may be a small group of patients, e.g. children, or those successfully treated patients with diffuse as opposed to nodular histologic appearances and bone marrow involvement, who should be considered for CNS prophylaxis (Young *et al.* 1979) with its associated significant toxicity. Examination of the CSF is an important preliminary staging procedure at presentation in such patients.

BURKITT'S LYMPHOMA

Burkitt's lymphoma is described in Chapter 6. In over half the cases where the lesions are disseminated the central nervous system is involved and it may be associated with paraplegia. Out of seventy-seven patients described by Ziegler *et al.* (1970) 46% presented or developed evidence of central nervous system involvement, including paraplegia, cranial neuropathy, altered levels of consciousness, and a malignant pleocytosis of the cerebrospinal fluid; 31% had neurological signs or symptoms at the time of presentation and almost half of these presented with spinal cord compression. As well as showing evidence of spinal cord compression, pathologically there may also be ischaemic changes and areas of demyelination on microscopic examination of the spinal cord. Tumour sometimes infiltrates the meninges and cranial nerve palsies are commonly seen. Ziegler *et al.* (1970) found that cranial nerve palsies were the commonest neurological complication after initial presentation, the third, fifth, sixth, seventh, ninth and twelfth cranial nerves being commonly affected. Patients with facial tumours were most likely to develop cranial nerve palsies; these usually result from a tumour spreading through the skull bones or foramina. The tumour may also extend from vertebral bodies into the extradural space, or paravertebral tumours may extend through the neural foramina.

Histologically, the pattern is that of an expanding nodular mass of undifferentiated lymphoreticular cells, best identified as large lymphocytes, 20 μm or more in diameter. The nuclei are best seen in smears as having finely stippled chromatin. There is marked cytoplasmic basophilia and pyroninophilia; Sudanophilic inclusions are seen in appropriately stained smears. The tissue contains numerous large non-neoplastic macrophages, variously loaded with cytoplasmic debris producing the 'starry sky' appearances.

LEUKAEMIA

The incidence of meningeal complications in childhood leukaemia rose about 10-fold during the period 1947–60 (Evans and Craig 1964), and by the early 1970s more than 50% of children with lymphoblastic leukaemia had evidence of central nervous system involvement (Evans *et al.* 1970; Price and Johnson 1973). During the early 1960s chemotherapy began to result in longer survival and until recently prophylactic nervous system therapy was not given. Once signs of CNS involvement had become manifest, very few were cured.

The rising incidence of meningeal complications prompted the use of a variety of prophylactic regimes including cranio-spinal irradiation and intrathecal chemotherapeutic agents.

The increased incidence of neurological complications associated with prolonged survival is seen in acute non-lymphoblastic leukaemias as well as acute lymphoblastic leukaemia. Complications occur within the nervous system as a result of several mechanisms including infiltration with leukaemic cells, haemorrhage, electrolytic disturbances, impaired cerebral circulation due to leucostasis, infection, and drug or irradiation therapy damage.

Leukaemic cells enter the nervous system mainly as a result of haematogenous spread. The cells first appear in the walls of veins and then migrate through the walls into the adjacent cerebral tissues (Fig. 7.9). In some cases the vessel wall may actually break down and release cells or cells may be released as a result of thrombocytopenic petechial haemorrhages or haemorrhages in relationship to intravascular coagulation (Figs 7.10 and 7.11). There may also be some direct invasion from the overlying meninges; invasion of the arachnoidal trabeculae results in their destruction and release of cells into the cerebrospinal fluid. In the early stages leukaemic cells are almost entirely restricted to the surface meninges and, even in the presence of very heavy surface infiltrates, the pia-glial membrane may prevent significant neural invasion (Fig. 7.12). Price and Johnson (1973) showed that infiltration of the deeper cerebral tissues occurs in about 15% of children with leukaemia, who die in relapse.

Leukaemic infiltrates may be found in any part of the nervous system and may be localised or diffuse (Figs 7.12 and 7.13). Lesions are usually diffuse within the overlying meninges and are often more localised within the deeper cerebral tissues. Localised lesions may, however, occur outside, within or beneath the dura mater. In some cases meningeal involvement may be so diffuse as to form a thick

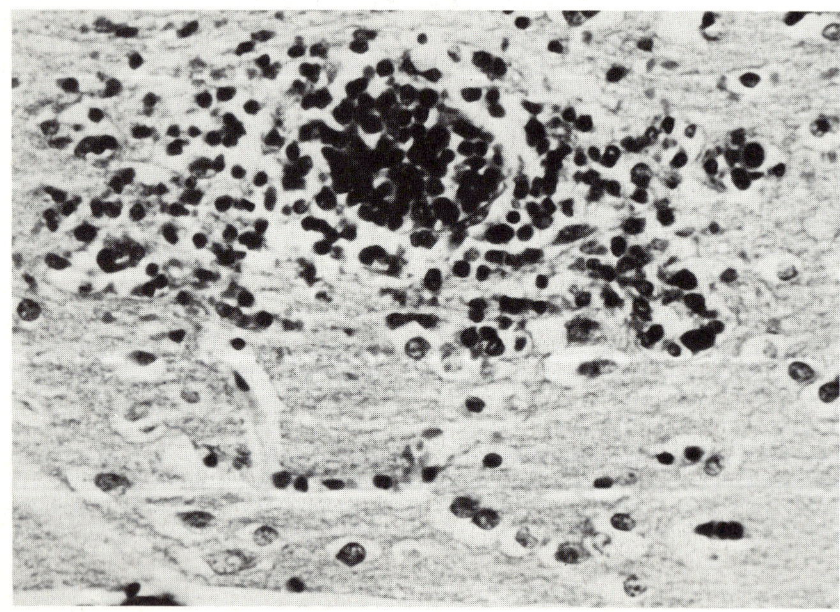

Fig. 7.9. Acute myeloid leukaemia showing infiltation of cerebral tissues adjacent to a small penetrating blood vessel. × 450.

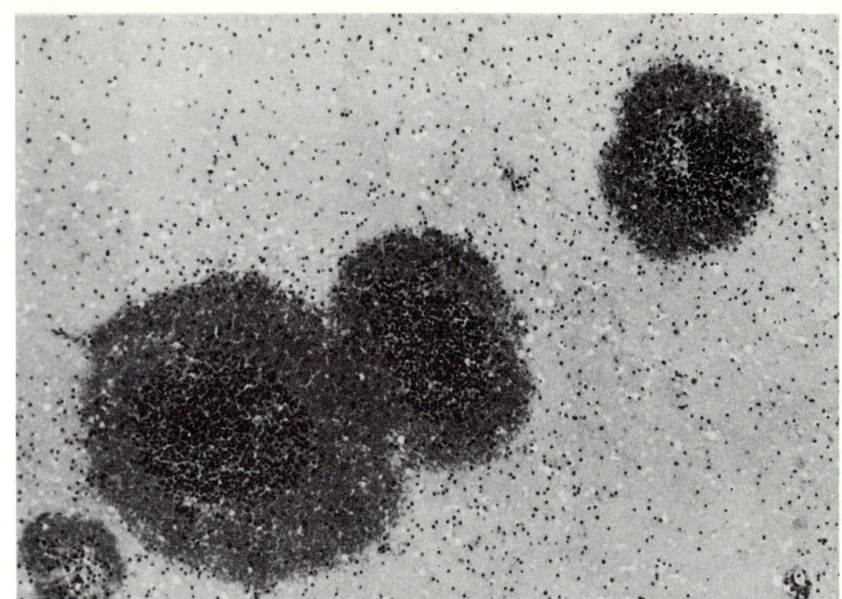

Fig. 7.10. Section of cerebral white matter showing petechial haemorrhages within which there are large numbers of leukaemic cells. × 180.

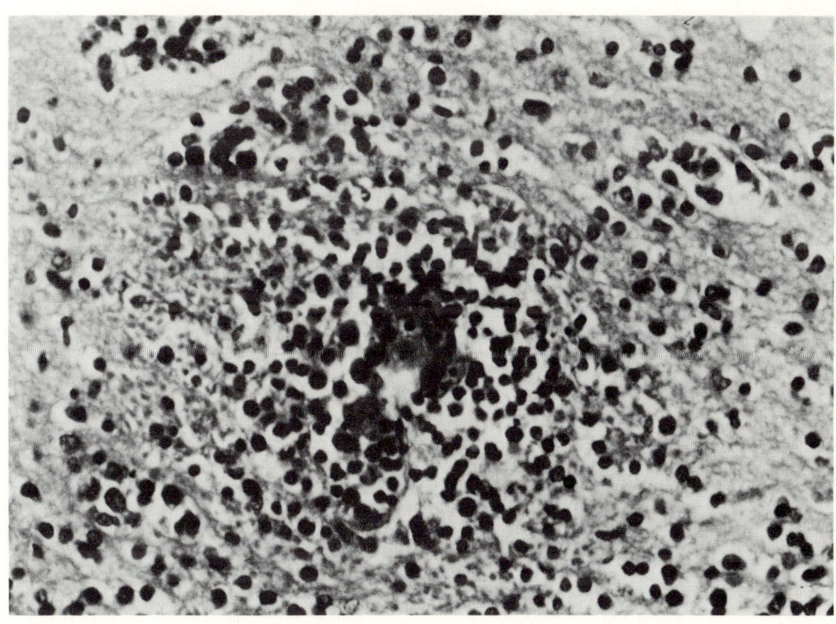

Fig. 7.11. Chronic granulocytic leukaemia. An area of infiltration by leukaemic cells is seen adjacent to a small blood vessel plugged with fibrin. Disseminated intravascular coagulation is sometimes seen in leukaemia and this can result in ischaemia of vessel walls with breakdown and release of leukaemic cells. × 450.

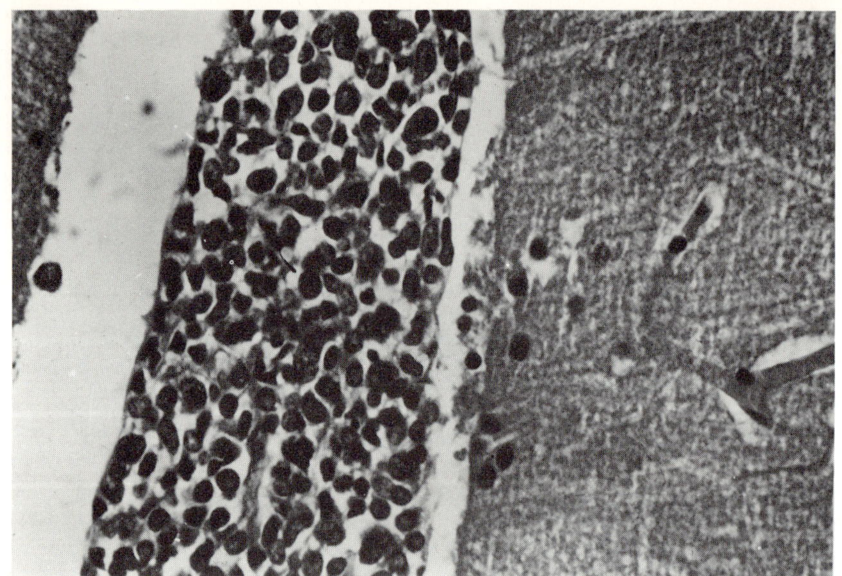

Fig. 7.12. Acute myeloid leukaemia showing heavy infiltrate of leukaemic cells within the subarachnoid space. This case showed diffuse involvement of the meninges but no evidence of invasion of cerebral tissues. ×640.

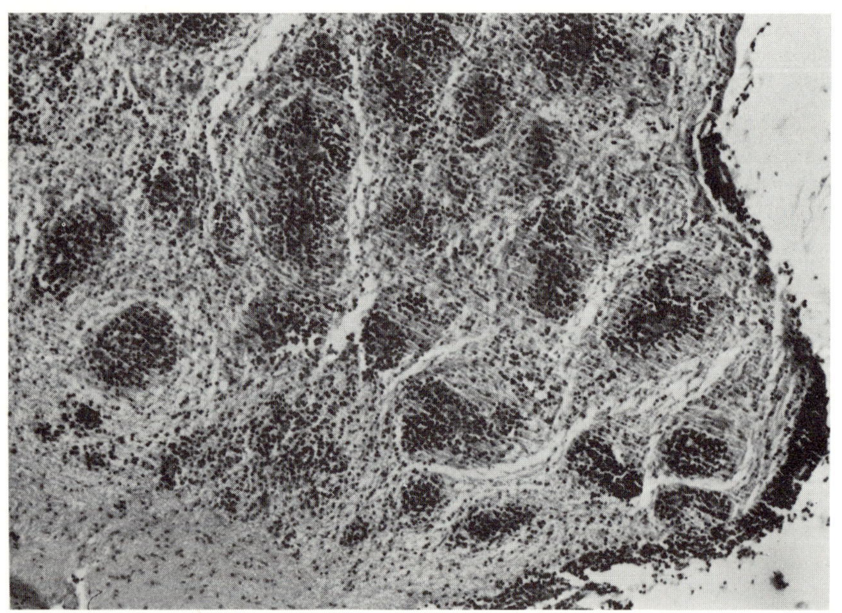

Fig. 7.13. Acute lymphoblastic leukaemia. Section of optic nerve showing numerous foci of infiltration by tumour cells. In this case leukaemic cells were localised to the region of the hypothalamus and optic nerves. ×180.

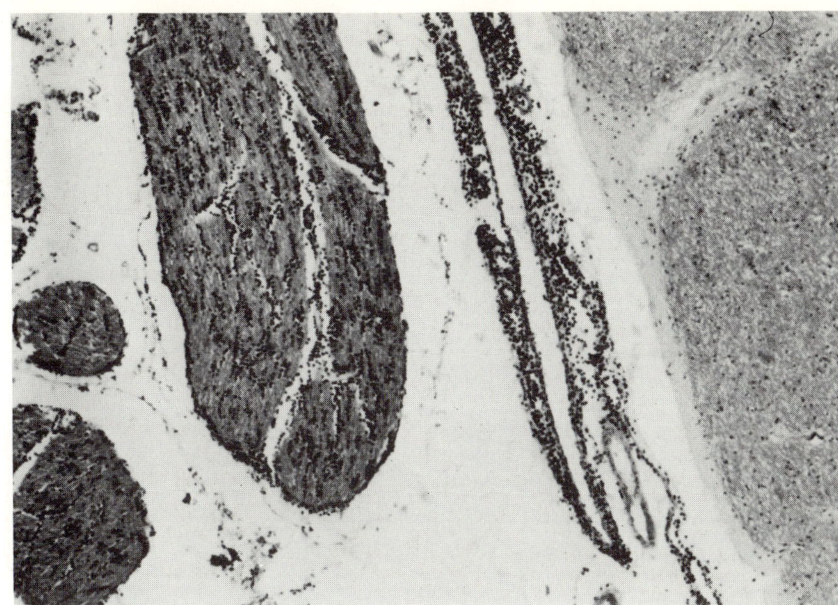

Fig. 7.14. Acute lymphoblastic leukaemia showing heavy infiltration of meninges and brain stem nerve roots. ×80.

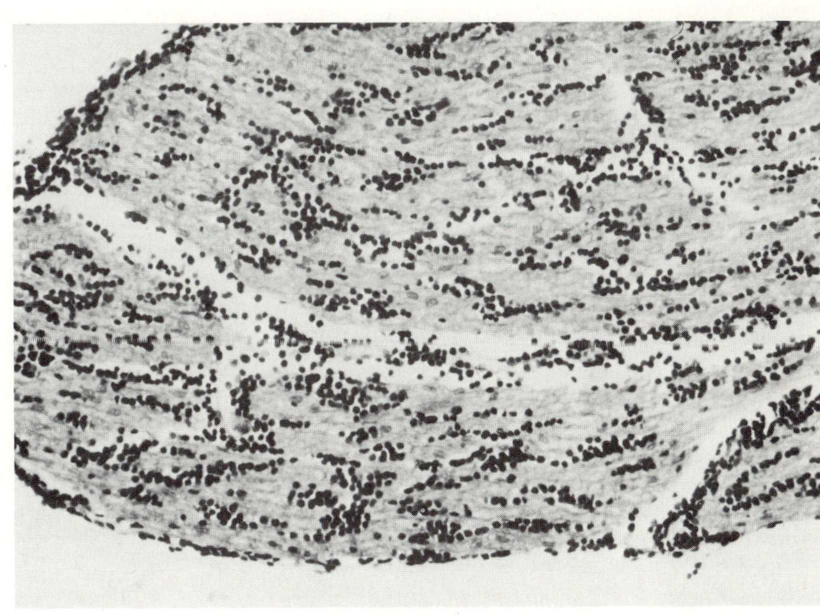

Fig. 7.15. Acute lymphoblastic leukaemia showing diffuse infiltration of nerve without destruction of axons. There were no clinical signs or symptoms relating to involvement of this nerve. ×300.

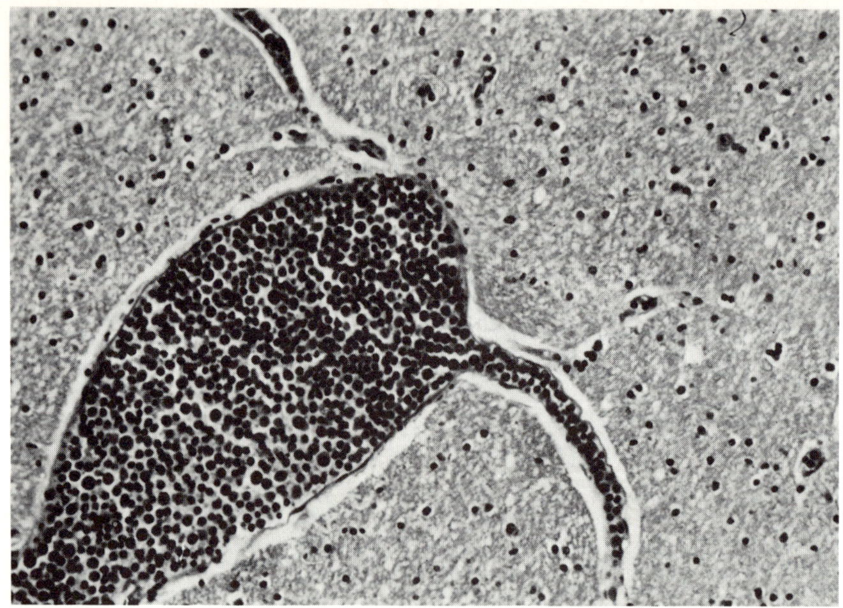

Fig. 7.16. Chronic myeloid leukaemia associated with the cellular hyperviscosity syndrome. Note that the blood vessel is almost entirely filled with leukaemic cells. ×450.

cuff over the surface of the brain, the brainstem, the cranial nerves, the spinal cord and peripheral nerve roots. This may result in blockage of the cerebrospinal fluid flow pathways, resulting in an obstructive form of hydrocephalus, or they may obstruct the re-absorptive pathways of the arachnoidal granulations, resulting in communicating hydrocephalus. It is important to realise that a considerable degree of infiltration of cranial nerves may occur without neurological abnormalities, since cells tend to infiltrate between nerve fibres without actually destroying myelin or axons (Figs 7.14 and 7.15); sometimes ischaemic lesions are produced as a result of pressure on feeding vessels (Price 1975).

It may be that some spread into the nervous system occurs through lymphatics. Graham-Pole and Willoughby (1975) showed that there were lymphatic connections with parts of the brain and that some cerebrospinal fluid is re-absorbed into the lymphatic pathways. West *et al.* (1972) also showed a significant association between involvement of lymphoid tissues elsewhere, including lymph nodes, spleen, and thymus gland, and involvement of the nervous system.

A wide variety of symptoms are seen in meningeal leukaemia, including nausea, vomiting, lethargy, irritability and headache, cranial or spinal nerve abnormalities, visual disturbances, convulsions, hemiplegia, speech, auditory or visual disturbances, or abnormalities of hypothalamic and pituitary function. The picture may be very similar to that of an infective meningitis; the diagnosis may be confirmed by examining the cerebrospinal fluid; leukaemic cells are present in about 90% of cases, but it is important to remember that the cerebrospinal fluid may be entirely normal. Sometimes the pleocytosis is associated with reduced sugar content and an elevated protein. The cerebrospinal fluid pressure is raised in the majority of cases, and there may be a 'dry tap' on lumbar puncture.

Direct invasion of the nervous system may occur in the absence of clinical signs and symptoms and the symptoms when present obviously vary considerably in relationship to the degree and site of involvement. The second, third, sixth, seventh and eighth cranial nerves are the commonest involved, although any may be affected. Lilleyman *et al.* (1979) described several cases of facial nerve involvement in acute lymphoblastic leukaemia of T cell type, and Davies-Jones *et al.* (1980) mentioned three cases of acute leukaemia with mental nerve involvement, producing sensory impairment of the lower lip and painless ulceration of the buccal mucosa of the lip. Hypothalamic and pituitary syndromes are not uncommon—obesity, somnolence, and change of behaviour pattern are the commonest. Some of these symptoms may be related to distension and atrophy of the floor of the third ventricle as a result of hydrocephalus, since not all cases are associated with evidence of infiltration by leukaemic cells.

Spinal cord problems may be a result of extradural

deposits, direct infiltration of nerve roots or the spinal cord itself, vascular occlusion, either by leukaemic cells, thrombus or a mixture of these two, or haemorrhage. A complete range of cord syndromes have been described, from complete transverse lesions with paraplegia, sensory abnormalities and abnormalities of rectal and bladder function, to partial cord syndromes and even isolated spinal nerve root lesions.

Localised deposits of leukaemic cells may occur sub-periosteally, usually in the cranial or facial bones, and these are usually attached to the dura mater. A variety of non-lymphoblastic leukaemia known as chloroma, due to its distinct greenish colour, is sometimes seen, more commonly in children than adults, and it seems likely that these tumours arise in the bone and spread outwards through the Haversian canals. They produce a variety of problems including exophthalmas, ophthalmoplegia, headaches, nausea and vomiting, papilloedema, cranial nerve palsies, seizures and hemiplegia. They rarely invade the cerebral tissues them-selves, but sometimes occur in the spinal extradural space where they may result in cord compression.

Rarely, neurological symptoms may be produced as a result of hyperviscosity in the presence of marked elevations in the white blood cell count (Preston *et al.* 1978) (Fig. 7.16). The syndrome is seen in all forms of leukaemia, acute or chronic, but neurological symptoms occur most commonly, and at lower white cell counts in patients with myeloid leukaemias than in patients with lymphocytic leukaemias. Symptoms and signs are very varied and include headaches, lethargy, impairment of consciousness, ataxia and impairment of auditory and visual function. Treatment by leucophoresis may produce rapid and complete reversal of symptoms. It is important to stress that blood transfusions may be hazardous in these patients since the additional red cell volume may further elevate blood viscosity, resulting in coma or death.

INTRACRANIAL HAEMORRHAGE

Bleeding usually occurs as a result of a haemorrhagic diathesis but may occur as an isolated event. Reduced platelet output by the bone marrow, either as a result of leukaemic infiltration or as a result of side effects of chemotherapeutic agents, is one of the main mechanisms of haemorrhage, but reduction of the platelet count as a result of platelet consumption (as may occur in disseminated intravascular coagulation) probably plays a part in some cases. It is unusual for bleeding to occur if

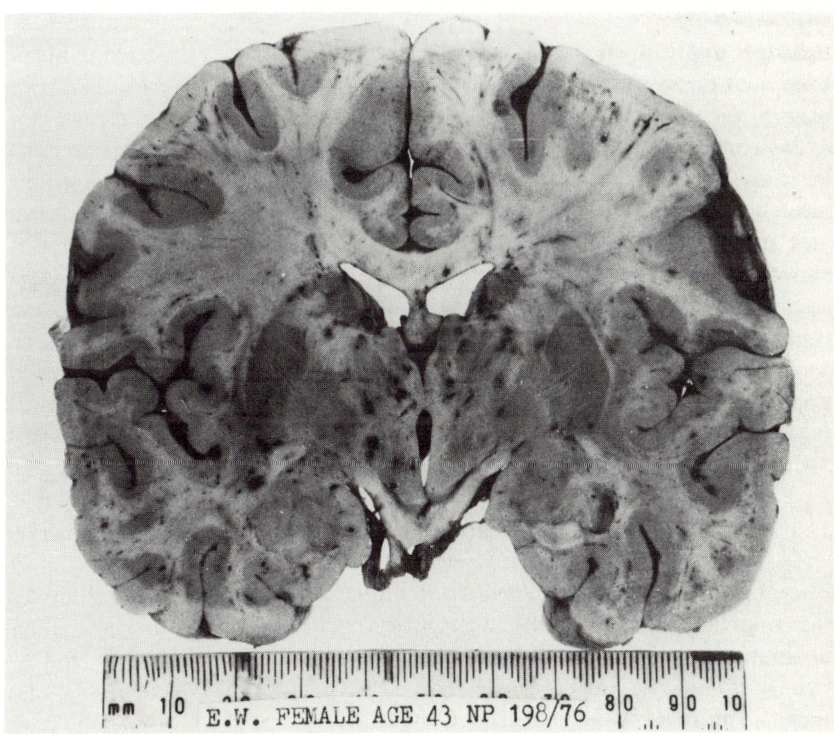

Fig. 7.17. Leukaemia. Coronal section of brain showing multiple small haemorrhages.

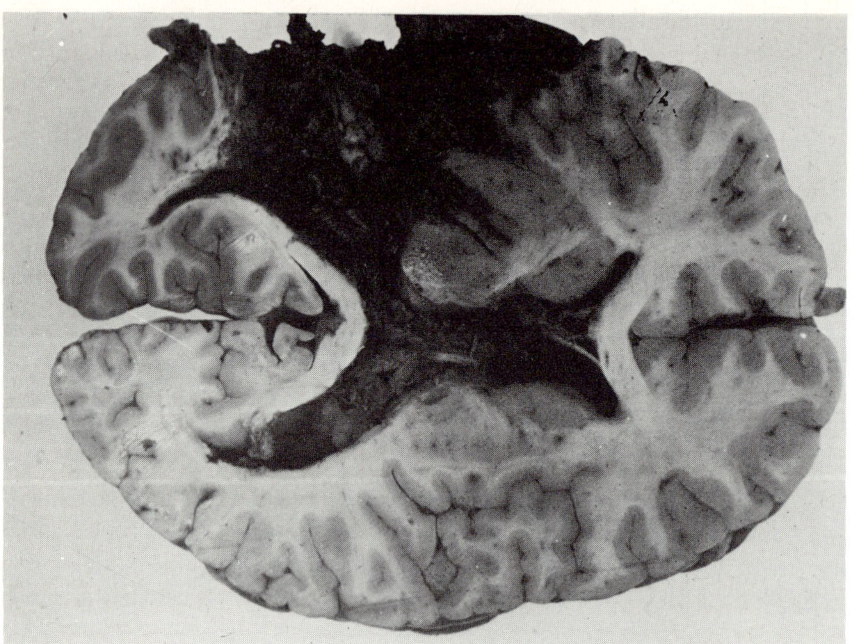

Fig. 7.18. Acute leukaemia. Horizontal section of brain showing massive haemorrhage into the left cerebral hemisphere rupturing both into the lateral ventricle and onto the surface of the brain.

the platelet count is above 20 000/cu mm in the absence of any other abnormality of coagulation; however, it may occur at any site within the nervous system or its surrounding meninges and it is often multifocal. The picture may vary from multiple small petechial haemorrhages to one or more massive haemorrhages (Figs 7.17 and 7.18).

Disseminated intravascular coagulation is seen commonly in promyelocytic leukaemia, probably due to the marked thromboplastic activity of intracytoplasmic granules (Gralnick and Abrell 1973). In other forms of leukaemia disseminated intravascular coagulation is particularly marked in cases with high white cells counts. Patients with a white cell count in excess of 100×10^9/l are particularly at risk. The risk is also greater at the stage of commencing chemotherapy, since this results in destruction of white cells and release of thromboplastic substances.

INFECTIONS IN LEUKAEMIA

There has been a marked increase in mortality due to infections in recent years, particularly since the introduction of intrathecal methotrexate and irradiation of the brain in the treatment of acute lymphoblastic leukaemia. Virus infections such as measles, *Herpes simplex*, varicella, mumps, and cytomegalia are often involved. In many cases the agent cannot be identified. Varicella-zoster meningoencephalitis carries a particularly high morbidity and mortality (Hattori *et al.* 1976). Measles encephalitis may be particularly difficult to diagnose since symptoms may be atypical and closely resemble subacute sclerosing panencephalitis. Almost any agent, viral, bacterial or fungal, may be involved (Figs 7.19 and 7.20) and the frequency of different types of organism varies from one part of the world to another. The incidence of bacterial infection is increased particularly following the use of intraventricular reservoirs.

From the diagnostic point of view blood cultures should always be carried out at the same time as a lumbar puncture, since these may sometimes be positive when no organisms are grown from the cerebrospinal fluid; if both are positive, this confirms the presence of bacteraemia as well as meningitis. A positive blood culture in the presence of a cerebrospinal fluid which fails to grow organisms is seen particularly in cases of infection due to *Listeria monocytogenes* (Gaya 1979). Gaya also suggests that a blood glucose estimation should be carried out at the same time as cerebrospinal fluid analysis since CSF glucose is usually about 70% of that of the blood, and an apparently normal cerebrospinal fluid glucose level in the presence of hyperglycaemia may suggest the presence of bacterial or mycotic infection. It is important to remember

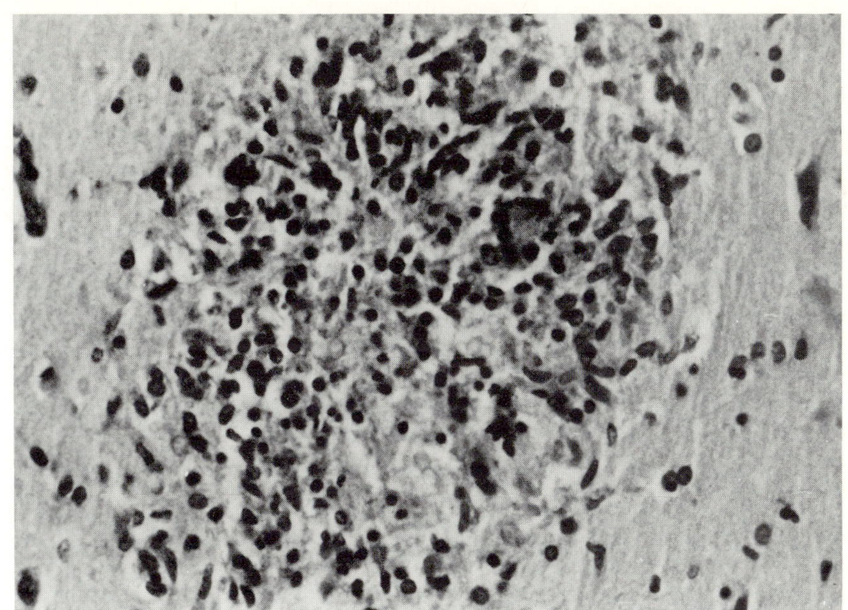

Fig. 7.19. Acute leukaemia. Small granuloma within the cerebral white matter due to *Candida albicans* infection. ×450.

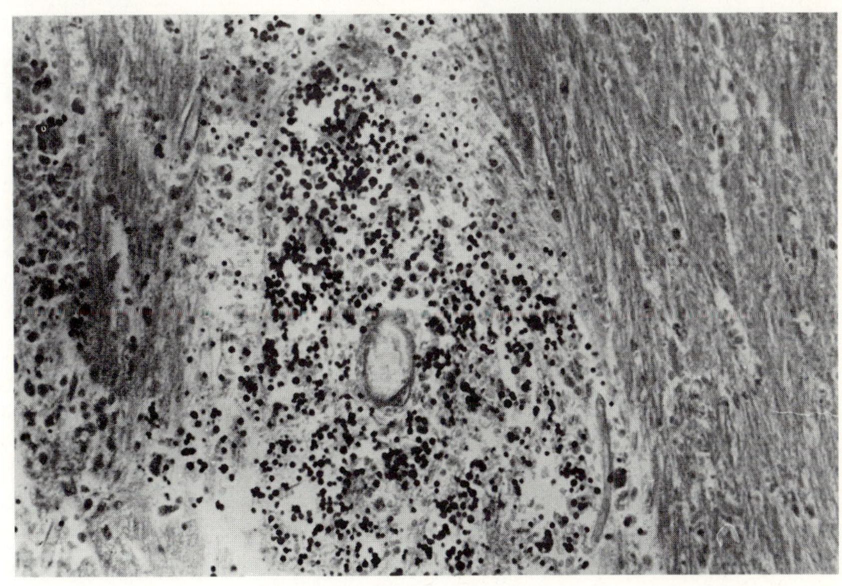

Fig. 7.20. Acute leukaemia. *Candida albicans* infection showing numerous yeasts within the perivascular spaces. Methenamine silver stain. ×138.

that the cell count may be unreliable since patients with severe leucopenia may not show the usual leucocyte response.

PROGRESSIVE MULTIFOCAL LEUCO-ENCEPHALOPATHY

Progressive multifocal leuco-encephalopathy is a rare disease associated with foci of demyelination. Lesions may be widespread within the central nervous system, occurring predominantly in the cerebral hemispheres, but they may also be found in the brainstem and cerebellum; occasionally, changes may even be found in the spinal cord. In contrast to disseminated sclerosis, the foci of demyelination are not particularly related to small blood vessels; they are surrounded by oligodendroglial cells showing abnormalities in the nuclei which become deeply basophilic and may contain inclusion bodies. Oligodendroglial cells are usually absent or markedly reduced in numbers in the centre of the lesions. Abnormalities are also found within the adjacent astrocytes; these may contain giant bizarre nuclei and some of the cells may be multinucleate, sometimes resembling neoplastic cells. As the disease progresses, new foci of demyelination continually appear.

Zu Rhein and Chou (1965) showed that the glial cell nuclei contained particles resembling Papova virus. A Papova virus was isolated from the brain of a patient with Hodgkin's disease (Padgett *et al.* 1971) and this virus was named JC virus, and then Weiner *et al.* (1972) isolated another virus antigenically similar to Simian virus-40 (SV-40).

Progressive multifocal leuco-encephalopathy complicates a variety of diseases involving the reticuloendothelial system, including various forms of leukaemia and lymphoma. It has also been described in association with tuberculosis, sarcoidosis and following renal transplant operations; it is rarely seen as an isolated phenomenon. It is almost certainly an opportunistic infection due to a variety of viruses affecting predominantly oligodendroglial cells and resulting in demyelination.

Progressive multifocal leuco-encephalopathy has an insidious onset, producing symptoms and signs which vary considerably from case to case, usually including disturbances of mental function, dementia, confusion, amnesia, disturbances of speech, vision, cerebellar function, pyramidal tract signs, cranial nerve abnormalities, and occasionally evidence of spinal cord involvement (Adams and Short 1965). There is no effective treatment and the disease usually progresses to death within a few months.

CENTRAL PONTINE MYELINOSIS

Adams *et al.* (1959) described a complication in chronic alcoholics who developed symmetrical patchy demyelination in the pons; they attributed this to malnutrition. The pattern of the demyelination differed from that of disseminated sclerosis in its anatomical situation and by its lack of relationship to blood vessels. Since then, a similar complication has been described in other systemic diseases including leukaemia and has been described in both adults and children (Rosman *et al.* 1966). A few cases have been reported in which areas of demyelination have been seen in other parts of the central nervous system as well as the pons. Histologically, the areas of demyelination are associated with the presence of numerous phagocytes distended with Sudanophilic lipids and there is relative sparing of nerve cells and axis cylinders. Oligodendroglial cells disappear from the areas of demyelination but there may be some reactive astrocytes present. The aetiology is unknown.

THERAPY AND ITS COMPLICATIONS IN LEUKAEMIA

Central nervous system involvement by leukaemia became a significant problem following the introduction of effective systemic therapy for childhood acute lymphoblastic leukaemia (Sansone 1954). The incidence of leukaemic involvement of the central nervous system in childhood acute lymphoblastic leukaemia has been reported as varying between 50 and 70% (Haghbin and Zuelzer 1965; West *et al.* 1972). Involvement of the nervous system may occur at any stage but frequently occurs during complete haematological remission (Sullivan 1957). Without additional local CNS therapy meningeal leukaemia recurs in about three months (Selawry and Odom 1968).

Most chemotherapeutic agents do not pass the blood–brain barrier and this requires the use of intrathecal or intra-ventricular therapy, usually with methotrexate or cytosine arabinoside. It seems unlikely that intrathecal drugs alone would reach leukaemic cells in the perivascular spaces in the deeper parts of the brain in effective concentration (Price and Johnson 1973); as a result combined therapeutic regimes, including intrathecally administered drugs, cranial irradiation, and systemic chemotherapy in high dosage have been employed. A variety of neurotoxic effects have been described in relationship to methotrexate therapy in particular, such as arachnoiditis (producing pain, radiating into one or other extremity), transient weakness and sensory disturbances; there may be evidence of a diffuse encephalopathy with intellectual impairment, ataxia and partial blindness (Kay *et al.* 1971); or there may be transient or permanent paraparesis or paraplegia. Similar complications have been described after the use of intra-ventricular cytosine arabinoside.

The principal pathological abnormalities found in leuco-encephalopathy associated with intensive CNS therapy are reactive astrocytosis, breakdown of myelin sheaths and neuronal processes and the release of nuclear and cytoplasmic glial debris into the neurophil. Lesions most commonly affect the fronto-parietal white matter but may also involve the occipital and temporal lobes to a lesser extent.

It seems likely that irradiation of small blood vessels results in increased permeability through the blood–brain barrier allowing methotrexate to cause white matter necrosis. Other factors must be involved since lesions do not develop in all children receiving CNS therapy.

Another form of pathological change seen following CNS therapy is mineralisation of small blood vessels and dystro-phic calcification of adjacent cerebral tissues. Distribution of the lesions differs from the demyelination process in that lesions are found particularly in the grey matter in these cases (Price and Birdwell 1978). The lentiform nucleus is affected early and lesions in the cerebral cortex and cerebellum appear later. Lesions are most marked in the 'watershed' areas of anastomosis between the anterior, middle and posterior cerebral arteries. These lesions are easily recognised on CAT scans (Fig. 7.21). Neurological abnormalities include focal seizures, ataxia, motor disabilities and behaviour disorders (Peylan-Ramu *et al.* 1978).

It seems likely that radiation is the main factor in the aetiology of these pathological abnormalities, although chemotherapy seems to play a part. Intravenous administration of cytotoxic drugs is probably particularly relevant since this results in high concentration of the drug in close contact with the endothelium exposed to irradiation, and MacIntosh *et al.* (1977) produced some evidence to suggest that intravenous methotrexate and cytosine arabinoside influence the development of these lesions.

The standard method of central nervous system prophy-

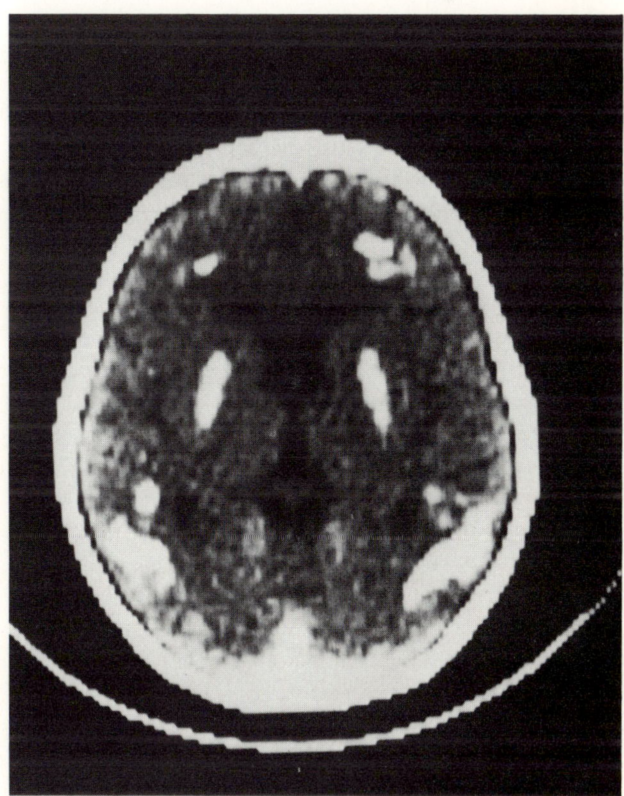

Fig. 7.21. CAT scan. Methotrexate encephalopathy showing foci of calcification within the lentiform nuclei and in the 'watershed' areas of anastomosis between the anterior, middle and posterior cerebral arteries.

laxis combines cranial radiation and intrathecal methotrexate. There is a 53% incidence of abnormal CT scans in asymptomatic children with acute lymphoblastic leukaemia, whose central nervous system prophylaxis consists of cranial radiation and either intrathecal methotrexate or intrathecal cytosine arabinoside (Peylan-Ramu *et al.* 1978). Ochs *et al.* (1980) carried out a study of forty-three asymptomatic children with acute lymphoblastic leukaemia in complete remission. In this series, ten were treated with intrathecal methotrexate alone, thirty-three were treated with intrathecal methotrexate combined with intermediate-dose intravenous methotrexate, and none were treated with cranial irradiation. Only one CT scan was clearly abnormal and this showed mildly dilated ventricles with visualisation of the cortical sulci. Seven more were classified as abnormal with borderline dilatation of the ventricles (three cases) and/or visualisation of cortical sulci (seven). None showed any evidence of calcification or decreased cerebral attenuation coefficient—findings that have previously been ascribed to methotrexate. Clinically, leuco-encephalopathy was not seen in any case. These results suggest that methotrexate alone is unlikely to produce structural central nervous system abnormalities.

The frequency of involvement of the central nervous system seems to increase with the dose of radiation and methotrexate, and the risk increase is in proportion to the immaturity of the brain (Arnold *et al.* 1978).

Vincristine is particularly neurotoxic and specifically affects peripheral nerves when given systemically (Casey *et al.* 1973). It produces sensory symptoms initially which, if the drug is not withdrawn, will progress to a significant sensory/motor neuropathy.

Sural nerve biopsies show axonal degeneration with or without evidence of segmental demyelination (McLeod and Penny 1969). No obvious abnormalities are seen on light-microscopial examination of muscle biopsies taken from painful proximal muscles, but electronmicroscopical changes may be seen in the myofibrils and there may be loss of Z-lines (Bradley *et al.* 1970). This fits in with the electrophysiological abnormalities described by Casey *et al.* (1973) who found myopathic units in some muscles as well as evidence of denervation.

REFERENCES

Adams J.H. & Short I.A. (1965) Progressive multifocal leuko-encephalopathy. *Scot. Med. J.* **10**, 195–202.

Adams R.D., Victor M. & Mancall E.L. (1959) Central pontine myelinolysis. *Arch. Neurol. Psychiat* (Chicago) **81**, 154–172.

Allison R.S. & Gordon D.S. (1955) Reticulosis of the nervous system simulating acute infective polyneuritis. *Lancet* **ii**, 120–122.

Arnold H., Kühne D., Franke H. & Grosch I. (1978) Findings in computed axial tomography after intrathecal methotrexate and radiation. *Neuroradiol.* **16**, 65–68.

Billingham M.E., Rawlinson D.G., Berry P.F. & Kempson R.L. (1975) The cytodiagnosis of malignant lymphomas and Hodgkin's disease in cerebro-spinal, pleural and ascitic fluids. *Acta Cytol.* **19**, 547–556.

Blanchard B.M. (1962) Peripheral neuropathy (non-invasive) associated with lymphoma. *Ann. Int. Med.* **56**, 774–778.

Bluming A.Z. & Zeigler J.L. (1971) Regression of Burkitt's lymphoma in association with Measles Infection. *Lancet* **ii**, 105–106.

Bradley W.G., Lassman L.P. & Pearce G.W. (1970) The neuro-myopathy of vincristine in man. *J. Neurol. Sci.* **10**, 107–131.

Brand M.M. & Marinkovich V.A. (1969) Primary malignant reticulosis of the brain in Wiscott–Aldrich syndrome. *Arch. Dis. Children* **44**, 536–542.

Buckley T.F. & Warwick F. (1968) Surgical management of intracranial Hodgkin's disease. *J. Neurol. Neurosurg. Psychiat.* **31**, 612–615.

Bunn P.A., Schein P.S., Banks P.M. & De Vita V.T., Jnr (1976) Central nervous system complications in patients with diffuse histiocytic and undifferentiated lymphoma: leukaemia revisited. *Blood* **47**, 3–10.

Casey E.B., Jellife A.M., Le Quesne P.M. & Millett Y.L. (1973) Vincristine neuropathy; clinical and electrophysiological observations. *Brain* **96**, 69–86.

Chernick N.L., Armstrong D. & Posner J.B. (1973) Central nervous system infections in patients with cancer. *Medicine* **52**, 562–581.

Chernick N.L., Armstrong D. & Posner J.B. (1977) Central nervous system infections in patients with cancer. *Cancer* **40**, 268–274.

Currie S. & Henson R.A. (1971) Neurological syndromes in the reticuloses. *Brain* **94**, 307–312.

Currie S., Henson R.A., Morgan H.G. & Poole A.J. (1970) The incidence of non-metastatic neurological syndromes of obscure origin in the reticuloses. *Brain* **94**, 307–312.

Davies-Jones G.A.B., Preston F.E. & Timperley W.R. (1980) *Neurological Complications in Clinical Haematology*, p 41. Blackwell Scientific Publications, Oxford.

Denny-Brown D. (1948) Primary sensory neuropathy with muscular changes associated with carcinoma. *J. Neurol. Neurosurg. Psychiat.* **11**, 73–87.

Evans A.E. & Craig M. (1964) CNS involvement in children with acute leukaemia. *Cancer* **17**, 256–258.

Evans A.E., Gilbert E.S. & Zandstra R. (1970) The increasing incidence of central nervous system leukaemia in children. *Cancer* **26**, 404–409.

Friedman M., Kim T.H. & Panahon A.M. (1976) Spinal cord compression in malignant lymphoma: treatment and results. *Cancer* **37**, 1485–91.

GAYA H. (1979) Central nervous system infections in neoplastic disease. In *CNS Complications of Malignant Disease*, pp. 251–257 (Eds Whitehouse J.M.A. & Kay H.E.M.) Macmillan Press Ltd. London and Basingstoke.

GENDELMAN S., RIZZO F. & MONES R.J. (1969) Central nervous system complications of leukaemic conversion of the lymphomas. *Cancer* 24, 676–682.

GRAHAM-POLE J. & WILLOUGHBY M.L.N. (1975) Leukaemia in the nervous system; factors in pathogenesis. In *Acute Childhood Leukaemia* (Modern Problems in Paediatrics Series 59). (Ed. Pochedly C.). Karger, Basel.

GRALNICK H.R. & ABELL E. (1973) Studies of the procoagulant and fibrinolytic activities of promyelocytes in acute promyelocytic leukaemia. *Brit. J. Haematol.* 24, 89–99.

GREGORY M.C. & HUGHES J.T. (1973) Intracranial reticulum cell sarcoma associated with immunoglobulin-A deficiency. *J. Neurol. Neurosurg. Psychiat* 36, 769–776.

GRIFFIN J.W., THOMPSON R.W., MITCHINSON M.J., DE KIEWIET J.C. & WELLAND F.H. (1971) Malignant lymphoma of the spinal epidural space. *Ann. Int. Med.* 74, 416–423.

GROSS S. (1971) Measles and leukaemia. *Lancet* i, 397.

GUNDERSSON C.H., MENRY J. & MALAMUD N. (1971) Plasma globulin determinations in patients with microglioma. *J. Neurosurg.* 35, 406–415.

HAGHBIN M. & ZUELZER W.W. (1965) A long-term study of cerebro-spinal leukaemia. *J. Paediat* 67, 23–28.

HATTORI A., IHARA T., IWASI T., KAMIYA H., SAKURAI M., IZAWI T. & TAKAHASLU M. (1976) Use of live varicella vaccine in children with acute leukaemia or other malignancies. *Lancet* ii, 210.

HENRY K. (1975) Electronmicroscopy in the non-Hodgkin's lymphomata. *Brit. J. Cancer* 31, Suppl 11, 73–93.

HENRY J.M., HEFFNER R.R., Jnr, DILLARD S.J., BARTE K.M. & DAVIES R.L. (1974) Primary malignant lymphomas of the central nervous system. *Cancer (Philadelphia)* 34, 1293–1302.

HOOVER R. & FRAUMENI J.F., Jnr (1973) Risk of cancer in renal transplant recipients. *Lancet* ii, 55–57.

HORVATH B., PENA C. & FISHER E.R. (1969) Primary reticulum cell sarcoma (microglioma) of the brain. *Arch. Path. (Chicago)* 87, 609–616.

HUTCHINSON E.C., LEONARD B.J., MAUDSLEY C. & YATES P.O. (1958) Neurological complications of the reticuloses. *Brain* 81, 75–92.

JELLINGER K., RADASZKIEWICZ T. & SLOWIK F. (1975) Primary malignant lymphomas of the central nervous system in man. *Acta Neuropath. Suppl.* 6, 95.

JELLINGER K. & RADASZKIEWICZ T. (1976) Involvement of the nervous system in malignant lymphomas. *Virchous Archiv. Path. Anat.* 370, 345–362.

JELLINGER K., SLOWIK F. & SLUGA E. (1979) Primary intracranial malignant lymphomas. A fine structural cytochemical and CSF immunological study. *Clin. Neurol. Neurosurg.* 81, 174–184.

JOHN H.T. & NABARRO J.D.H. (1955) Intracranial manifestations of malignant lymphoma. *Brit. J. Cancer* 9, 386–400.

JOHNSON P.C. (1975) Ultrastructural study of two central nervous system lymphomas. *Acta Neuropath. (Bev.)* Suppl. VI, 155–160.

KAY H.E., KNAPTON P.J. & O'SULLIVAN J.P. (1971) Severe neurological damage associated with methotrexate therapy. *Lancet* ii, 542.

KINNEY T.D. & ADAMS R.D. (1943) Reticulum cell sarcoma of the brain. *Arch. Neurol. Psychiat. (Chicago)* 50, 552–558.

LAW I.P., DICK F.R., BLOM J. & BERGEVIN P.R. (1975) Involvement of the central nervous system in non-Hodgkin's lymphoma. *Cancer* 36, 225–231.

LILLEYMAN J.S., ANTONION A.G. & SUGDEN P.J. (1979) Facial nerve palsy in acute leukaemia. *Scand. J. Haematol.* 22, 87–90.

McINTOSH S., FISHER D., ROTHMAN S.G., ROSEFELD N., LEBEL J.F. & O'BRIEN R.T. (1977) Intracranial calcification in childhood leukaemia. *J. Paediat.* 91, 909–913.

McLEOD J.G. & PENNY R. (1969) Vincristine neuropathy; an electrophysiological and histological study. *J. Neurol. Neurosurg. Psychiat.* 32, 297–304.

MULLINS G.M., FLYNN J.P.G., EL-MAHDI A.M., McQUEEN J.D. & OWENS A.H. (1971) Malignant lymphoma of the spinal epidural space. *Ann. Int. Med.* 74, 416–423.

NATHWANI B.N., KIM H. & RAPPAPORT H. (1976) Malignant lymphoma, lymphoblastic. *Cancer* 38, 964–983.

NEAULT R.W., VAN SCOY R.E., OKAZAKI H. & MacCARTY C.S. (1972) Uveitis associated with isolated reticulum cell sarcoma of the brain. *Amer. J. Ophthalmol.* 73, 431–436.

OCHS J.J., BERGER P., BRECHER M.L., SINKS L.F., KINKEL W. & FREEMAN A.I. (1980) Computed tomography brain scans in children with acute lymphocytic leukaemia receiving methotrexate alone as central nervous system prophylaxis. *Cancer* 45, 2274–2278.

PADGETT B.L., WALKER D.L., ZU RHEIN G.M. & ECHROADE R.J. (1971) Cultivation of papova-like virus from human brain with progressive multifocal leukoencephalopathy. *Lancet* i, 1257–1258.

PEYLAN-RAMU N., POPLACK D.G., PIZZO P.A., ADORNATO B.T. & DI CHIRO G. (1978) Abnormal CT scans in children with ALL following CNS prophylaxis. *New. Engl. J. Med.* 298, 815–819.

PRESTON F.E., SOKOL F., LILLEYMAN J.S., WINFIELD D.A. & BLACKBURN E.K. (1978) Cellular hyperviscosity as a cause of neurological symptoms in leukaemia. *Brit. Med. J.* 1, 476–478.

PRICE R.A. (1975) Histopathology of central nervous system in leukaemia. In *Acute Childhood Leukaemia* (Modern Problems in Paediatrics Series 80) (Ed. Pochedly C.). Karger, Basle.

PRICE R.A. & BIRDWELL D.A. (1978) The central nervous system in childhood leukaemia. *Cancer* 42, 717–728.

PRICE R.A. & JOHNSON W.W. (1973) The central nervous system in childhood leukaemia. *Cancer* 31, 520–533.

ROSMAN N., KAKULAS B. & RICHARDSON E. (1966) Central pontine myelinolysis in a child with leukaemia. *Arch. Chicago Neurol.* 14, 273–280.

RUSSEL D.S. & RUBINSTEIN L.J. (1976) *Pathology of Tumours of the Nervous System* (4th edn). Blackwell Scientific Publications, London.

SANSONE G. (1954) Pathomorphosis of acute infantile leukaemia treated with modern therapeutic agents; meningoleukaemia and Frolich's obesity. *Ann. Paediatrici* 183, 33–41.

SCHAUMBERG H.H., PLANCK C.R. & ADAMS R.D. (1972) The reticulum cell sarcoma-microglioma group of brain tumours. *Brain* 95, 199–212.

SCHNECK S.A. & PENN I. (1971) *De novo* brain tumour in renal transplantation recipients. *Lancet* i, 983–984.

SELAWRY O.S. & ODOM S. (1968) On eradication of leukaemia meningopathy. *Proc. Am. Ass. Cancer. Res.* 9, 62–69.

SKARIN A.T., ROSENTHAL D.S., MOLONEY W.C. & FREI E. (1977) Combination chemotherapy of advanced non-Hodgkin lymphoma with bleomycin, adriamycin, cyclophosphamide, vincristine and prednisolone. *Blood* 49, 759–770.

SKARIN A.T., ZUCKERMAN K.S., PITMAN S.W., ROSENTHAL D.A., MOLONEY W., FREI E. & CANELLOS G.P. (1977) High dose methotrexate with folinic acid in the treatment of advanced non-Hodgkin lymphoma including CNS involvement. *Blood* 50, 1039–1047.

SPARLING H.J., ADAMS R.D. & PARKER F. (1947) Involvement of the nervous system by malignant lymphomas. *Medicine* 26, 285–332.

SULLIVAN M.P. (1957) Intracranial complications of leukaemia in children. *Paediatrics* 20, 757–781.

TAYLOR C.R., RUSSELL R., LUKES R.J. & DAVIES R.J. (1978) An immunohistological study of immunoglobulin content of primary central nervous system lymphomas. *Cancer (Philadelphia)* 41, 2197–2205.

ULRICH J. & WUTHRICH R. (1974) Multiple sclerosis: reticulum cell sarcoma of the nervous system in a patient treated with immunosuppressive drugs. *Europ. Neurol.* 12, 65–78.

WALTON J.N., TOMLINSON B. & PEARCE G.W. (1968) Subacute poliomyelitis and Hodgkin's disease. *J. Neurol. Sci.* 6, 435–445.

WEBB H.E., MOLOMUT N., PADNOS M. & WETHERLEY-MEIN G. (1975) The treatment of eighteen cases of malignant disease with an arenavirus. *Clin. Oncol.* 1, 157–169.

WEINER L.P., HERNDON R.H. & NARAYAN O. (1972) Isolation of virus related SV-40 from patients with progressive multifocal leukoencephalopathy. *New Engl. J. Med.* 286, 385–390.

WEST R.J., GRAHAM-POLE J., HARDISTY R.M. & PIKE M.C. (1972) Factors in pathogenesis of central nervous system leukaemia. *Brit. Med. J.* 3, 311–314.

YOUNG R.C., HOWSER D.M., ANDERSON T., JAFFE E. & DE VITA V.T. (1979) CNS infiltration: a complication of diffuse lymphomas. In *CNS Complications of Malignant Disease* (Eds Whitehouse J.M.A. & Kay H.E.M.). Macmillan, London.

ZIEGLER J.L., BLUMING A.Z., MORROW R.H., FASS L. & CARBONE P.P. (1970) Central nervous system involvement in Burkitt's lymphoma. *Blood* 36, 718–728.

ZIMMERMAN H.M. (1975) Malignant lymphomas of the nervous system. *Acta. Neuropath. (Berl.)* Suppl. VI, 69–74.

ZU RHEIN G.M. & CHOU S.M. (1965) Particles resembling papova viruses in human cerebral demyelinating disease. *Science* 148, 1477–1479.

Chapter 8

Histiocytosis. Reticuloendotheliosis and other miscellaneous lymphoreticular disorders

The term histiocytosis comprises a miscellaneous group of rare disorders, ranging from systemic rapidly fatal neoplasia to solitary benign focal granulomatous lesions. Their unity is that they are proliferative disorders of the macrophage/mononuclear phagocyte/histiocyte (see Groopman and Golde 1981, for review). The term has the disadvantage of grouping together lesions which behave in a widely dissimilar manner. Two lesions are considered for convenience here which may not be or are not of macrophage origin—leukaemic reticuloendotheliosis and mastocytosis. These lesions may be classified as follows:

1 Progressive systemic malignant neoplasms.

(a) Malignant histiocytosis (synonyms—malignant reticulosis, histiocytic medullary reticulosis of Robb-Smith).

(b) Malignant histiocytosis of childhood (Letterer–Siwe) and allied conditions—the familial reticuloendotheliosis.

(c) Leukaemic reticuloendotheliosis (LRE—hairy cell leukaemia).

(d) Systemic mastocytosis.

2 Disseminated lesions accompanied by if not actually caused by abnormal storage of metabolic products.

(a) Hand–Schuller–Christian disease.

(b) Gaucher's disease.

(c) Niemann–Pick disease.

(d) Sea-blue histiocytosis.

(e) Xanthomatosis.

(f) Xanthogranulomatosis.

(g) Multicentric reticulohistiocytosis.

The term histiocytosis X, suggested by Lichtenstein to cover eosinophilic granuloma of bone, Hand–Schuller–Christian disease and Letterer–Siwe disease, attempts to categorize together disorders of widely differing course and prognosis.

3 Systemic reactive histiocytosis

Malignant histiocytosis

This was first clearly described by Scott and Robb-Smith (1939) and its pathology further described by Marshall

(1956). The literature has been admirably surveyed by Abele and Griffin (1972) and Warnke et al. (1975). It is an acute progressive invariably fatal disease of adults (mean age 36 years, range 1–78 years) characterized usually by weakness, malaise and weight loss, fever, hepatosplenomegaly, often by oedema, skin rashes, ascites and pleural and pericardial effusions, in about half of cases by lymphadenopathy and rather less often jaundice and soft tissue masses. Anaemia is always present and less often thrombocytopenia and leucopenia. Haematological investigation shows abnormalities in the peripheral blood in 15% of all cases, usually a few abnormal normoblasts, metamyelocytes and myelocytes and occasionally abnormal histiocytes. Occasionally the condition may present with leucocytosis and eosinophilia (Ballard et al. 1975) and rarely with massive splenomegaly (Vardman et al. 1975). The latter presentation may be associated with a more chronic form of the disease. Some workers, e.g. Isaacson et al. (1979), believe that a significant number of gut lymphomas are, in fact, variants of malignant histiocytosis.

The outstanding histological finding is a diffuse proliferation of abnormal histiocytes in lymph nodes, spleen and liver. The histiocytes are large cells with pale vesicular nuclei and abundant eosinophilic cytoplasm usually containing phagocytosed erythrocytes and other particles. Some cells are smaller without evidence of phagocytosis, while others are larger and multinucleate and may resemble Reed–Sternberg cells. Gross nuclear and cytoplasmic pleomorphism is obvious in the neoplastic cells. At least in the early stages of the lesion tumour cells tend to infiltrate and expand sinusoids rather than destroying tissue architecture (Fig. 8.1). Some of the cells may contain cholesterol crystals or Sudanophil lipid. Histochemical and immunohistochemical studies yield conflicting results, probably dependent on the degree of differentiation of the malignant cells; non-specific esterase and sometimes lysozyme are present (Mendelsohn et al. 1980; Carbone et al. 1981). Membrane marker studies of these cells show retention of a true histiocytic marker (Green et al. 1975). Purpuric or necrotic skin lesions are common and show nodular arrangement of neoplastic cells in the deep dermis

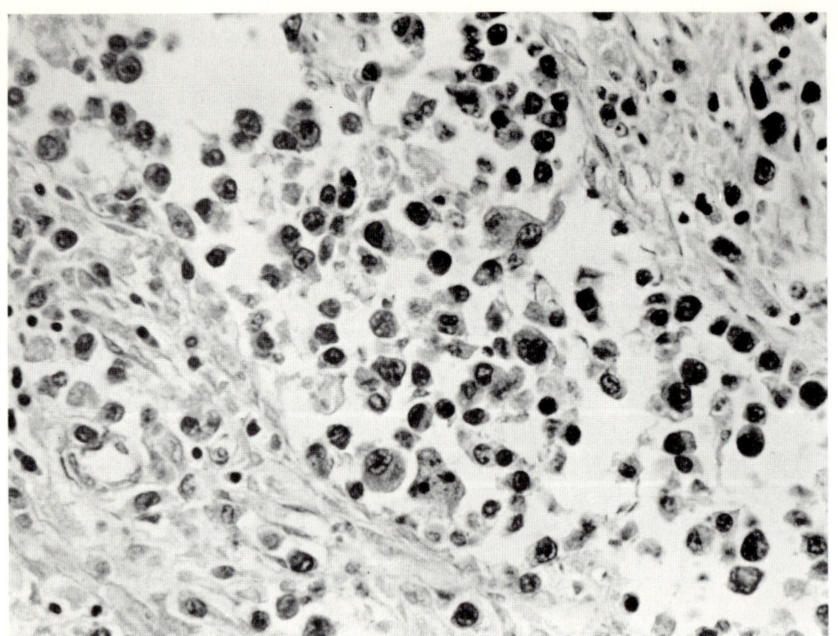

Fig. 8.1. Lymph node sinusoid filled with a mixed population of cells, some evidently histiocytic and several clearly malignant, from a lymph node of a 19 year old girl who died of malignant histiocytosis within 6 months of diagnosis. Elsewhere this node and other lymphoreticular tissues were diffusely infiltrated with malignant cells. ×216.

and around skin appendages. This condition has sometimes been regarded as a rare variant of non-Hodgkin's lymphoma and treatment with combination cytotoxic chemotherapy given; the outcome is usually fatal, nevertheless.

Malignant histiocytosis of childhood (Letterer–Siwe disease) and allied conditions

This syndrome was described by Letterer (1924) and Siwe (1933) as an acute febrile and fatal disorder of childhood, characterized by histiocytic infiltrates in lymphoreticular organs and bones. It occurs usually in children under 3 years old and more commonly in males. Liver, spleen and lymph nodes are usually enlarged, anaemia is frequent. There is a characteristic skin lesion—usually brown scaling papules which often ulcerate. Destructive osteolytic lesions and miliary infiltrations of lung are also seen. Lymph nodes are infiltrated by well-differentiated histiocytes with eosinophilic cytoplasm and ovoid or reniform nuclei with fine chromatin. The cytoplasm is vacuolated, less often foamy, and may contain phagocytized inclusions and haemosiderin. Erythrophagocytosis is uncommon and there may be a few giant cells. Total destruction of the node is seen only late in the disorder. Similar infiltrates are found in liver and spleen and character-

istically in bones and skin. Infiltrates in the skin are characteristically found in the superficial part of the dermis (Figs 8.2 and 8.3). A curious ultrastructural finding in the malignant histiocytes of Letterer–Siwe disease is an elongated membrane bound inclusion, characteristically 42 nm in external diameter with an electron dense core 11 nm in diameter which may show a repeating density (Cancilla *et al.* 1967). This structure probably also occurs in ordinary malignant histiocytosis (Imamura *et al.* 1971) and is similar or identical to the 'Langerhans granules' of cutaneous Langerhans cells. These structures are probably endocytic; their nature, importance and specificity is doubtful. The rare occurrence of Letterer–Siwe disease in young adults demonstrates that this syndrome is very similar or identical to malignant histiocytosis of adults (Shahani and Ward 1973).

The familial reticuloendothelioses of childhood

Several rare familial disorders have been described. The earliest of these, the familial haemophagocytic reticulosis of Farquar and Claireaux (1952) and Bell *et al.* (1968), appears to be similar to malignant histiocytosis but occurs in the first years of life. Nezelof and Eliachar (1973) described a similar lesion occurring in three siblings in which the cellular

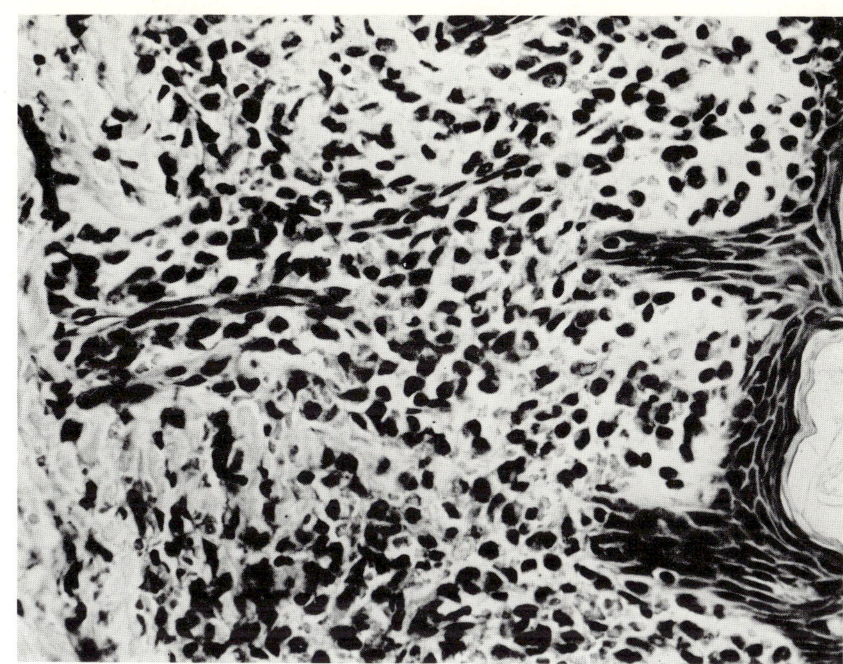

Fig. 8.2. Skin from patient with Letterer–Siwe disease showing infiltration of the dermis with lymphoreticular cells. ×216.

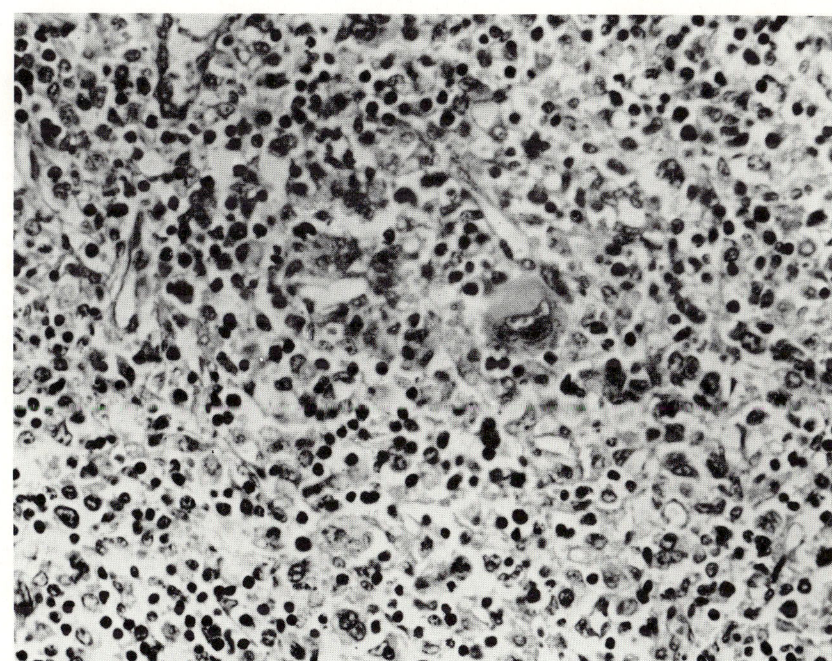

Fig. 8.3. Lymph node from patient with Letterer–Siwe disease showing infiltration with histiocytic cells and a tumour giant cell. × 216.

infiltrates in lymphoreticular organs included blast cells, monocytes and histiocytes with erythrophagocytosis. Falletta *et al.* (1973) described in 17 pre-school aged boys a fatal X linked recessive reticuloendothelial syndrome with hyperglobulinaemia, fever, hepatomegaly, purpura and anaemia, characterized by infiltration with immature mononuclear cells. Farber (1952) described a similar fatal disorder in infants (disseminated lipogranulomatosis) in which the infiltrating histiocytes contained lipid. These and other descriptions refer to a group of essentially similar conditions which differ little from malignant histiocytosis. Ford *et al.* (1962) describe a condition of familial lipochrome histiocytosis in 3 adult sisters with splenomegaly, arthritis, pulmonary infiltrates and a high susceptibility to bacterial infection, associated with hyperglobulinaemia.

In the majority of children with the above progressive and systemic histiocytoses, cytotoxic chemotherapy using alkylating agents, vinca alkaloids, antibiotics, steroids or various combination regimes may give remission (Horton 1977) though the outlook remains poor especially in the young child; death usually occurs as a result of infection in association with multi-organ involvement.

Leukaemic reticuloendotheliosis

The term leukaemic reticuloendotheliosis was first used by Ewald (1923) to refer to a progressive, but usually slowly progressive, proliferative disorder in which abnormal reticulum cells are found in bone marrow, blood and spleen. The early literature is reviewed by Bouroncle *et al.* (1958). Characteristic hairy cells have been described in the blood (Schrek and Donnelly 1966; Ghadially and Skinnider 1972) giving rise to the alternative description 'hairy cell leukaemia'. Such cells contain a tartrate-resistant acid phosphatase. Since the lesion often is not accompanied by a large number of circulating abnormal white cells the term 'leukaemic reticuloendotheliosis' (LRE) appears preferable. Numerous current ultrastructural, cytochemical and immunocytochemical studies on these cells have failed to demonstrate unequivocally whether they are of lymphocytic or monocytic origin. The current balance of evidence marginally favours the view that they are of the monocyte–macrophage series (Green *et al.* 1975).

The condition characteristically presents with pallor, fatigue, fever and weight loss. The spleen is enlarged, sometimes grossly and the liver is often enlarged. The blood shows anaemia usually normocytic and normochromic, and thrombocytopenia. Initial white cells counts from 400 to 13000 cmm have been reported and the white cell count characteristically falls as the disease progresses. The hairy cells in the blood have long thin cytoplasmic processes sometimes visible in ordinary smears but best seen with the EM.

The spleen may be slightly or grossly enlarged (up to 4600 g) and show diffuse infiltration and widening of the pulp cords by uniform mononuclear cells with no evidence of mitosis. The infiltration encroaches upon or may actually obliterate the white pulp, though not the splenic capsule or fibrous trabeculae. Individual cells at the light microscope level have ovoid, sometimes indented, sometimes elongated, pointed nuclei with finely stippled nuclear chromatin (Fig. 8.4). The cells in tissue sections are not seen as 'hairy' without electron microscopy. The spleen cells also contain tartrate-resistant acid phosphatase. Similar appearances are seen in lymph node, marrow and liver. Occasionally in the marrow the lesion may have the appearance of a uniform fibroblastic proliferation.

Some difficulties may arise in distinguishing LRE in the spleen from leukaemia, and non-Hodgkin lymphomas. Characteristically non-Hodgkin lymphomas primarily involve the white pulp and expand in a nodular manner. LRE primarily involves red pulp and expands in a diffuse manner. The cells of small lymphocytic lymphomas are smaller and rounder than those of LRE with more coarsely clumped chromatin, while those of large lymphocytic lymphomas have relatively less cytoplasm and more nuclear hyperchromatism and pleomorphism. Histiocytic lymphomas involve both red and white pulp non-preferentially and have larger more pleomorphic cells with more mitosis. The cells of malignant histiocytosis are bigger and more pleomorphic with more nuclear hyperchromasia and bigger nuclei than those of LRE; mitosis is frequent and the malignant histiocytes may show evidence of phagocytosis.

The prognosis in LRE is relatively good: of 21 patients of Burke *et al.* (1974), 4 died, 3, 41, 54 and 60 months after diagnosis. Splenectomy is held by many to improve prognosis and steroid treatment may make it worse chiefly due to the increased chance of a lethal infection.

Systemic mastocytosis

This lesion is considered here for completeness though it does not fit neatly into any classification of lymphoreticular disease.

Mastocytosis, an abnormal proliferation of tissue mast cells, involves skin, lymph nodes, viscera, bones and the entire

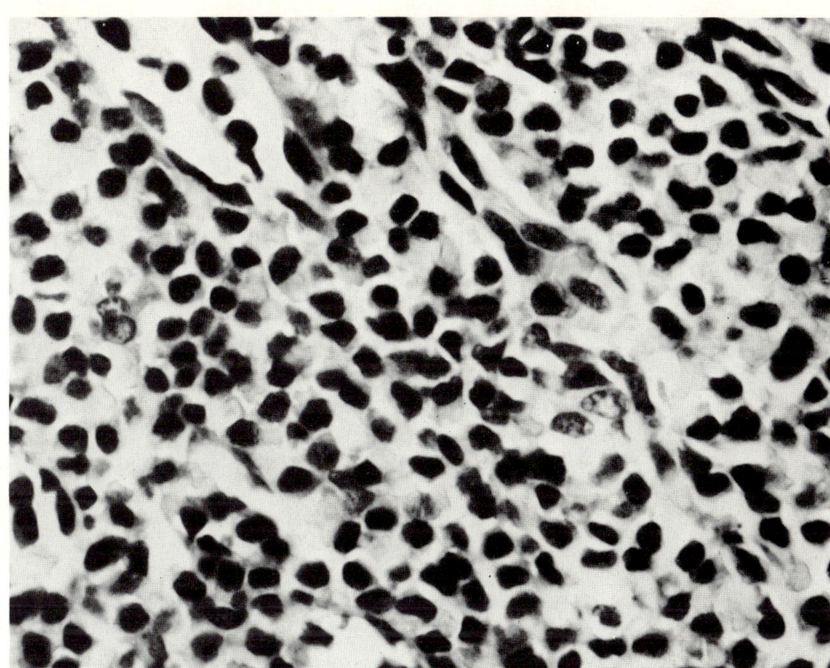

Fig. 8.4. Spleen from patient with hairy cell leukaemia showing diffuse infiltration with small cells with round, ovoid or sometimes pointed nuclei. ×450.

reticuloendothelial system. Histologically the typical cells of mastocytosis differ from normal mast cells (Gonella 1967) in that they may contain several nuclei of bizarre shapes and the cytoplasmic granules may vary in size, number and distribution. Spherical intracytoplasmic virus like particles are sometimes present and there are also certain biochemical differences particularly in polysaccharide content.

The characteristic skin change is of urticaria pigmentosa; successive urticarial eruptions followed by persistent pigmented lesions which urticate on irradiation.

Lymph node involvement may be regional or generalized (Havard and Bodley Scott 1959). Para-aortic lymph node abnormalities have been demonstrated on lymphography (Munro et al. 1969; Hancock et al. 1976). Hepatomegaly and splenomegaly occur with widespread mast cell infiltration of the reticuloendothelial system. Haematological changes are common and anaemia, leucopenia, monocytosis, thrombocytopenia, bleeding diastheses and mast cell leukaemia have all been described (Sagher and Even-Paz 1960). Bony lesions are not uncommon; radiological examination usually shows sclerotic changes.

We have treated a patient with systemic mastocytosis who developed mixed pyramidal and neuro-myopathic signs as a remote effect of her disease (Hancock et al. 1976).

Systemic mastocytosis with reticuloendothelial involve-

ment may be progressive and fatal. Corticosteroid therapy may give temporary benefit but antimitotic drugs and radiotherapy have not proved helpful.

Disseminated lipid histiocytosis (Hand–Schuller–Christian disease)

In 1893 Hand described a 3 year old boy with hepatosplenomegaly, lymphadenopathy, exophthalamos, polyuria and osteolytic lesions in the skull and later (1921) he described a second similar case and reviewed others independently described by, among others, Schuller and Christian. Recent reviews are those of Lieberman et al. (1969); Lucaya (1971); Vogel and Vogel (1972). Lichtenstein (1964) grouped this lesion together with Letterer-Siwe disease and eosinophilic granuloma of bone as an entity—histiocytosis. This term is not useful because of the widely varying prognosis of these lesions.

The term Hand–Schuller–Christian disease is currently best used to described a systemic, often febrile, slowly progressive, often but not always fatal disorder of childhood, in which there are granulomatous lesions in bone, notably skull, liver, spleen and lymph nodes and lungs, associated with normal plasma cholesterol levels and variable anaemia. Skin lesions are present in about one-third of cases. The

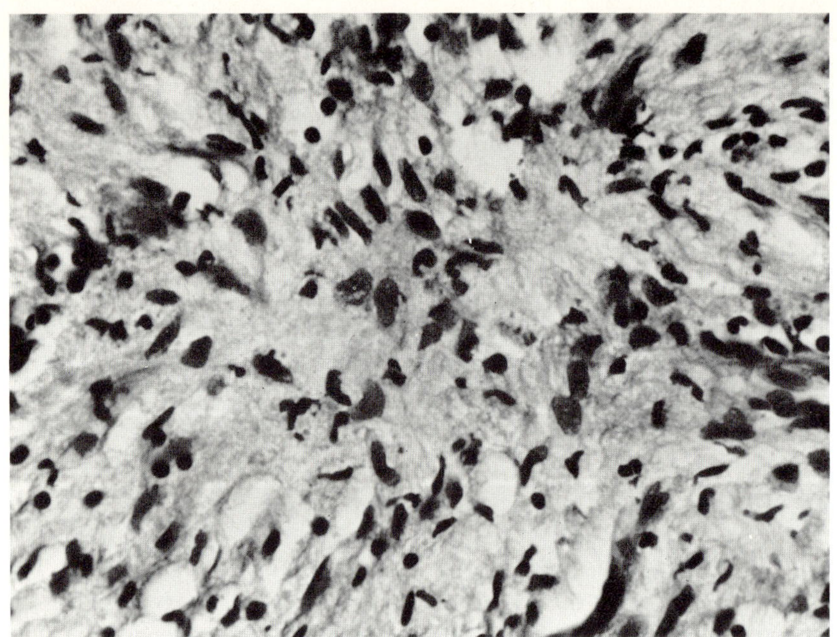

Fig. 8.5. Lesion from skull of patient with Hand–Schuller–Christian disease showing tissue infiltration with large poorly eosinophilic histiocytes. Few eosinophils are present in the lesion. ×450.

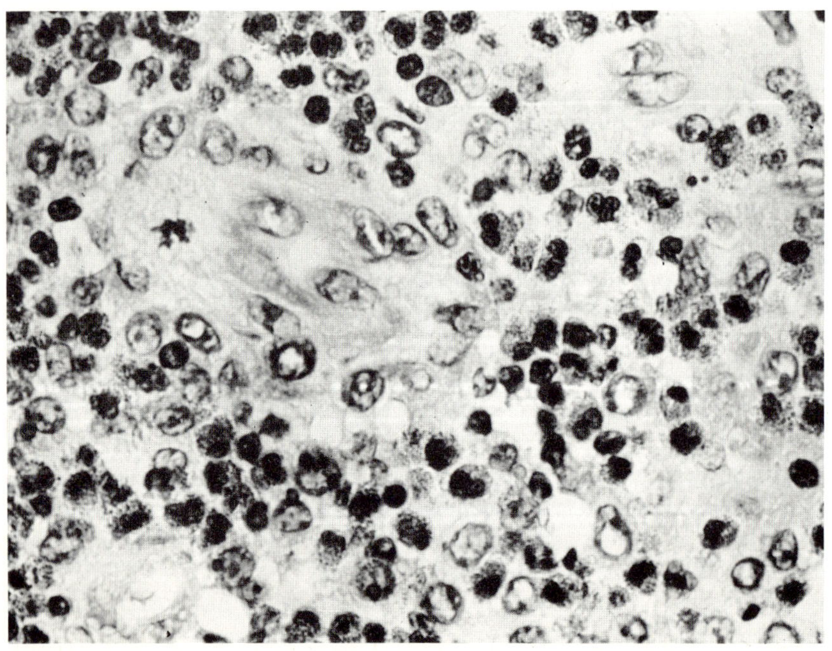

Fig. 8.6. Bone infiltrated by large histiocytes devoid of atypia and showing only rare mitotic figures and by eosinophil leucocytes. Eosinophilic granuloma of bone. ×450.

manifestations of the classical triad—cranial bone granulomas, exophthalmos and diabetes—may not become obvious till late in the disease. The prominent histological features of these lesions are large macrophages laden with cholesterol, and eosinophil leucocytes (Fig. 8.5). These macrophages have been shown with the EM to contain Langerhans granules—similar to those seen in Letterer–Siwe disease (Basket and Nezelof 1970; Imamura and Muroya 1971). At the light microscopic level the cells have much eosinophilic cytoplasm and a round, oval or reniform nucleus. Mitosis may be present.

The prognosis depends on the degree of dissemination. At the benign end of the spectrum, solitary bone lesions often behave in an entirely benign fashion. The prominent histological feature of these lesions is the eosinophil—from which they take their name of eosinophilic granuloma of bone (see review by Cline and Golde 1973). Prominent lymphadenopathy is uncommon (Freund and Ripps 1941).

Eosinophilic granuloma is manifested by isolated, and occasionally multiple, osteolytic lesions, usually in older children and young adults. There is little systemic disturbance though occasionally lung (Engelbreth-Holm et al. 1944) and cutaneous lesions are seen. Histologically the early lesion resembles an inflammatory granuloma. Histiocytic proliferation and eosinophilic infiltration is seen. In later stages the eosinophils disappear and are replaced by 'foam' cells and fibroblasts—fibrosis then becomes extensive. The lesions usually remain localized and may heal spontaneously over 2–3 years (Fig. 8.6).

Gaucher's disease

This is the best known of a group of rare congenital disorders in which due to enzyme defects, sphingolipids accumulate in cells. In most of these disorders—(see Volk et al. 1972 for review) lipid accumulates throughout many organs, including often the CNS; the lymphoreticular system is either spared or not specifically affected. In Gaucher's disease the accumulation is characteristically in lymphoreticular cells; the lesion will accordingly be briefly described here.

The disease often starts in infancy and is characterized by enlargement of spleen and liver and infiltration of these organs with large (20–80 μm) abnormal histiocytes containing abundant delicate interlacing fibrils, which stain with PAS and Sudan Black B, and at the EM level show elongated rod-shaped structures—Gaucher bodies—0.5–3.0 mm long, containing smooth walled tubules. Occasionally Gaucher cells are found in lymph nodes and bone marrow (Fig. 8.7).

In the progressive, invariably fatal form found both in infancy and less often in youth there are in addition disseminated CNS lesions resulting in severe mental deterioration and progressive lesions in many organs including liver,

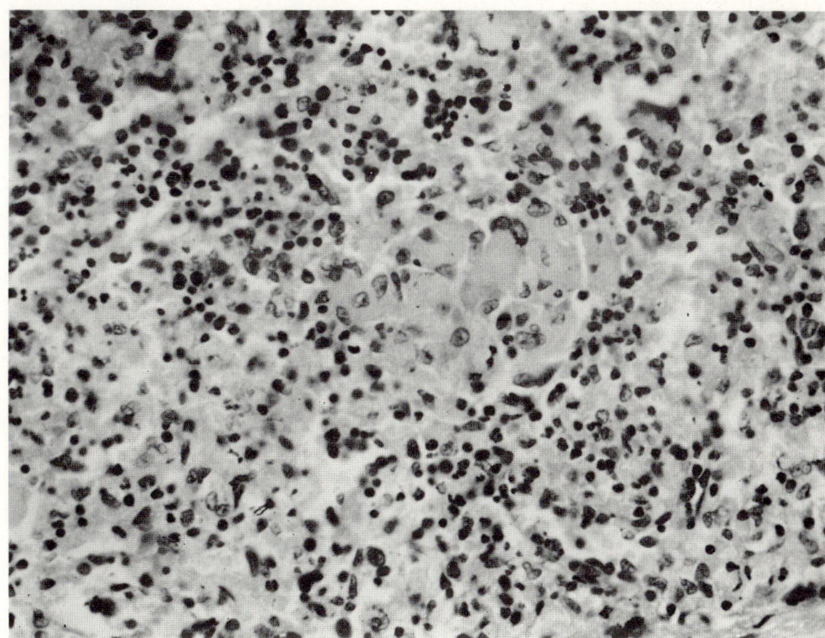

Fig. 8.7. A section of lymph node showing infiltration by large pale mature histiocytes in Gaucher's disease. ×216.

lymph nodes and bone. The prognosis is better if signs of disease develop in later life.

The biochemical lesion is a defect in the enzyme responsible for breaking down glucocerebrosides derived from red cells. Local symptoms respond to low dose radiotherapy; multiple lesions in progressive disease indicate the need for cytotoxic chemotherapy with prolonged follow-up if remission is achieved.

Niemann–Pick disease

A similar enzyme defect leads to diffuse accumulation of sphingomyelin in many organs, among them liver, spleen and lymph nodes where macrophages store the lipid and appear as foam cells in H & E sections. They stain poorly with fat stains such as Sudan III but positively with acid haematin. For full details of this and other rarer storage disorders the review of Volk *et al.* (1972) should be consulted.

The sea-blue histiocyte syndrome

It seems (Sawitsky *et al.* 1954; Silverstein *et al.* 1970; Sawitsky *et al.* 1972; Silverstein and Ellefson 1972), that there is a range of clinical conditions characterized by infiltration of lymphoreticular tissues by cells which stain 'sea-blue' with Romanowsky stains; this has been called the sea-blue histiocyte syndrome.

The syndrome occurs throughout life in a variety of races; the mean age of incidence is 21 years and most patients have an enlarged liver and spleen and less often mild or moderate lymphadenopathy. Other manifestations include streaky pulmonary infiltrates radiologically resembling tuberculosis or sarcoidosis, skin pigmentation, occasionally gut involvement, and sometimes, when the lesion manifests itself in early life, a progressive neurological disorder with ataxia, dementia and epilepsy. Thrombocytopenia is nearly universal, purpura common and massive gastrointestinal bleeding less common. In most patients the disease runs a benign course; much less often, particularly in children and young people, there is progressive pulmonary and hepatic failure and sometimes a progressive neurological disorder. The condition is clearly familial, probably inherited as an autosomal recessive.

The diagnosis is made by identifying large histiocytes or macrophages in the marrow. These cells have a nucleus with fairly dense chromatin and a recognizable nucleolus and the cytoplasm is packed with granules which stain sea-blue (or blue-green) with Wright Giemsa stain; other macrophages have fewer smaller granules in a foamy cytoplasm. The cells do not label *in vitro* with tritiated thymidine; they stain positively with PAS and Sudan Black B, are autofluorescent and probably contain sphingomyelin and glycosphingolipids. It is likely that the hereditary form of sea-blue histiocytosis is a new and distinct lipidosis; the metabolic abnormality involved is uncertain. Increased urinary mucopolysaccharide levels have been noted.

The spleen in the cases examined was large (1 385–1 875 g) and showed foamy histiocytes throughout the red pulp both between and lining sinusoids. Lesions have also been identified in lymph nodes, usually in medullary sinuses and in liver.

Variants of the syndrome have been described. Blankenship *et al.* (1973) recorded 3 siblings with splenomegaly, peripheral neuropathy, cafe-au-lait spots and an elevated serum acid phosphatase. Ghosh (1972) noted the presence of hepatic porphyria in a case of the sea-blue histiocyte syndrome. Rywlin *et al.* (1971) described 'ceroid histiocytosis' of the spleen in a patient with hyperlipoproteinaemia, type 5. The patient had an enlarged spleen showing many macrophages containing 'wax-like' material insoluble in lipid solvent, but staining with Sudan Black B, oil red O and PAS and showing acid fast staining with basic fuchsin and methylene blue.

The syndrome may be a primary entity or may be a non-specific manifestation of a storage disorder, occurring in, e.g. Tay–Sachs disease, Niemann–Pick disease, Gaucher's disease, chronic granulocytic leukaemia, idiopathic thrombocytopenic purpura, sickle cell anaemia and the malabsorption syndrome. Clark and Davidson (1972) point out that lipofuscin accumulates in the marrow in large amounts in patients suffering from illnesses where there is marked fever and leucocytosis. Dosik *et al.* (1972) note that in 10 of a group of 60 patients with chronic granulocytic leukaemia abnormal macrophages are present in the bone marrow which resemble either sea-blue histiocytes or Gaucher cells. They suggest that excessive cell destruction leads to accumulation of an excess of glucocerebroside and sphingomyelin, overloading the enzyme systems available for the destruction of these substances and leading to an accumulation of these substances in macrophages. It now seems likely that the phenomenon is much more often secondary than primary (Varela-Duran *et al.* 1980).

Xanthomatosis

In a number of disorders where there is prolonged elevation of

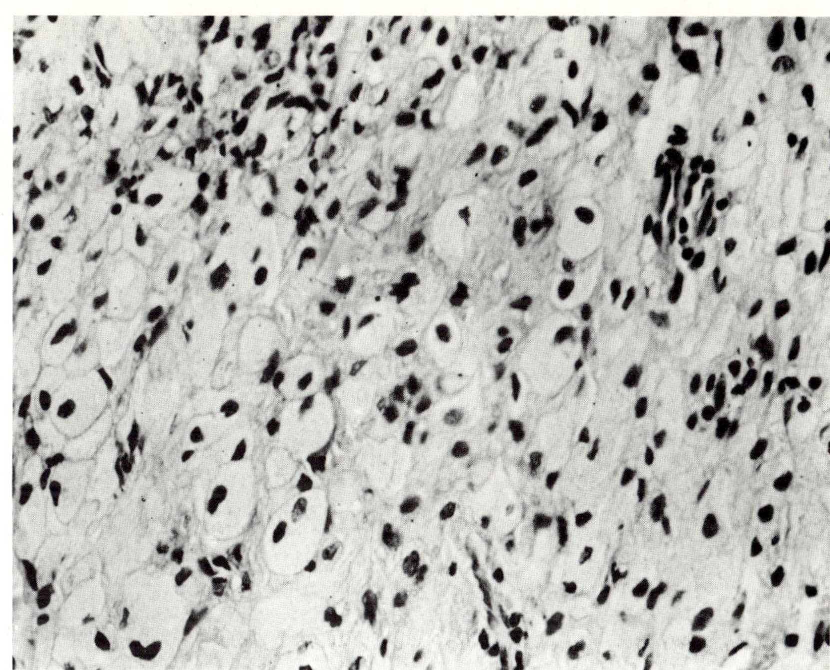

Fig. 8.8. Skin showing the large foamy histiocytes in the skin in cutaneous xanthomatosis. ×216.

plasma lipid levels yellowish plaques are found in the skin, notably of the face and eyelids. These are composed of macrophages heavily laden with Sudanophilic triglyceride lipid and also cholesterol (Fig. 8.8).

Juvenile xanthogranuloma

These are single or multiple reddish papules appearing in the first year of life lasting for a year or two and then regressing. In this lesion there is a dense infiltration of the deeper part of the dermis with small or medium-sized macrophages, usually non-vacuolated but containing some birefringent lipid with a number of lymphocytes and eosinophils and spindle-shaped fibroblasts. Giant cells with a ring of nuclei are prominent (Helwig and Hackney 1954; Mihm *et al.* 1974).

Multicentric reticulohistiocytosis

This condition is characterized by multiple papular brown skin and mucosal lesions and a destructive arthritis. The lesions show numerous large altered mononuclear or multi-nucleate histiocytes with muddy rose-coloured cytoplasm. These are PAS positive, stain for fat and may have a foamy appearance. Interspersed among these are other mixed inflammatory cells. There is commonly a considerable sys-temic upset, with fever, weight loss, and weakness; the disease is one of relapse and remission, and ultimately leaves severe joint deformity (Barrow and Holubar 1969; Mihm *et al.* 1974).

Systemic reactive histiocytosis

This is rare. A febrile illness has recently been described in which viral infection is associated with diffuse histiocytosis—the 'virus-associated hemophagocytic syndrome' of Risdall *et al.* (1979). The patient is usually a child, or renal transplant patient, severely ill, prostrate and febrile. Manifestations include coagulation defects and cytopenia, skin rashes, pulmonary infiltrates and enlargement of liver, spleen and lymph nodes. The associated virus is usually the herpes virus, rarely an adenovirus. The lymph nodes show florid histiocytic hyperplasia and haemophagocytosis without cellular atypia, and there is little destruction of sinusoidal architecture. 13 of 19 patients recovered.

REFERENCES

ABELE D.C. & GRIFFIN J.B. (1972) Histiocytic medullary reticulosis. *Arch. Derm.* **106**, 319–329.
BALLARD J.O., BURDER R.A., RATH C.E. & POWELL D. (1975)

Malignant histiocytosis in a patient presenting with leukocytosis, eosinophilia and lymph node granuloma. *Cancer* **35**, 1444–1448.

BARROW M.V. & HOLUBAR M.D. (1969) Multicentre reticulohistiocytosis. *Medicine* **48**, 287–305.

BASKET E. & NEZELOF C. (1970) Recent progress in the knowledge of histiocytosis. *Arch. Dis. Child.* **45**, 150–151.

BELL R.J.M., BRADFIELD A.J.E., BARNES N.D. & FRANCE N.E. (1968) Familial haemophagocytic reticulosis. *Arch. Dis. Child.* **43**, 601–606.

BLANKENSHIP R.M., GREENBER B.R., LUCAS R.N., REYNOLDS R.D. & BEUTLER E. (1973) Familial sea-blue histiocytes with acid phosphataemia. *J. Amer. Med. Ass.* **225**, 54–56.

BOURONCLE B.A., WISEMAN B.K. & DOAN C.A. (1958) Leukaemic reticuloendotheliosis. *Blood* **13**, 609–630.

BURKE J.S., BYRNE G.E. & RAPPAPORT H. (1974) Hairy cell leukaemia (leukaemic reticuloendotheliosis). *Cancer* **33**, 1399–1410.

CANCILLA P.A., LAHEY M.E. & CARNES W.H. (1967) Cutaneous lesions of Letterer–Siwe disease electron microscopic study. *Cancer* **20**, 1986–1991.

CARBONE A., MICHEAU C., CAILLAUD, J.M. & CARLU C. (1981) A cytochemical and immunohistochemical approach to malignant histiocytosis. *Cancer* **47**, 2862–2871.

CLARK K.G.A. & DAVIDSON W.M. (1972) Bone marrow lipofuscin. *J. Clin. Path.* **25**, 947–950.

CLINE M.J. & GOLDE D.W. (1973) A review and re-evaluation of the histiocytic disorders. *Amer. J. Med.* **55**, 49–60.

DOSIK H., ROSNER F. & SAWITSKY A. (1972) Acquired lipidosis: Gaucher-like cells and blue cells in chronic granulocytic laeukaemia. *Sem. Haemat.* **9**, 309–316.

ENGELBRETH-HOLM J., TEILUM G. & CHRISTENSEN E. (1944) Eosinophil granuloma of bone, Schuller–Christian's disease. *Acta. Med. Scand.* **118**, 292.

EWALD O. (1923) Die leukaemische reticuloendotheliosis. *Deutsche Arch. Klin. Med.* **142**, 222.

FALLETTA J.M., FERNBACH D.J., SINGER D.B., SOUTH M.A., LANDING B.H., HEATH C.W., SHORE N.A. & BARRETT F.F. (1973) A fatal x-linked recessive reticuloendothelial syndrome with hyperglobulinaemia. *J. Pediatr.* **83**, 549–566.

FARBER S. (1952) A lipid metabolic disorder—disseminated 'lipogranulomatosis'—a syndrome with similarity to and important difference from Niemann–Pick and Hand–Schuller–Christian disease. *Amer. J. Dis. Child.* **84**, 499–500.

FARQUAR J.W. & CLAIREAUX A.E. (1952) Familial haemophagocytic reticulosis. *Arch. Dis. Child.* **27**, 519–525.

FORD D.K., PRICE G.E., CULLING C.F. & VASSAR P.S. (1962) Familial lipochrome pigmentation of histiocytes with hyperglobulinaemia, pulmonary infiltration, splenomegaly, arthritis and susceptibility to infection. *Amer. J. Med.* **33**, 478–489.

FREUND M. & RIPPS M.L. (1941) Hand–Schuller–Christian Disease. A case in which lymphadenopathy was a predominant feature. *Amer. J. Dis. Child.* **61**, 759–769.

GHADIALLY F.N. & SKINNIDER L.F. (1972) Ultra-structure of hairy cell leukaemia. *Cancer* **29**, 444–452.

GHOSH ML.L (1972) The sea-blue histiocyte syndrome with hepatic porphyria and infectious mononucleosis. *J. Clin. Path.* **25**, 945–946.

GONELLA J.S. (1967) Mast cell disease. *Prog. Clin. Cancer* **3**, 281–293.

GREEN I., JAFFE E.S., SHERACH E.M., EDELSON R.L., FRANK M.M. & BERARD C.W. (1975) Determination of the origin of malignant reticular cells by the use of surface membrane markers. In Rebuck J.W., Berard C.W. & Abell M.R. (eds.), *The Reticuloendothelial System*, pp. 282–300. Williams and Wilkins, Baltimore.

GROOPMAN J.E. & GOLDE D.W. (1981) The Histiocytic Disorders: A pathophysiologic analysis. *Ann. Int. Med.* **94**, 95–107.

HANCOCK B.W., DANDONA P., CUMBERLAND D.C. & JARRETT J.A. (1976) Systemic mastocytosis, central nervous system features and lymphographic demonstration of lymph node involvement. *Postgrad. Med. J.* **52**, 659–662.

HAND A. (1921) Defects of membranous bones exophthalmos and polyuria in childhood. Is it dyspituitarism? *Amer. J. Med. Sci.* **162**, 509.

HAVARD C.W.H. & BODLEY SCOTT R. (1959) Urticaria pigmentosa with visceral and skeletal lesions. *Quart. J. Med.* **28**, 459–470.

HELWIG E.B. & HACKNEY V.C. (1954) Juvenile xanthogranuloma (nevoxanthoendothelioma). *Amer. J. Path.* **30**, 625.

HORTON J. (1977) The lymphomas—Histiocytosis. In *Clinical Oncology* (Eds Horton J. & Hill G.J.), pp. 709–712. Saunders, Philadelphia.

IMAMURA M. & MUROYA N. (1971) Lymph node ultrastructure in Hand–Schuller–Christian disease. *Cancer* **27**, 956–964.

IMAMURA M., SAKAMOTO S. & HANAZONO H. (1971) Malignant histiocytosis; a case of generalised histiocytosis with infiltration of Langerhans granule-containing histiocytes. *Cancer* **28**, 467–475.

ISAACSON P., WRIGHT D.M., JUDO M.A. & MEPHAM B.L. (1979) Primary gastrointestinal lymphomas. A classification of 66 cases. *Cancer* **43**, 1805–19.

LETTERER E. (1924) Aleukaemische reticulose. *Frankfurt Z. Path.* **30**, 377.

LICHTENSTEIN L. (1964) Histiocytosis X (eosinophilic granuloma of bone, Letterer–Siwe disease and Schuller–Christian disease). *J. Bone Joint Surg.* **46**, 76–90.

LIEBERMAN P.M., JONES C.R., DARGEON H.W.K. & BEGG C.F. (1969) A reappraisal of eosinophilic granuloma of bone, Hand–Schuller–Christian syndrome and Letterer–Siwe syndrome. *Medicine (Baltimore)* **48**, 375–400.

LUCAYA J. (1971) Histiocytosis X. *Amer. J. Dis. Child.* **121**, 289–295.

MARSHALL A.G.E. (1956) Histiocytic medullary reticulosis. *J. Path. Bact.* **71**, 61–71.

MENDELSOHN G., EGGLESTON J.C. & MANN R.B. (1980) Relationship of lysosome (muramidase) to histiocytic differentiation in malignant histiocytosis. An immunohistochemical study. *Cancer* **45**, 273–279.

MIHM M.C., CLARK W.M. & REED R.J. (1974) The histiocytic infiltrates of the skin. *Hum. Path.* **5**, 45–54.

MUNRO D.D., CRAY O. & FEIWEL M. (1969) Lymphangiography in dermatology. *Brit. J. Dermatol.* **81**, 652–660.

NEZELOF C. & ELIACHAR E. (1973) La lyphohistiocytose familiale. Review génerale á propos de trois observations. Liens éventuels avec les syndromes secondaries. *Nouv. Rev. Franç Hemat.* **13**, 319–338.

RISDALL R.J., MCKENNA R.W., NESBIT M.E., KRIVIT W., BALFOUR H.H., SIMMOND R.L. & BRUNNING R.D. (1979) Virus associated hemophagocytic syndrome. A benign histiocytic proliferation distinct from malignant histiocytosis. *Cancer* **44**, 993–1002.

RYWLIN A.M., LOPEZ-GOMEZ A., TACHMES P. & PARDO V. (1971) Ceroid histiocytosis of the spleen in hyperlipemia. *Amer. J. Clin. Path.* **56**, 572–579.

SAGHER F. & EVEN-PAZ Z. (1960) Mastocytosis (Urticaria Pigmentosa). In Bluefarb S.M. (ed.), *Cutaneous Manifestations of Reticulo-endothelial Granulomas*, Chapter 4, pp. 268–436. Charles C. Thomas, Illinois.

SAWITSKY A., HYMAN G.A. & HYMAN J.B. (1954) An unidentified reticuloendothelial cell in bone marrow and spleen. *Blood* **9**, 977–985.

SAWITSKY A., ROSNER F. & CHODSKY S. (1972) The sea blue histiocyte syndrome: A review: genetic and biochemical studies. *Sem. Haematol.* **9**, 285–297.

SCHREK R. & DONNELLY W.J. (1966) 'Hairy cells' in blood in lymphoreticular neoplastic disease and 'flagellated' cells of normal lymph nodes. *Blood* **27**, 199–211.

SCOTT R.B. & ROBB-SMITH A.H.T. (1939) Histiocytic medullary reticulosis. *Lancet* **2**, 194.

SHAHANI R.T. & WARD A.M. (1973) Letterer–Siwe disease in a young adult. *Brit. J. Derm.* **89**, 313–316.

SILVERSTEIN M.D., ELLEFSON R.D. & AHERN E.J. (1970) The syndrome of the sea-blue histiocyte. *N. Engl. J. Med.* **282**, 1–4.

SILVERSTEIN M.N. & ELLEFSON R.D. (1972) The syndrome of the sea-blue histiocyte. *Sem. Haematol.* **9**, 299–307.

SIWE S.A. (1933) Die reticuloendotheliose—ein neues Krankeitbild unter den hepatosplenomegalien. *Z. Kinderheilk.* **55**, 212–247.

VARDMAN J.W., BYRNE G.E. & RAPPAPORT H. (1975) Malignant histiocytosis with massive splenomegaly in asyptomatic patients. A possible chronic form of the disease. *Cancer* **36**, 419–427.

VARELA-DURAN J., ROHOLT P.C. & RATCLIFF N.B. (1980) Sea-blue histiocyte syndrome. A secondary degenerative process of macrophages. *Arch. Path. Lab. Med.* **104**, 30–4.

VOGEL J.M. & VOGEL P. (1972) Idiopathic histiocytosis; A discussion of eosinophilic granuloma, the Hand–Schuller–Christian syndrome, and the Letterer–Siwe syndrome. *Sem. Haematol.* **9**, 349–369.

VOLK B.W., ADAEHI M. & SCHNECK L. (1972) The pathology of sphingolipidoses. *Sem. Haematol.* **9**, 317–348.

WARNKE R.A., KIM H. & DORFMAN R.F. (1975) Malignant histiocytosis (histiocytic medullary reticulosis). 1. Clinicopathologic study of 29 cases. *Cancer* **35**, 215–230.

Leukaemia is a neoplastic proliferation of haemopoietic cells with widespread involvement of the bone marrow, and is usually associated with the presence in the peripheral blood of varying numbers of the abnormal cells. Leukaemic infiltrates may occur in other tissues apart from the bone marrow, and are indeed common, in the early phase of the chronic leukaemias, in the haemopoietic organs such as spleen and lymph nodes. In the past, leukaemic involvement of other tissues was invariably seen during the course of the disease; with the introduction of aggressive therapy this is less common and generally only occurs terminally when all therapies have failed. Conversely, with the new therapies prolonging life, the incidence of leukaemic involvement of the so-called sanctuary areas (such as the central nervous system) is now of major importance. The nature of the extramedullary tissue involved, and the amount of infiltrate depends mainly on the type of leukaemia. The massively enlarged spleen of chronic myeloid leukaemia or 'hairy cell' leukaemia (Bouroncle 1979; Catovsky *et al.* 1974) and the symmetrical lymph node enlargement of chronic lymphocytic leukaemia (Wintrobe 1974) are all part of the well-known and expected physical findings in these diseases. The involvement of other organs is rare, but almost any organ can be involved, and the alert clinician must be aware of these occurrences to explain unusual symptoms arising in the course of the disease.

The organs involved in leukaemia can be considered under:

1 the haemopoietic organs, which are invariably involved to some degree (the spleen, liver and lymph nodes)

2 the pharmacological sanctuary sites, particularly the central nervous system

3 other organs, which are usually involved only later in the disease and when, but not always, the leukaemic cell mass is great.

1 HAEMOPOIETIC ORGANS

Spleen

The spleen is invariably involved in the chronic leukaemias (Wintrobe 1974) and is often massive in chronic granulocytic leukaemia and hairy cell leukaemia (Wintrobe 1974; Bouroncle 1979; Catovsky *et al.* 1974) (Fig. 9.1). The organ is symmetrically involved with a diffuse infiltrate so that its normal shape is preserved. In chronic granulocytic leukaemia the reported incidence of splenomegaly at time of diagnosis varies from 40% to 70% (Wintrobe 1974). Increasing splenomegaly generally parallels increasing peripheral white cell counts, and reduction in spleen size follows therapy. In uncontrolled chronic myeloid leukaemia the spleen reaches massive size, with average weights of 1500 g (Amromin 1968) and 1696 g (Krumbhaar and Stengel 1942) being reported in autopsy studies. Myeloid metaplasia is prominent in this condition and the splenic pulp contains large numbers of mature and immature cells of the granulocyte series. Infarction of the spleen is common (Krumbhaar and Stengel 1942) and in advanced cases fibrosis may be seen. In chronic myelomonocytic or chronic monocytic leukaemia splenomegaly is not so marked (Miescher and Farquet 1974; Geary *et al.* 1975; Skinnider *et al.* 1977). In chronic lymphocytic leukaemia the presence of splenomegaly, usually associated with lymphadenopathy, at the time of diagnosis is an important prognostic indicator. Rai *et al.* (1975) reported a 71 months median survival time with splenomegaly with or without lymphadenopathy (Stage 2) compared with 150 months with no splenomegaly or lymphadenopathy (Stage 0). Binet *et al.* (1977) identified a small group (8 patients) with an excellent prognosis; these patients had splenomegaly without peripheral lymphadenopathy. This, however, is not in keeping with other studies (Galton *et al.* 1974) and in our review of 745 cases, there were 35 cases of splenomegaly without lymphadenopathy where the median survival was 6.6 years (Skinnider *et al.* 1982). Splenomegaly is a prominent feature of hairy cell leukaemia (Bouroncle 1979; Catovsky *et al.* 1974)

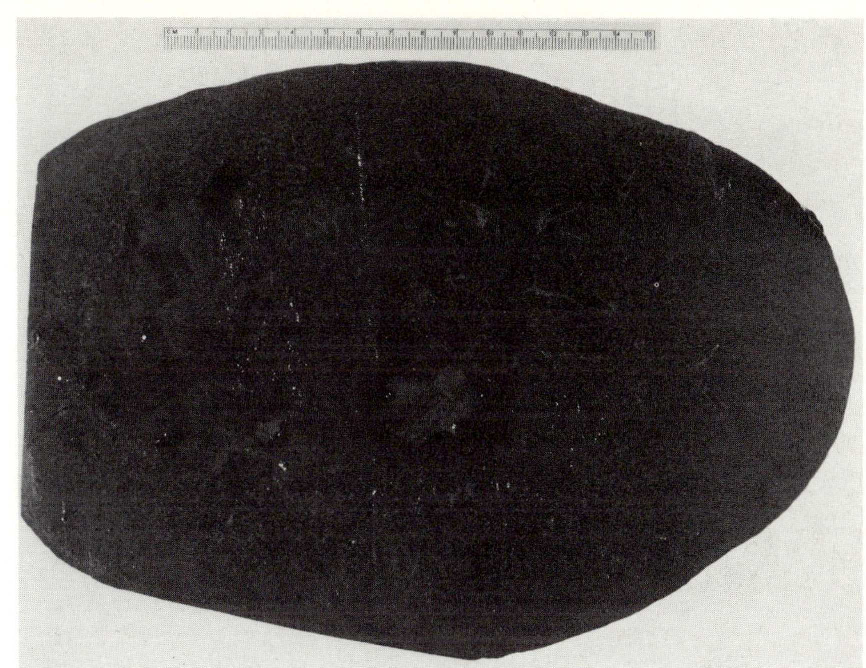

Fig. 9.1. Massively enlarged spleen weighing 3614 g from a 43-year-old lady with 'hairy' cell leukaemia who presented with pancytopenia and splenomegaly.

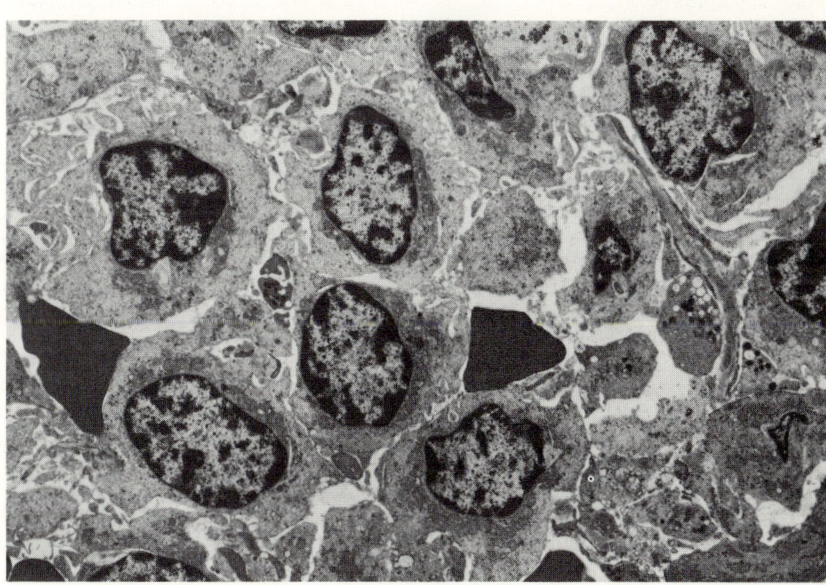

Fig. 9.2. Electron micrograph of packed cells in the spleen of a 55-year-old male with 'hairy' cell leukaemia. × 3280.

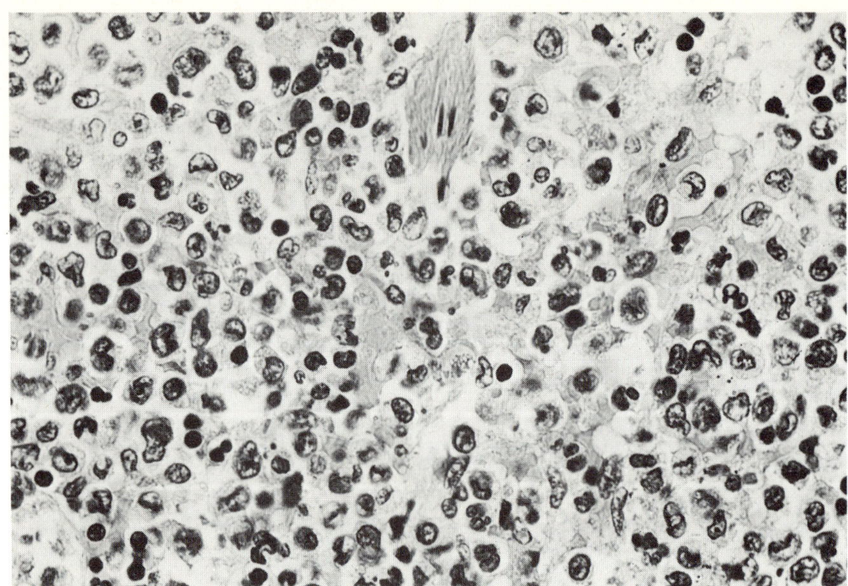

Fig. 9.3. Splenic infiltration throughout the pulp both within and outside the sinusoids in acute myelomonocytic leukaemia in a 56-year-old female. × 328.

and often the diagnosis in this condition is first made by splenectomy (Fig. 9.2) in cases of pancytopenia and spleno-megaly, especially when the typical hairy cells are absent or have been missed in the peripheral blood. The cellular morphology is sufficiently different from chronic lymphocytic leukaemia to allow a diagnosis to be made and the presence of tartrate-resistant acid phosphatase in the leukaemic cells generally confirms the diagnosis (Katayama and Yang 1977; Janckila *et al.* 1978).

Early in the acute leukaemias splenomegaly is not a prominent feature (Gunz and Baikie 1974), although it may be seen in acute lymphoblastic leukaemia and, if marked, is associated with a poorer prognosis (Simone 1975). Infiltration in myeloid leukaemias is generally throughout the pulp, both intra and extrasinusoidal (Fig. 9.3), capsular invasion is often present and haemorrhage from associated thrombocytopenia may be an accompanying feature. In the acute monocytic leukaemias which may supervene on malignant histiocytosis, splenomegaly is prominent (Byrne and Rappaport 1973).

Liver

Like the spleen, significant involvement of this organ is seen in the chronic leukaemias. Involvement is diffuse and the liver retains its normal shape and smooth appearance. In chronic myeloid leukaemia, infiltration of the cells occurs in the sinusoids, while in chronic lymphocytic leukaemia, it is characteristically in and around the portal tracts. Involvement of the liver is usually minimal in the early stages of acute leukaemia. The association of a sinusoidal involvement in acute myeloid leukaemia (Fig. 9.4) and a predominantly portal tract infiltration in acute lymphoblastic leukaemia generally holds true, but is not as clear as in the chronic leukaemias (Gunz and Baikie 1974). Infiltration may be massive (Fig. 9.5) and cause liver necrosis and resulting abnormal liver function tests. Liver enlargement at time of diagnosis in acute lymphoblastic leukaemia in childhood is a poor prognostic sign (Simone 1975).

Lymph nodes

If lymph node enlargement is present in a leukaemia it is most likely a lymphatic leukaemia, although involvement of lymph nodes can occur in granulocytic leukaemia, either acute or chronic. Significant lymphadenopathy is seen in chronic lymphocytic leukaemia where symmetrical enlargement of the lymph nodes is a common clinical finding. Out of 745 cases of chronic lymphocytic leukaemia in our study (Skinnider *et al.* 1982) 70% had enlarged lymph nodes at the time of diagnosis. The pattern of involvement is usually symmetrical and this may help to distinguish cases of diffuse well-differentiated lymphocytic lymphoma where involvement may be quite focal. Microscopically, one sees the normal architecture replaced by a diffuse infiltrate of generally

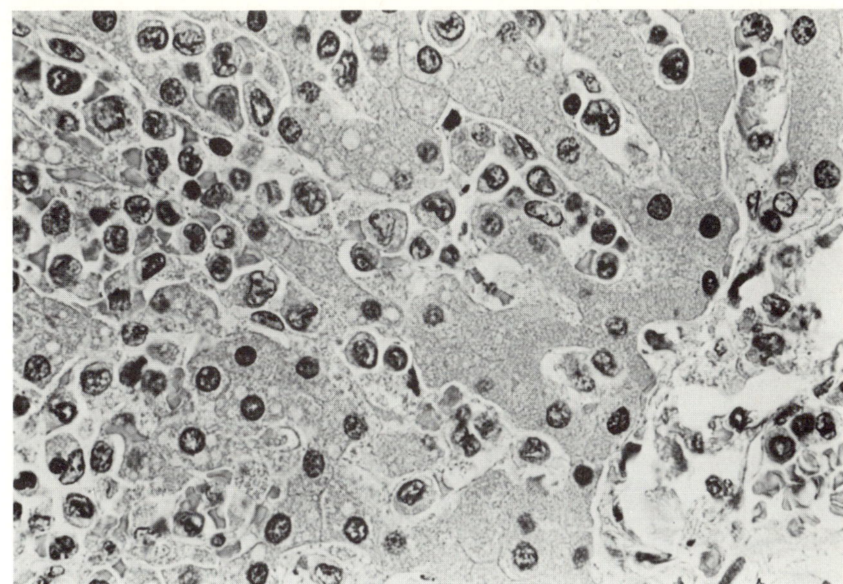

Fig. 9.4. Sinusoidal infiltrate of liver seen in acute myelogenous leukaemia. × 523.

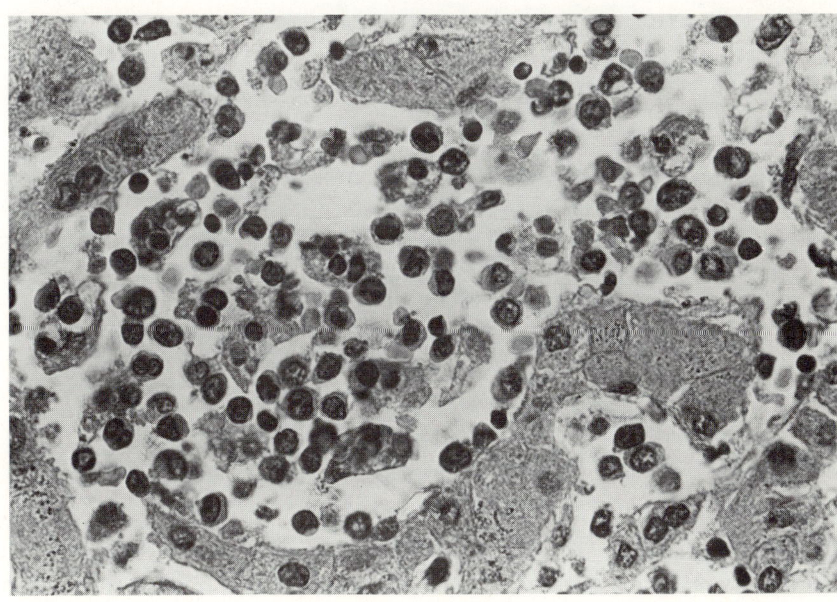

Fig. 9.5. Degeneration and necrosis of hepatic cells caused by massive accumulation of blasts in acute myelogenous leukaemia. × 533.

well-differentiated lymphocytes, while in granulocytic leuk-aemias the primary follicles persist with the leukaemic infiltrate mainly in the sinusoids and interfollicular area. In considering leukaemic involvement of lymph nodes one must also remember that certain types of lymphoma are particularly prone to develop a leukaemic phase. This is especially so in lymphomas occurring in the younger age group. Bone marrow involvement with spill into the peripheral blood is found in a considerable percentage of Burkitt's lymphoma, and the lymphoblastic lymphoma (T cell type) of the mediastinum is notorious for this evolution (Hausner *et al.* 1977).

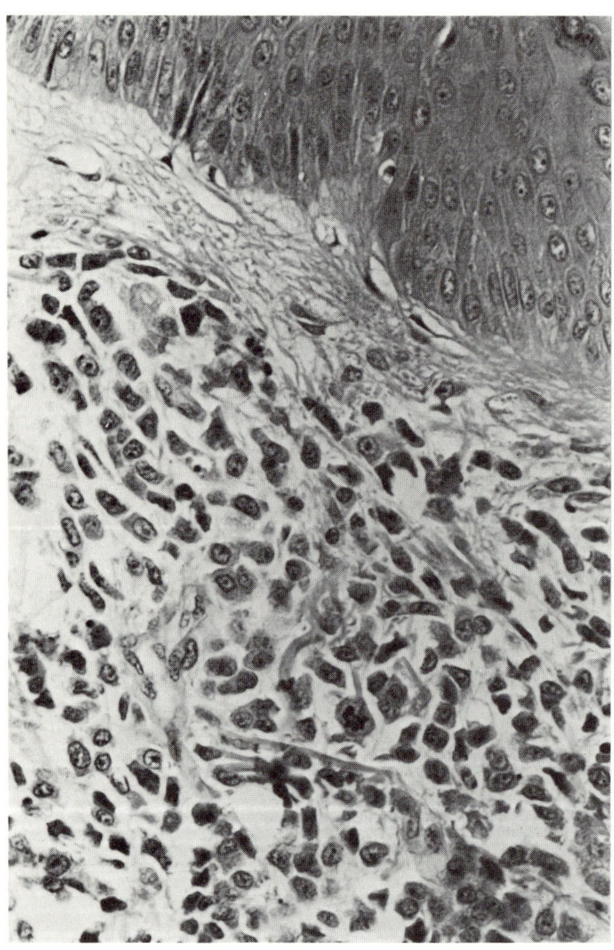

Fig. 9.6. Infiltration of the dermis by histiocytic cells in a woman in whom acute monocytic leukaemia became manifest four months later. At the time of the skin biopsy the peripheral blood was normal and the marrow did not show evidence of leukaemia. ×405.

Other extramedullary sites

By and large leukaemic infiltrations in other tissues were seen frequently in the past as the disease progressed inexorably towards its end. One exception is the skin manifestations in acute monocytic leukaemia (Schilling type) where extramedullary infiltrates may antedate obvious marrow or peripheral blood involvement (Fig. 9.6). As therapy in those days was generally ineffective this involvement did not pose any special management problem. With the introduction of the newer chemotherapeutic regimens for acute lymphoblastic and adult acute non-lymphoblastic leukaemias soft tissue infiltrates are much less common and usually occur in situations where relapse and resistance to therapy has occurred.

2 PHARMACOLOGICAL SANCTUARY SITES

The important exceptions to the above are the so-called 'pharmacological sanctuary' sites where leukaemic blasts may appear even though the patient is in complete haematological remission. The most important site for this type of recurrence is the central nervous system, but it occasionally occurs in the ovary or testis. Relapse in the lymph nodes and the bone have been reported while the bone marrow was in remission but in both cases within one month marrow relapse was already evident (Hustu and Aur 1978). It is the type of infiltrate occurring in the 'sanctuary' sites that is of tremendous clinical importance and is worthy of more detailed discussion. The other types of infiltrate usually seen in advanced and resistant disease are of more academic interest. They do not alter the prognosis, nor do they require any different treatment apart from perhaps local radiotherapy for symptomatic relief.

Central nervous system

Even prior to modern chemotherapy the CNS was one of the commonest sites of extramedullary involvement. Incidences of 50–70% have been reported in acute lymphoblastic leukaemia (Evans 1964; Evans *et al.* 1970; Haghbin and Zuelzer 1965; West *et al.* 1972). In the older literature, autopsy findings (Schwab and Weiss 1935; Leidler and Russell 1945) showed meningeal involvement of the cerebral hemispheres, basal ganglia, brain stem and cerebellum to be most common, involvement of the spinal cord less so. Cranial

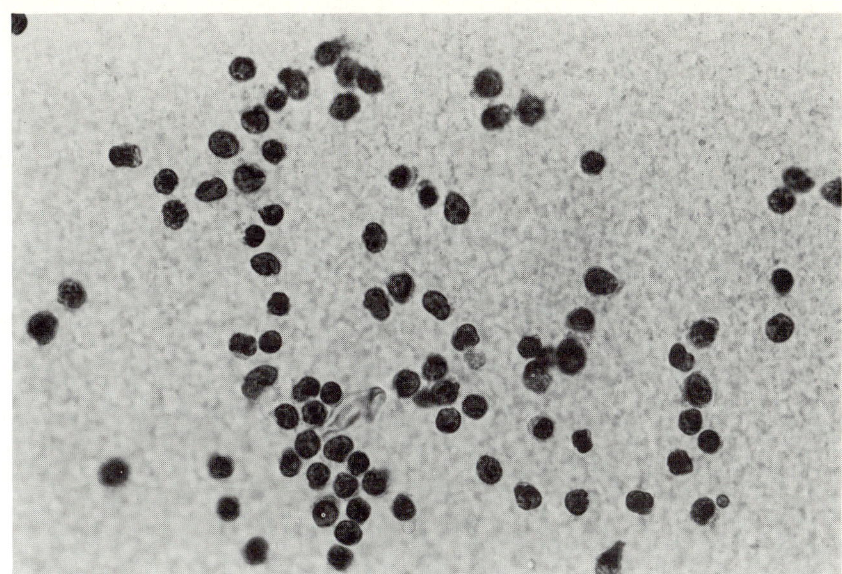

Fig. 9.7. Blast cells in the cerebrospinal fluid of a 6-year-old boy presenting with headache and vomiting 20 months after remission of acute lymphoblastic leukaemia. The CSF was aspirated onto a Nucleopore filter and stained with H&E. ×541.

nerves were affected more frequently than spinal nerves (Phair *et al.* 1964). Previously CNS leukaemia was diagnosed only when neurological signs and symptoms developed, but now the diagnostic criterion is the presence of excessive numbers of blasts in the cerebrospinal fluid (Nies *et al.* 1965). With the advent of prolonged remissions with chemotherapy the incidence of CNS involvement increased, and occurred often when the child was still in complete haematological remission (Hardisty and Norman 1967).

The implications, treatment and prophylaxis of this complication have been reviewed by Hustu and Aur (1978). Without prophylactic treatment, the likelihood of a CNS relapse is greater in those patients with high peripheral blast counts (George *et al.* 1968; Melhorn *et al.* 1970), and also the CNS relapse occurs within a shorter period of time (6.5 months with peripheral counts >20,000/cmm as against 18 months with counts <20,000/cmm (Hustu and Aur 1978)). With prophylactic treatment the frequency of CNS relapse is the same regardless of the initial peripheral blast count, but if CNS relapse does occur it does so within shorter time with the higher counts (Hustu and Aur 1978). The diagnosis depends on identification of blasts in the CSF. This can be done by examining a film prepared from a centrifuged specimen (a Shandon Cytocentrifuge is a suitable machine) or by passing the CSF through a small filter (Millipore or Nucleopore) (Kline 1962; Wertlake *et al.* 1972) (Fig. 9.7). Aspiration onto a filter can be done at the time of lumbar puncture by attaching a Swinney filter to the aspirating syringe (Burechailo and Cunningham 1974). The blasts can easily be identified by this method.

Testicular and ovarian leukaemia

Leukaemic involvement of the gonads is frequent in advanced disease. At autopsy testicular involvement has varied 29–92% (Sullivan and Hrgovic 1973; Haggar *et al.* 1969) and ovarian involvement has been reported at 24% (Sullivan and Hrgovic 1973). In Hustu's (1978) series testicular involvement at autopsy was 53.3% and ovarian involvement was 30 per cent. More recently testicular involvement appears to be occurring with increased frequency and appears to be related to the increased survival times. It now occurs often while the patient is in haematological remission (Fig. 9.8), and a good percentage have never had a previous relapse (Stoffel *et al.* 1975; Kuo *et al.* 1976). This, of course, raises the question of prophylactic treatment of the gonads, but most centres balk at preventive irradiation of these organs.

3 OTHER ORGANS

Involvement of other extramedullary sites does not occur while the patient is in haematological remission and thus it is

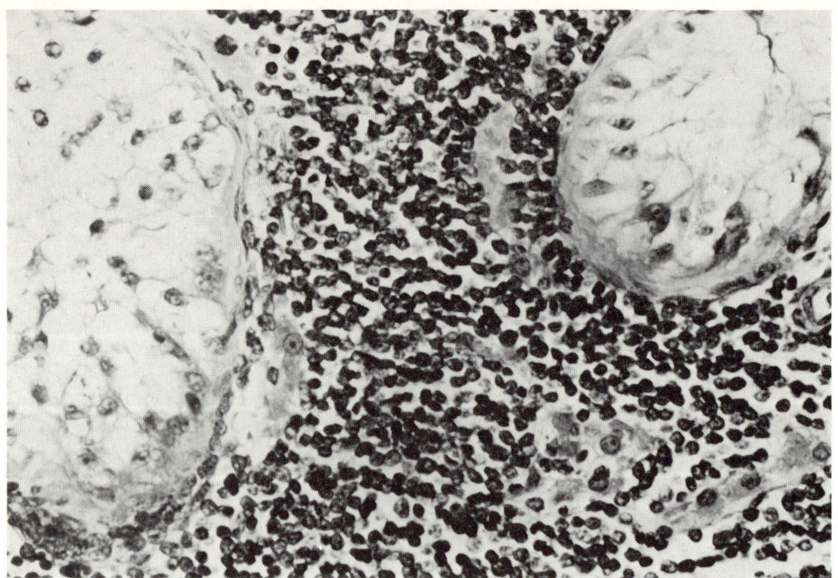

Fig. 9.8. Section from a testicular biopsy from a 10-year-old boy who had been treated for acute lymphoblastic leukaemia 2 years previously. He was still in haematological remission but the section shows a massive infiltrate of acute leukaemia blast cells. × 328.

usually only seen occasionally at presentation, or in advanced or resistant disease. Infiltration of other organs is commonly found at autopsy where the leukaemia has been out of control for some time with very high peripheral counts. This is to be expected when one considers the mass of leukaemic blasts to be at 10^{12} or 10^{13} cells. Where the patient has died during aggressive chemotherapy leukaemic cells may be considerably diminished. The nature of involvement and percentage of cases found involved at autopsy are reviewed by Amromin (1968). This type of involvement is generally of little importance in the management of the patient but a few exceptions to this rule should be noted, where involvement of tissues at the initial presentation of the disease may provide valuable clinical signs and symptoms. These tissues are the skin, bones and joints. Involvement of the lung, particularly in chronic lymphocytic leukaemia, may also cause clinical problems during the course of the disease.

Skin

Occasionally skin lesions may present as the first sign of disease and there may even be some time between the skin lesion and the development of the classical bone marrow and peripheral blood involvement (See Fig. 9.6). This type of presentation usually occurs only with acute monocytic leukaemia. These cases present problems in management as initially they may be diagnosed and treated as a localised lymphoma. Skin lesions are also common during the course of monocytic and other leukaemias, especially lymphocytic (Javier *et al.* 1967). The lesions vary considerably in appearance and may be localised or generalised. They must be distinguished from skin rashes associated with leukaemia which are also quite common and which include generalised pruritus, scaly lichenoid lesions and exfoliative dermatitis (Davies 1955). The solid leukaemic lesions may be dermal or in the subcutaneous tissue, and may be quite large. We have noticed cutaneous leukaemic infiltrates at the sites of intravenous infusions in the brachial and neck veins.

Mouth

Lesions in the mouth and throat are usually ulcerative and infective and are the results of the neutropenia from the disease itself or from the chemotherapy (Epstein and MacEachern 1937). Fungal opportunistic infection is common. Leukaemic lesions *per se* are also seen, and the gingival hypertrophy due to leukaemic infiltration occurs most frequently in acute monocytic leukaemia. It should be noted, however, that gingival hypertrophy may also occur as a result of infection alone (Gunz and Baikie 1974).

Bones and joints

Lesions in the bones and joints at time of presentation of the

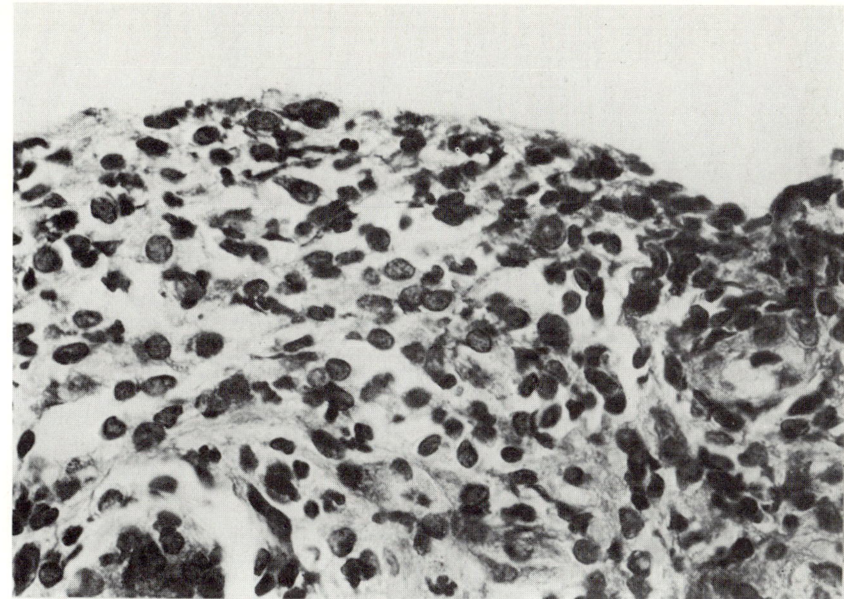

Fig. 9.9. Biopsy from synovial membrane from the elbow joint of a 69-year-old man showing infiltrate with numerous blast cells. His presenting symptom was severe joint pain in right elbow with a leucocytosis of 36000. × 533.

disease are commoner in children, but can occur in adults (Gunz and Baikie 1974). As they are often part of the presenting symptoms and may simulate other diseases such as rheumatic fever (Duffy and Driscoll 1958) bone infiltrates are more important clinically than other sites, apart from the CNS and testis or ovary. In children, bone and joint pains are a frequent part of the initial symptoms and the radiological appearance provides valuable diagnostic features (Poynton and Lightwood 1932; Baty and Vogt 1935). Radiological changes have been reported in two thirds of cases; the changes are of several types and consist of:

1 transverse lines of lessened density at the metaphyseal end of the long bones. Above the age of two they are very suggestive of acute leukaemia (Baty and Vogt 1935)

2 subperiosteal new bone formation found mainly in the long bones and due to the leukaemic infiltrate elevating the periosteal layer. This is quite common (Willson 1959)

3 osteolytic lesions seen early in the disease, generalised osteoporosis tends to occur later and may be partly related to steroid therapy (Amromin 1968)

4 osteosclerotic lesions which are much rarer (Kellerhouse and Limarzi 1965).

The above varieties of lesions are more common in the acute lymphoblastic leukaemia in children but can occur also in the adult acute non-lymphoblastic type. When osteolytic lesions do occur in the adult variety, one must remember that

occasionally multiple myeloma and adult acute leukaemia can present together (Videbaek 1971). With chronic leukaemias osteosclerosis may occur when myelofibrosis supervenes during the course of chronic myeloid leukaemia (Wintrobe 1974); bone lesions are rare. The joints are occasionally involved in acute leukaemia and symptoms related to them may form part of the presenting picture, the patient actually presenting with arthritis. This is illustrated by the following case of a 69-year-old man who was referred to a rheumatology clinic with severe joint pain in the right elbow and forearm, of three weeks duration. The elbow joint was swollen and red. Laboratory data was as follows—Hb 12.1 g/dl, WBC 36000/cmm, the differential count showed a granulocytosis with a marked shift to the left but the most striking feature was an absolute monocytosis of 5300/cmm. Synovial biopsy showed a leukaemic infiltrate (Fig. 9.9). The joint fluid however contained mainly granulocytes. Bone marrow examination confirmed the diagnosis of myelomonocytic leukaemia.

Lung

As with other organs leukaemic infiltrates are common in advanced cases and have been found at autopsy in 27–62% of cases (Green and Nichols 1959; Bodey *et al.* 1966) (Fig. 9.10). Occasionally some of the presenting symptoms are related to

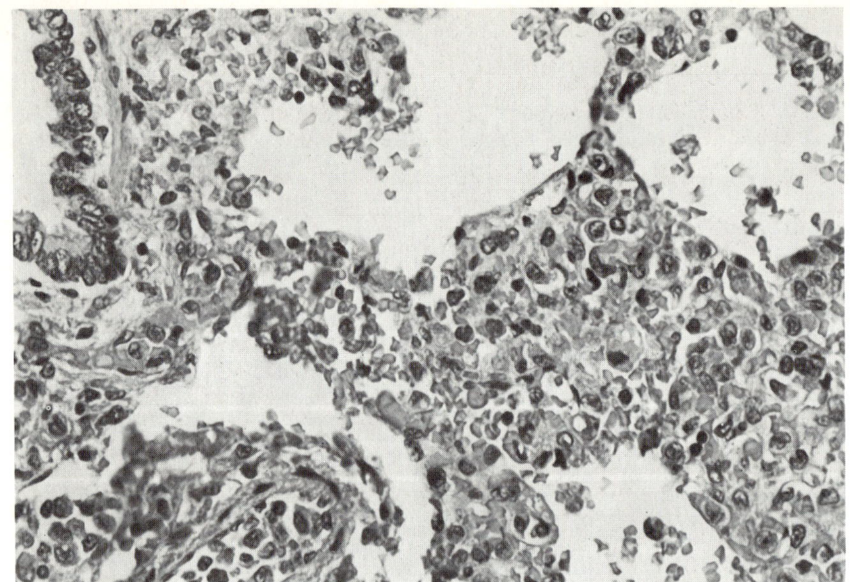

Fig. 9.10. Leukaemic infiltrate in the lung of an infant with acute undifferentiated leukaemia. × 328.

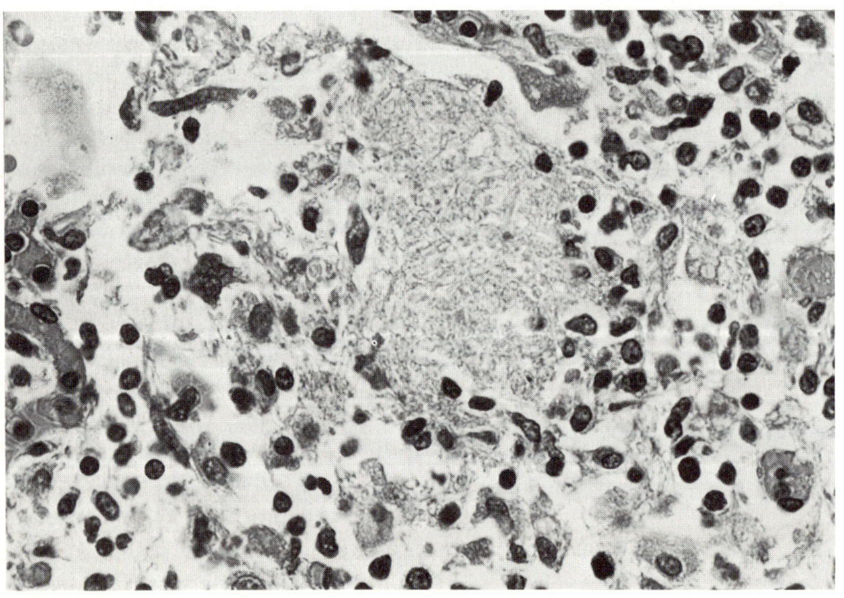

Fig. 9.11. Section of lung biopsy from a 65-year-old patient with chronic lymphocytic leukaemia treated with prednisone and chlorambucil for 6 months. The patient had increasing dyspnoea, slight fever and X-ray showed infiltrates throughout both lung fields. Section shows infiltrate of small well differentiated lymphocytes with intra-alveolar, eosinophilic amorphous material on H&E section. × 533.

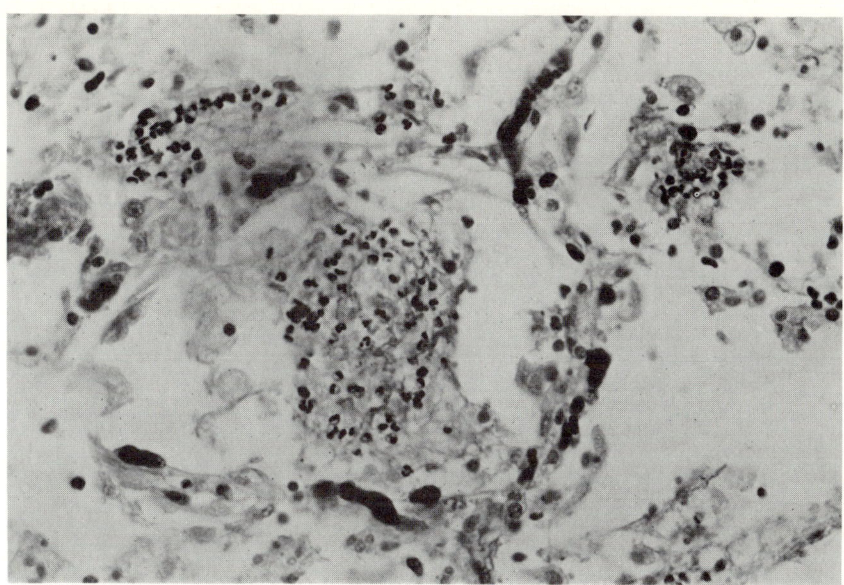

Fig. 9.12. Section from same case as Fig. 9.11 stained with methenamine silver showing *Pneumocystis carinii* (arrows). × 390.

lung involvement, and in one unusual case following an unsatisfactory marrow interpretation in a child with pancytopenia and an abnormal chest X-ray, a lung biopsy was performed and the diagnosis was made in this manner. Pulmonary infiltrates occurring during the course of leukaemias, whether acute or chronic present some diagnostic problems. The infiltrates may derive from the leukaemic cells; this occurs in the acute leukaemias and in chronic lymphocytic leukaemia and requires special management, particularly in the latter condition. It must be remembered, however, that certain types of chemotherapy cause lung damage with resultant symptoms and radiological changes in the lung (Green 1977; Sostman *et al.* 1977). Bleomycin has a specific lung toxicity (DeLena *et al.* 1972; Aso *et al.* 1976) and busulphan used in chronic granulocytic leukaemia may also cause lung damage (Podoll and Winkler 1974); chlorambucil (Rose 1973) and melphalan (Taetle *et al.* 1978) are less often implicated. Lastly, leukaemic patients on chemotherapy are prone to opportunistic lung infection, fungi and *Pneumocystis carinii*; these may prove difficult to diagnose (Masur and Jones 1980). Thus when pulmonary symptoms arise and infiltrates are evident radiologically, thorough investigation, often including lung biopsy, is necessary before a correct diagnosis can be reached (Figs 9.11 and 9.12).

Other tissues

As previously indicated any organ in the body can be involved with leukaemic infiltrates, and where the mass of leukaemic cells is high, as is seen in terminal cases resistant to treatment, leukaemic infiltrates are widespread. Occasionally they may give rise to symptoms in the gastrointestinal tract (Fig. 9.13). However, symptoms and complications are more likely to arise from the chemotherapy rather than leukaemic infiltrates *per se* (Cornes *et al.* 1961; Prolla and Kirsner 1964). Cardiac signs and symptoms such as heart block have sometimes been attributed to leukaemic infiltrates (Aronson and Leroy 1947; Bregnani and Perrotta 1960) but again it is difficult to know whether other causes, such as infection and microabscesses (Roberts *et al.* 1968) or chemotherapy such as adriamycin (Young *et al.* 1981), may be the underlying factor. Renal involvement is seen commonly at autopsy (Norris and Wiener 1961) but does not usually present any specific therapeutic problem.

Ocular manifestations may be due to the leukaemic infiltrates themselves and may involve the retina, choroid, conjunctiva and ocular muscles (Ridgway *et al.* 1976; Murray *et al.* 1977). However, many ophthalmic symptoms and signs are related to haemorrhages from thrombocytopenia; papilloedema is usually related to central nervous system infiltration and meningeal leukaemia.

Considering the nature of the leukaemic cell, its evident loss of adhesiveness and its circulation by the blood throughout the entire body, it is not surprising that extramedullary leukaemic infiltrates are common. The infiltrates, however, are generally diffuse, and solitary solid tumour masses are

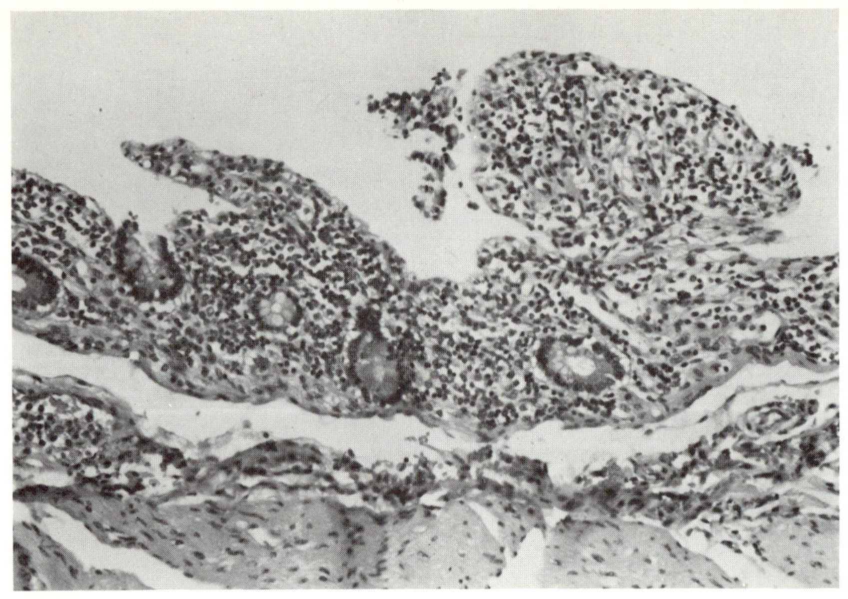

Fig. 9.13. Sections from the small bowel of a patient with acute myelomonocytic leukaemia showing infiltration of the mucosa and submucosa with leukaemic blast cells. × 144.

relatively rare. At present their main significance is limited to involvement of the sanctuary sites in acute lymphoblastic leukaemia in children, but as treatment of adult leukaemia improves, this type of involvement is also likely to assume great clinical importance.

REFERENCES

Amromin G.D. (1968) *Pathology of Leukemia*. Hoeber. New York.

Aronson S.F. & Leroy E. (1947) Electrocardiographic findings in leukemia. *Blood* **2**, 356–62.

Aso Y., Yoneda K. & Kikkawa Y. (1976) Morphologic and biochemical study of pulmonary changes induced by bleomycin in mice. *Lab. Invest.* **35**, 558–68.

Baty J.M. & Vogt E.C. (1935) Bone changes of leukemia in children. *Am. J. Roentgenol.* **34**, 310–14.

Binet J.L., Leporrier M., Dighiero G., Charron D., D'Athis P., Vaugier G., Beral H.M., Natali J.C., Raphael M., Nizet B. & Follezon J.V. (1977) A clinical staging system for chronic lymphocytic leukemia. *Cancer* **40**, 855–64.

Bodey G.P., Powell R.D. Jr., Hersh E.M., Yeterian A. & Freireich E.J. (1966) Pulmonary complications of acute leukemia. *Cancer* **19**, 781–93.

Bouroncle B.A. (1979) Leukemic reticuloendotheliosis (hairy cell leukaemia). *Blood* **53**, 412–36.

Bregnani P. & Perrotta P. (1960) The heart in leukemia. Clinical and electrocardiographic aspects. *Folia Cardiol.* **19**, 193–207.

Burechailo F. & Cunningham I.A. (1974) Counting cells in cerebrospinal fluid collected directly on membrane filters. *J. Clin. Path.* **27**, 101–5.

Byrne G.E. & Rappaport H. (1973) *Malignant Histiocytosis in Malignant Diseases of the Hematopoietic System*, Gann Monograph No. 5, University Park Press, Baltimore.

Catovsky D., Petit J.E., Galton D.A.G., Spiers A.S.D. & Harrison C.V. (1974) Leukaemic reticuloendotheliosis (hairy cell leukemia): a distinct clinico-pathological entity. *Br. J. Haematol.* **26**, 9–27.

Cornes J.S., Jones J.G. & Fisher G.B. (1961) Gastroduodenal ulcerations and massive hemorrhage in patients with leukemia, multiple myeloma and malignant tumors of lymphoid tissue. *Gastroenterology* **41**, 337–334.

Davies J.H.T. (1955) Dermatological aspects of blood diseases. In *Modern Trends in Blood Diseases*, p. 66 (ed. Wilkinson J.F.) Hoeber, New York.

DeLena M., Guzzow A., Monfardini S. & Bonadonna G. (1972) Clinical, radiologic and histopathologic studies on pulmonary toxicity induced by treatment with bleomycin. *Cancer Chemother. Rep.* **56**, 343–355.

Duffy J.H. & Driscoll E.J. (1958) Oral manifestations of leukemia. *Oral Surg.* **11**, 484–90.

Epstein E. & MacEachern K. (1937) Dermatologic manifestations of the lymphoblastoma—leukemia group. *Arch. Intern. Med.* **60**, 867–875.

Evans A.A., Gilbert E.S. & Zandstra R. (1970) The increasing incidence of central nervous system leukemia in children. *Cancer* **26**, 404–409.

Evans A.E. (1964) Central nervous system involvement in children with acute leukemia. A study of 921 patients. *Cancer* **17**, 256–8.

Galton D.A.G., Goldman J.M., Wiltshaw E., Catovsky D., Henry K. & Goldenberg G.J. (1974) Prolymphocytic leukemia. *Br. J. Haematol.* **27**, 7–23.

Geary C.G., Catovsky D., Wiltshaw E., Milner G.R., Scholes M.C., Van Noorden S., Wadsworth L.D., Muldal S.,

MacIver J.E. & Galton D.A.G. (1975) Chronic myelomonocytic leukaemia. *Br. J. Haematol.* **30**, 289–302.

George P., Hernandez K., Hustu H.O., Borella L., Holton C. & Pinkel D. (1968) A study of total therapy of acute lymphocytic leukemia in children. *J. Ped.* **72**, 399–408.

Green M.R. (1977) Pulmonary toxicity of antineoplastic agents. *West. J. Med.* **127**, 292–8.

Green R.A. & Nichols N.J. (1959) Pulmonary involvement in leukemia. *Am. Rev. Resp. Dis.* **80**, 833.

Gunz F. & Baikie A.G. (1974) *Leukemia* (3rd edn). Grune and Stratton, New York.

Haggar R.A., MacMillan A.B. & Thompson D.G. (1969) Leukemic infiltration of testis. *Can. J. Surg.* **12**, 197–201.

Haghbin M. & Zuelzer W.W. (1965) A long-term study of cerebrospinal leukemia. *J. Ped.* **67**, 23–28.

Hardisty R.M. & Norman P.M. (1967) Meningeal leukemia. *Arch. Dis. in Childhood* **42**, 441–447.

Hausner R.J., Rosas-Uribe A., Wickstrum D.A. & Smith P.C. (1977) Non-Hodgkin's lymphoma in the first two decades of life. *Cancer* **40**, 1533–1547.

Hustu H.O. & Aur R.J.A. (1978) Extramedullary leukemia. In *Clinics in Hematology*, Vol. 7, pp. 313–337 (ed. Simone J.V.) W.B. Saunders Ltd., London.

Janckila A.J., Li C.Y., Lam K.W. & Yam L.T. (1978) The cytochemistry of tartrate-resistant acid phosphatase. *Am. J. Clin. Path.* **70**, 45–55.

Javier B.V., Yount W.J., Crosby D.J. & Hall T.C. (1967) Cardiac metastases in lymphoma and leukemia. *Dis. Chest* **52**, 481–4.

Katayama I. & Yang J.P.S. (1977) Reassessment of a cytochemical test for differential diagnosis of leukemic reticuloendotheliosis. *Am. J. Clin. Path.* **68**, 268–273.

Kellerhouse L. & Limarzi L.R. (1965) Bone manifestations of hematologic disorders. *Med. Clin. N. Amer.* **49**, 203–228.

Kline T.S. (1962) Cytological examination of the cerebrospinal fluid. *Cancer* **15**, 591–597.

Krumbhaar E.B. & Stengel A. (1942) The spleen in the leukemias. *Arch. Pathol.* **34**, 117–132.

Kuo T., Tschang T. & Chu J. (1976) Testicular relapse in childhood acute lymphocytic leukemia during bone marrow remission. *Cancer* **38**, 2604–2612.

Leidler F. & Russell W.O. (1945) The brain in leukemia. *Arch. Pathol.* **40**, 14–33.

Masur H. & Jones T.C. (1980) Protozoal and helminthic infections. In *Infections in the Abnormal Host*, pp. 414–18 (ed. Grieco M.H.) Yorke Medical Books, United States.

Melhorn D.K., Gross S., Fisher B.J. & Newman A.J. (1970) Studies on the use of 'prophylactic' intrathecal amethopterin in childhood leukemia. *Blood* **36**, 56–60.

Miescher P.A. & Farquet J.J. (1974) Chronic myelomonocytic leukemia in adults. *Semin. Hematol.* **11** (2), 129–139.

Murray K.H., Paolino F., Goldman J.M., Galton D.A.G. & Grindle C.F.J. (1977) Ocular involvement in leukemia. *Lancet* **ii**, 829–831.

Nies B.A., Malmgren R.A., Chu E.W., Del Vecchio P.R., Thomas L.B. & Freireich E.J. (1965) Cerebrospinal fluid cytology in patients with acute leukemia. *Cancer* **18**, 1385–1391.

Norris H.J. & Wiener J. (1961) The renal lesions in leukemia. *Am. J. Med. Sci.* **241**, 512–517.

Phair J.P., Anderson R.E. & Namiki H. (1964) The central nervous system in leukemia. *Ann. Intern. Med.* **61**, 863–875.

Podoll L.N. & Winkler S.S. (1974) Busulphan lung. *Am. J. Roentgenol.* **120**, 151–156.

Poynton F.J. & Lightwood R. (1932) Lymphatic leukemia with infiltration of the periosteum, simulating acute rheumatism. *Lancet* **i**, 1192–1194.

Prolla J.C. & Kirsner J.B. (1964) The gastrointestinal lesions and complications of the leukemias. *Ann. Intern. Med.* **61**, 1084–1103.

Rai K.R., Sawitsky A., Cronkite E.P., Chanana A.D., Levy R.N. & Pasternack B.S. (1975) Clinical staging of chronic lymphocytic leukemia. *Blood* **46**, 219–234.

Ridgway E.W., Jaffe J. & Walton D.S. (1976) Leukemic ophthalmopathy in children. *Cancer* **38**, 1744–1749.

Roberts W.C., Bodey G.P. & Wertlake P.T. (1968) The heart in acute leukemia. A study of 420 autopsy cases. *Am. J. Cardiol.* **21**, 388–412.

Rose M.S. (1973) Busulphan toxicity syndrome caused by chlorambucil. *Br. Med. J.* **2**, 123.

Schwab R.S. & Weiss S. (1935) The neurologic aspect of leukemia. *Am. J. Med. Sci.* **189**, 766.

Simone J.V., Aur R.J. & Hustu H.O. (1975) Combined modality therapy of acute lymphocytic leukemia. *Cancer* **35**, 25–35.

Skinnider L.F., Card R.T. & Padmanabh S. (1977) Chronic myelomonocytic leukemia—an ultrastructural study by transmission and scanning electron microscopy. *Am. J. Clin. Path.* **67**, 339–346.

Skinnider L.F., Tan L., Schmidt J. & Armitage G. (1982) Chronic lymphocytic leukaemia. A review of 745 cases and assessment of clinical staging. *Cancer* **50**, 2951–5.

Sostman H.D., Matthay R.A. & Putman C.E. (1977) Cytotoxic drug-induced lung disease. *Am. J. Med.* **62**, 608–615.

Stoffel T.J., Nesbitt M.E. & Levitt S.H. (1975) Extramedullary involvement of the testes in childhood leukemia. *Cancer* **35**, 1203–1211.

Sullivan M.P. & Hrgovic M. (1973) Extramedullary leukemia. In *Clinical Pediatric Oncology* (2nd edn.) pp. 371–96 (Eds Sutow W.W., Vietti T.J. & Fernbach D.J.) Mosby, St. Louis.

Taetle R., Dickman P.S. & Feldman P.S. (1978) Pulmonary histopathologic changes associated with melphalan therapy. *Cancer* **42**, 1239–1245.

Videbaek A. (1971) Unusual cases of myelomatosis. *Brit. Med. J.* **2**, 326.

Wertlake P.T., Markovits B.A. & Stellar S. (1972) Cytologic evaluation of cerebrospinal fluid with clinical and histologic correlation. *Acta Cytol.* **16**, 224–239.

West R.J., Graham-Pole J., Hardisty R.M. & Pike M.C. (1972) Factors in pathogenesis of central nervous system leukemia. *Br. Med. J.* **3**, 311–314.

Willson J.K.V. (1959) The bone lesions of childhood leukemia. A survey of 140 cases. *Radiology* **76**, 672–81.

Wintrobe M.M. (1974) *Clinical Hematology*. Lea & Febiger, Philadelphia.

Young R.C., Ozols R.F. & Myers C.E. (1981) The anthracycline antineoplastic drugs. *N. Eng. J. Med.* **305**, 139–53.

Chapter 10

Myelomatosis and other monoclonal gammopathies

The early story of myelomatosis revolves around three separate descriptions over a period of 40 years. Dalrymple (1846) described as 'mollities et fragilitas ossium' the bony lesions found at autopsy on the patient who inspired both MacIntyre (1850) and Bence Jones (1847) to write about the extraordinary properties of a new protein which the former had found in the urine of a patient. The intensive chemical analysis and characterization of the protein was, however, performed by Bence Jones and thus it is his name which attains first recall in the story of myelomatosis.

The name multiple myeloma is the result of observations made by Rustizky (1873); he described a tumour of cancellous bone and bone marrow which he found as a multicentric tumour at autopsy. Numerous other reports followed, but it was Kahler (1889) who eventually published the full clinical picture of what we recognize as myelomatosis. The patient had first complained of pain ten years previously, in 1879. This was transient but exacerbations returned with increasing frequency as the disease progressed. Bence Jones protein was detected in the urine in 1881, and from then until the patient's death in 1887 the classical triad of bone pain, secondary infection, and skeletal destruction was relentlessly progressive. Kahler recognized the relationship between the skeletal softening, the Bence Jones protein, and the myeloma and he concluded his descriptive paper with the words 'marked albuminosuria must be a frequent symptom of this bone marrow disease, i.e. myeloma'.

Recent reviews of the field are those of Azar and Potter (1973); Snapper and Kahn (1975); and Salmon (1982).

MYELOMATOSIS

Myelomatosis is a chronic, progressive and invariably fatal disorder involving an unrestrained proliferation of plasma cells or plasma cell precursors which infiltrate the bone marrow and occasionally other tissues. It is uncommon but not rare, and is being recognized with increasing frequency. The pathological and clinical features of myelomatosis are due to tissue infiltration by the myeloma cells and to the disturbance of protein metabolism resultant on the proliferation of a single clone of immunoglobulin producing cells.

CLINICAL FEATURES

Myelomatosis is essentially a disease of middle and old age with a maximal incidence in the sixth and seventh decades. It is uncommon under the age of 40 years. The majority of patients present with bone pain, the symptoms of anaemia, tumour formation, spontaneous fractures or increasing skeletal deformities. Less commonly they may present with haemorrhagic states, nervous system involvement or recurrent infections, whilst 10% present in renal failure.

Bone pain is the commonest presenting feature, and in many patients is the outstanding symptom. Pain is characteristically aching and may be aggravated by movement or coughing; it may be fluctuant in intensity. Tenderness of the bones on palpation is common. Pathological fracture is frequent: compression fracture of the vertebrae and fracture of ribs being the most common. Fractures often follow trauma or strain and may be the cause of severe deformity. Tumour formation may occur on any bone, but is especially noted on the ribs. The tumours vary in size, and can be quite large; they are generally firm and tender, although when the cortical bone is excessively thin 'egg-shell' crackling can be elicited and the tumours appear fluctuant. Anaemia to some degree occurs in the vast majority of patients and is severe in advanced cases. It is, however, an uncommon presenting feature. Haemorrhagic states are common, and include epistaxes, gingival haemorrhage and excessive bruising. Melaena, haematuria and retinal haemorrhages may also occur. Recurrent infections, particularly pulmonary, are common and are not infrequently the presenting feature. Pneumonia is often the immediate cause of death. Nervous system involvement is usually due to spinal cord compression from compression fracture of vertebrae, but other factors such as peripheral neuritis and hyperviscosity may also be involved. Renal insufficiency is a common feature at some stage in the course of the disease and is a not uncommon presenting feature. Myelomatosis should be considered in cases of chronic renal insufficiency where the blood pressure remains normal. Acute renal failure is a less common presenting feature.

DIAGNOSIS

Diagnosis of myelomatosis depends on the ability to satisfy any two of three criteria (Medical Research Council 1973):

1 An absolute increase in plasma cells or their precursors in the bone marrow.
2 A skeletal abnormality, either osteolytic lesions, generalized osteoporosis, or a pathological fracture.
3 A protein abnormality in the serum or urine.

Bone marrow

Bone marrow aspiration usually reveals a diffuse proliferation of plasma cells, but on occasions the lesions are focal and poor results are obtained from a single attempt at aspiration. The marrow fragments are usually hypercellular with less than the usual component of fat. Myeloma cells usually constitute 10–40% of the nucleated cell population, although higher proportions may be seen if a localized tumour nodule is aspirated. The myeloma cells vary considerably in morphology from small, well-differentiated, plasma cells to large undifferentiated cells of 20–30 μm in diameter (Fig. 10.1). Multinucleate cells are not uncommon, but in themselves are not diagnostic of malignancy. The cytoplasm of the myeloma cell shows variable basophilic staining depending on the overall maturity of the cell—the basophilia increasing with the degree of maturity. Immunofluorescent staining of the bone marrow smears with antisera, specific for the individual immunoglobulin heavy and light chains, shows a single heavy and light chain population—a monoclonal population.

Many variations in the cytoplasmic characteristics of myeloma cells have been described, but, despite attempts to correlate the appearances with immunochemical class or prognosis of the disease, these have not proved reliable. Mott, morula or grape cell (Stich *et al.* 1955) describes the myeloma cells in which the cytoplasm is filled with vacuoles. The walls of the vacuoles stain deeply with pyronin and electron microscopy identifies them as dilatations of the endoplasmic reticulum. Although vacuolated plasma cells may be found in hyperimmunization states in animals, the grape cell is virtually never seen in man except in myelomatosis. The thesaurocyte (Maldonado *et al.* 1965) or 'flaming' plasma cell describes the myeloma cell with an acidophilic cytoplasm. The reddish cytoplasm is loculated by basophilic strands.

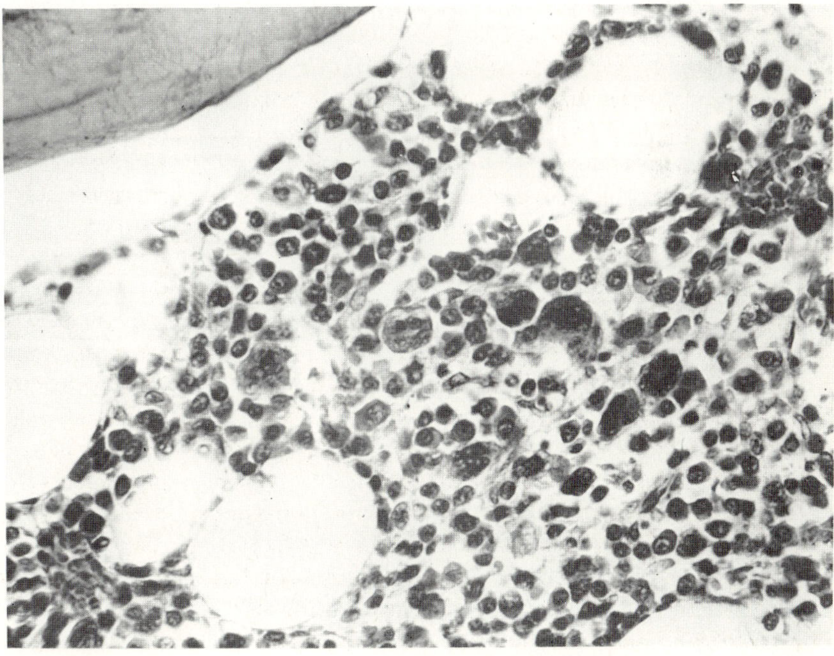

Fig. 10.1. Section of bone from a patient with malignant myeloma showing diffuse infiltration with typical and atypical plasma cells. × 400.

This appearance is associated with immunoglobulins rich in carbohydrate residues and tends to be more common in IgA myelomatosis. Inclusion bodies of the Russell body type are seen in myelomatosis in relation to areas of medullary necrosis. Large numbers of Russell bodies have been described in rapidly progressive myelomatosis but this is an inconsistent feature, and their recognition depends largely on the staining technique employed.

Erythropoiesis and myelopoiesis are variable, and may be normal in the early stages although hypoplasia is more usual in advanced cases. Megakaryocyte maturation is usually unaffected despite the occasional finding of thrombocytopenia.

Increased numbers of plasma cells may be seen in the bone marrow in certain other disorders. These include rheumatoid arthritis, lupus erythematosus, sarcoid, secondary carcinoma and chronic infection. These are, however, usually mature plasma cells, and rarely exceed 10% of the nucleated cell population. Immunofluorescent staining of the bone marrow will reveal polyclonal plasma cell proliferation with more than one immunoglobulin heavy chain and both light chains represented.

Skeletal abnormalities

The bone changes in myelomatosis include osteolytic lesions, pathological fractures, and a profound osteoporosis with generalized diffuse decalcification. In only 10% of cases are bone changes absent.

As myeloma cells proliferate predominantly in active red bone marrow, the osteolytic lesions are found in the axial skeleton—the vertebral column, ribs, skull and pelvis. The localized osteolytic lesions appear as multiple, rounded, discrete, punched out areas with no peripheral sclerosis.

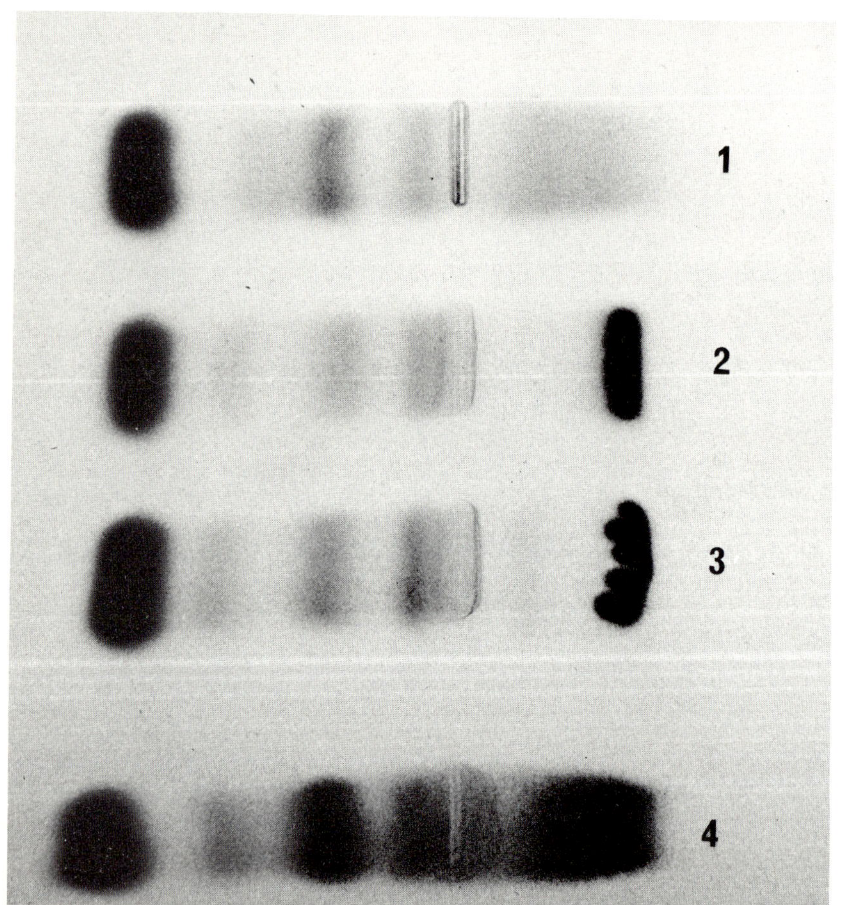

Fig. 10.2. Zone electrophoresis on cellulose acetate membrane pH 8.6.
1 Normal serum.
2 Myeloma.
3 Myeloma.
4 Inflammatory disease.

With progressive decalcification the skeleton becomes brittle and pathological fractures are common. Far the most common are compression fractures of the vertebral bodies, followed by fractures of ribs, sternum, pelvis, and long bones. Myelomatosis is the most likely cause of fractures of the ribs and sternum when trauma is not involved.

In most patients with myelomatosis the profuse proliferation of myeloma cells within the marrow leads to a generalized thinning of the cortical bone and decalcification. This leads to an overall increase in radiolucency of the skeleton and the radiological diagnosis of osteoporosis.

Immunochemistry (Figs 10.2 and 10.3)

Neoplastic proliferation of a single clone of plasma cells leads to the production of a quantity of identical immunoglobulin molecules which migrate on electrophoresis as a discrete, abnormal band. This has been variously termed Paraprotein, M—component, where the M can stand for Myeloma or Macroglobulinaemia, or Monoclonal component (MIg), the protein produced by a single clone of immunoglobulin producing cells. Unbalanced immunoglobulin chain production leads to the synthesis of excess light chains which appear in the urine as monoclonal component which often has the characteristic thermolabile properties of Bence Jones protein. In addition to the presence of the monoclonal serum component there may also be a general reduction in level of the normal immunoglobulins, and in some cases this immune paresis may be the sole protein abnormality.

Myelomatosis can be classified according to the immunochemical type of protein produced (Hobbs 1969) as seen in Table 10.1.

Table 10.1 Myelomatosis classified according to immunoglobulin type

		% with Bence Jones protein
IgG	56%	60
IgA	24	70
IgM	1	100
IgD	2	100
IgE	<1	100
Light chain only	14	100
Biclonal	1	70
No abnormal protein	1	Nil

IgG and IgA myelomatosis

These two varieties represent the 'classic' myelomatosis and together represent about 80% of all cases.

IgD myelomatosis

This variant tends to present at a younger age, to be associated with a high incidence of extramedullary tumour involvement, and to be more rapidly progressive than the classic IgG or IgA myelomatosis (Fahey 1968). Almost exclusively associated with Bence Jones proteinuria, there is a high incidence of renal impairment. The monoclonal component is rarely more than a moderate one, and an MIg of 10 g/l represents a tumour size equivalent to that of a 30–40 g/l IgG monoclone.

IgM myelomatosis

This rare form of myelomatosis tends to obscure the differences between myelomatosis and macroglobulinaemia; clinical features include elements of both diseases, although the bone marrow plasmacytosis and osteolytic bone lesions confirm its classification as myelomatosis. The monoclonal IgM is invariably of 7s sedimentation coefficient and represents IgM in its monomeric form.

IgE myelomatosis

This, the most rare variant, was first described by Johansson and Bennich (1967). Their case, and later cases, have shown no osteolytic bone lesions, a peripheral blood picture of plasma cell leukaemia, a monoclonal IgE component in the serum, and Bence Jones proteinuria type λ.

Light chain myelomatosis

Like IgD myelomatosis, this tends to occur at a younger age, and to be associated with a high degree of renal impairment. It has been suggested (Hobbs 1971) that the production of free light chains represents biochemical dedifferentiation paralleling malignant dedifferentiation. This myelomatosis variant tends to be less well-differentiated cytologically, and to be more rapidly progressive.

Biclonal myelomatosis

Although uncommon, a number of cases of myelomatosis in which there is more than one monoclonal component have

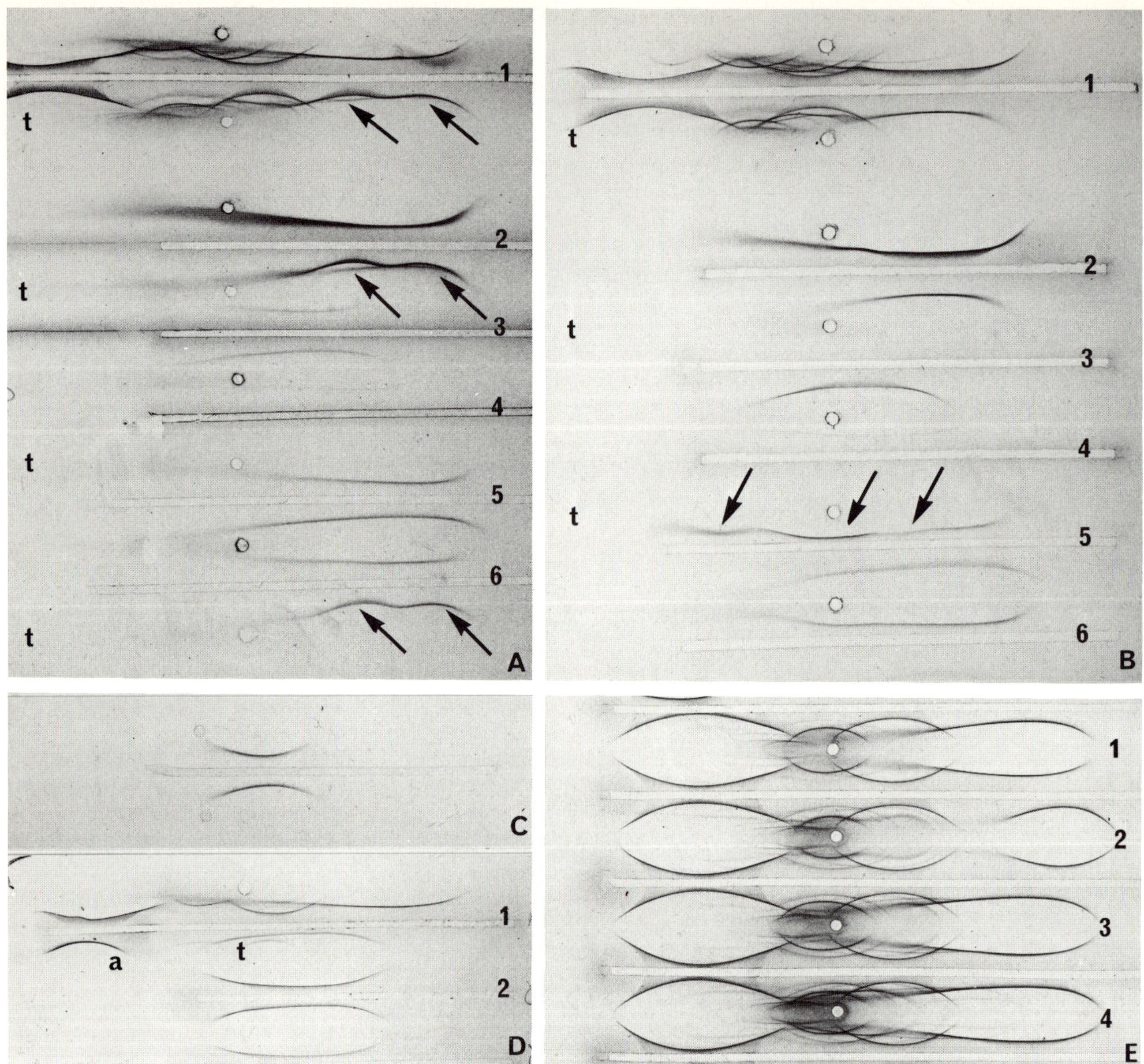

Fig. 10.3. Immunoelectrophoresis of serum and urine

A Immunoelectrophoresis of serum from a biclonal IgG lambda myeloma. Test samples applied to wells marked t, alternate wells containing a normal control serum.

Antisera:

1 anti whole human serum.   4 anti μ chain.
2 anti γ chain.   5 anti κ chain.
3 anti α chain.   6 anti λ chain.

The anomalous arcs produced by the tumour-related protein are indicated with the arrows. Note the reduced IgA arc and the absent IgM arc.

B Immunoelectrophoresis of serum from a light chain or micro-molecular myeloma with free light chains (Bence Jones Protein) in the serum.

Test samples applied to wells marked t, alternate wells contain a normal control serum.

Antisera:

1 anti whole serum.   4 anti μ chain.
2 anti γ chain.   5 anti κ chain.
3 anti α chain.   6 anti λ chain.

been described; the MIgs are rarely immunochemically identical. The series reported by Ballieux *et al.* (1968); Fateh Moghadem *et al.* (1968) and Miller and Korngold (1966) show 12 different immunoglobulin combinations in 19 cases (Table 10.2). Although the biclonal protein production usually represents two independent malignant cell lines, occasional cases have been reported (Rudders *et al.* 1973) where the two abnormal proteins appear to originate from the same cell line.

Non-secretory myelomatosis

The complete absence of abnormal protein from the serum and urine is a rare event in myelomatosis; in some cases, however, the true immunochemical class can be ascertained by immunofluorescent examination of the bone marrow aspirate (Loeffler *et al.* 1967). In the case reported by River *et al.* (1972) the bone marrow immunofluorescent studies were also negative.

THE KIDNEY IN MYELOMATOSIS

Renal failure is a common complication and a not infrequent cause of death in myelomatosis (Medical Research Council 1973), there being a continuous spectrum of changes from minimal functional impairment to acute oliguric renal failure. The proportion of myelomatosis deaths due directly or indirectly to renal failure used to be in the order of 30%, but modern cytotoxic therapy has reduced this to 15%. 10% of cases still present, however, with irreversible renal failure and die within the first two months of treatment. A high blood urea and low serum albumin are poor prognostic signs (Peto 1971). The major causes of renal impairment in myelomatosis are summarized in Table 10.3.

Hypercalcaemia no longer carries the poor prognosis that it used to. Although it rarely responds to cortisone therapy and

Table 10.2. Immunochemical MIg type in 19 cases of biclonal myelomatosis

IgG κ and IgG κ	2
IgG κ and IgG λ	2
IgG κ and IgA κ	3
IgG κ and IgA λ	1
IgG κ and IgM κ	1
IgG κ and λ	1
IgG λ and IgA λ	3
IgA κ and IgA λ	1
IgA κ and IgM κ	2
IgM κ and IgM κ	1
IgM κ and IgM λ	1
IgM κ and IgA λ	1
	19

Table 10.3. Possible causes of renal impairment in myelomatosis

	% of patients
Hypercalcaemia	45
Pyelonephritis	30
Coagulation anomalies	25
'Myeloma Kidney'	15
Amyloidosis	10
Myelomatous invasion of the kidney	10
Hyperviscosity	5
Hyponatraemia	4
'Minimal change' nephrosis	2
Hyperuricaemia	< 1
Fanconi syndrome	< 1

Fig. 10.3 (*cont.*) The anomalous arcs produced by the polymerized free light chains are indicated by the arrows. Note the restricted IgG arc and the apparent absence of IgA and IgM arcs.
C Immunoelectrophoresis of urine samples containing free immunoglobulin light chains—Bence Jones Protein.
  Antiserum: anti κ chain.
D Immunoelectrophoresis of urine sample from a patient with heavy chain disease.
  Antisera:
1 anti whole human serum.
2 anti γ chain.

Note that the urine contains albumin (a), a trace of transferrin (t) and a large arc which can be identified as γ heavy chain. No light chain or Fab determinants were detected.
E Immunoelectrophoresis of patients' serum developed with anti whole human serum.
  Sample:
1 Normal serum.
2 IgG monoclonal gammopathy.
3 Inflammatory.
4 Inflammatory.

is aggravated by bed rest and low fluid intake, the hypercalcaemia usually responds rapidly to intravenous cytotoxic therapy. Nephrocalcinosis, deposition of calcium salts in renal tubular epithelium, and renal stones are common findings.

Pyelonephritis as a feature of the immune paresis and susceptibility to infection is common and is found in 30% of all cases of myelomatosis.

Coagulation anomalies play an, as yet, incompletely understood role in the genesis of renal failure in myelomatosis. Recent studies (Preston and Ward 1974) have shown the deposition of fibrin within renal glomerular capillaries and in intertubular capillaries.

'Myeloma kidney' (Fig. 10.4) describes the classical renal lesion in myelomatosis. Histological examination shows dense eosinophilic, often laminated, casts in the proximal and distal convoluted tubules with an attendant syncytial cellular reaction. The presence of giant cells is not, however, specific as they may also be found, albeit rarely, around protein casts in other renal diseases. The presence of dense tubular casts causes atrophy of the related tubular cells and further decrease in the reabsorptive capacity of the nephron. This classic appearance is seen in only 15% of cases despite Bence Jones proteinuria in 80%, and is apparently unrelated to the quantity of paraproteinuria, to immunochemical type or to blood urea. The appearance can, however, be mimicked by radio-contrast procedures (Gross *et al.* 1968) and then be a cause of acute oliguric renal failure.

Amyloid deposition occurs in the kidney in 10% of all cases. Amyloid shows a pericollagenous distribution in relation to the glomerular capillary loops and to the tubular basement membranes. Renal amyloidosis is almost invariably associated with Bence Jones proteinuria. A rare finding is that of amyloid deposition within the renal tubular lumen; such a case was described by Friman *et al.* (1970); the patient with an IgD myelomatosis presented with uraemia. Renal biopsy showed a fibrotic interstitium with periglomerular fibrosis. The glomeruli were apparently normal, but the tubules were atrophic and contained laminated casts which stained strongly for amyloid. Syncytial reaction to the casts was present but was not considered a prominent feature.

Myelomatous invasion of the kidney occurs in 10% of cases, predominantly those of IgD or Bence Jones type. Hyperviscosity and cryoglobulinaemia occurs in 5% of cases of myelomatosis and, in these, renal failure is a common feature. The glomerular capillary occlusion may be relieved by plasmapheresis therapy. The histological appearances are inconstant but may include a thickening of the capillary loops in the glomerulus.

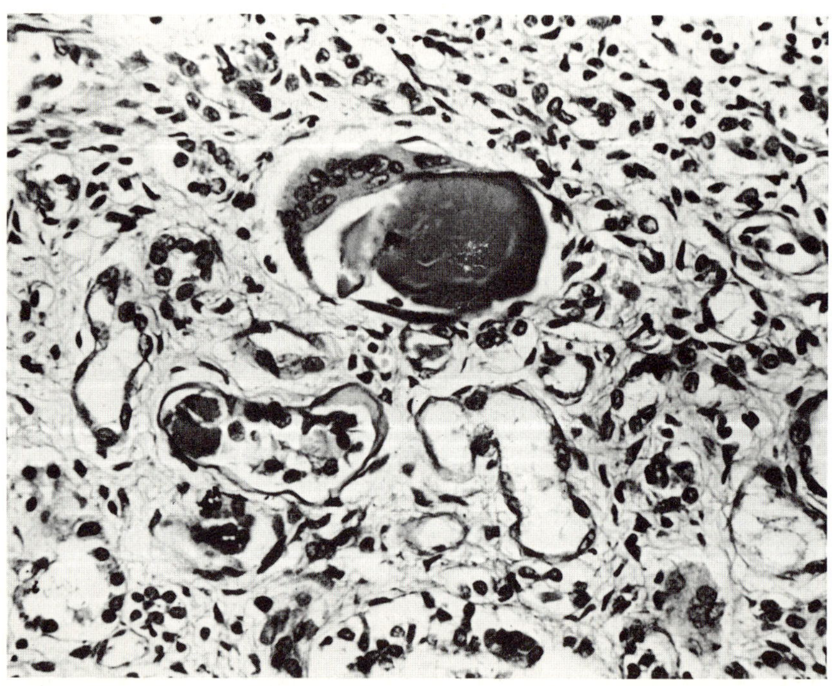

Fig. 10.4. Myeloma kidney showing tubular degeneration, interstitial fibrosis, accumulation of proteinaceous casts within tubules and giant cell formation around the tubules. ×216.

Hyponatraemia, which occurs in 4% of cases, is due predominantly to a high monoclonal protein concentration (IgG levels in excess of 60 g/l) displacing plasma water, increasing plasma osmotic pressure, and binding anions. Infusion of saline can have a deleterious effect and is contraindicated.

'Minimal change' nephrosis is a rare renal complication of myelomatosis; it usually responds to tumour orientated cytotoxic therapy, proteinuria being reduced in parallel with the monoclonal immunoglobulin and reappearing with relapse of the tumour.

Hyperuricaemia is associated with high levels of tumour-kill in rapidly progressive myelomatosis.

Fanconi syndrome is another rare renal complication of myelomatosis. Bence Jones proteinuria and the re-absorption of the abnormal protein by proximal tubular cells can lead to a degree of damage to the functional capacity of those tubular cells such that they become incapable of re-absorbing aminoacids, phosphates and glucose. This aminoaciduria and hyperphosphaturia with its attendant osteomalacia forms the basis of the adult Faconi syndrome.

The occurrence of this complication of myelomatosis was first reported in 1949 and a further 10 cases at least have been reported since that time (Horn *et al.* 1969).

EXTRAMEDULLARY PLASMACYTOMA

Despite the widespread distribution of plasma cells throughout the tissues of the body, plasma cell tumours most commonly occur within the bone marrow, and extramedullary plasma cell tumours are rare. 75% of those described occur in the submucosa of the upper respiratory tract, and are often multifocal. Major immunoglobulin disturbances and monoclonal gammopathies are rare although immunoglobulin production, in particular half molecule production, can be demonstrated on critical examination of many cases. The growth and mode of spread resemble that of histiocytic lymphoma, and are characterized by the rapid invasion of local lymph nodes and subsequent blood-borne dissemination to other sites. Even when the disease has disseminated widely, however, bone marrow involvement is unusual. Primary plasmacytoma of lymph nodes is a rare occurrence.

It would appear that extramedullary plasmacytomas are quite distinct from solitary plasmacytomas of bone and rarely develop into myelomatosis. Prognosis is generally good, and they respond well to surgical excision and radiotherapy with a low recurrence rate.

Solitary plasmacytomas of bone

In myelomatosis the well-demarcated osteolytic lesions seen on radiological examination represent multiple plasmacytomata. In other patients one or more such lesions may develop in the absence of overt myelomatosis. These solitary plasmacytomas of bone consist of proliferating myeloma cells supported by a thin connective tissue stroma. Diagnosis of solitary plasmacytomas of bone should only be made when all of the following criteria can be satisfied:

1 multiple bone marrow aspirations at different sites do not reveal any plasma cell abnormality
2 the serum electrophoretic pattern is within normal limits
3 there is no Bence Jones proteinuria.

Certain rare exceptions do, however, occur, and minor monoclonal immunoglobulin components, both intact molecules and fragments have been recorded. A final diagnosis can only be made after a long period of observation; the majority of cases disseminate after a period of as long as 24 years to give rise to overt myelomatosis.

A study of the reported cases of solitary plasmacytoma of bone shows that, in regard to age at presentation, mode of spread and the lack of extramedullary lesions, solitary plasmacytoma of bone is a variant of myelomatosis and distinct from the extramedullary plasmacytoma. It may present at any age from 14 years upwards with a median in the sixth decade. The most frequent sites affected are femur (20%), pelvis (20%) and a vertebra (20%). Dissemination is by widespread involvement of active haematopoetic tissue when myeloma cells can be found on the bone marrow aspiration in almost all cases.

HEAVY CHAIN DISEASES

Increased understanding and knowledge of immunoglobulin structure has led to more widespread characterization of the proteins in serum and urine of patients with proliferative disorders of lymphocytes and plasma cells. These disorders are now frequently classified according to the protein produced, and emphasis is laid on the fact that there may be balanced synthesis of immunoglobulin, leading to the production of only the homogenous molecule, or unbalanced synthesis leading to the synthesis of free light, or, more rarely, heavy chains additional to or even instead of the intact molecule. This increase in knowledge has led to the description of new syndromes associated with anomalies of immunoglobulin synthesis. Notable amongst these are the heavy chain diseases.

Three immunochemical types of heavy chain disease have been described corresponding to the heavy chains of IgG (γ), IgA (α) and IgM (μ). The anomalous protein produced in all three diseases shows a deletion in the constant region of the Fd fragment of the heavy chain, synthesis of the chain recommencing at the hinge region which represents the start of the Fc region. Deletion at this point in the molecule would involve the cysteic acid residue, which has been shown to be the point of linkage of the heavy and light chains of the immunoglobulin molecule.

GAMMA HEAVY CHAIN DISEASE

First described in 1963 (Franklin *et al.* 1964), some 25 cases have now been reported (Zawadzki *et al.* 1969; Bloch *et al.* 1973). The disease occurs in the middle aged and elderly and shows no sex discrimination. The features are more those of non-Hodgkin's lymphoma than myeloma, with lymphadenopathy, often fluctuating, a common feature. The lymphoid structures of Waldeyer's ring are characteristically involved with associated palatal oedema and an unusual orange hue to the tonsils. Hepatosplenomegaly is present in most cases, whilst bone lesions are rare. Almost all of the patients have had repeated febrile episodes as a result of recurrent infections and septicaemia, overwhelming infection being the usual cause of death. Laboratory findings include anaemia, eosinophilia, leucopenia and hyperuricaemia. Bone marrow examination is not diagnostic, although the infiltrate of lymphocytes and plasma cells may resemble that seen in macroglobulinaemia. Lymph node biopsy also reveals a rather pleomorphic picture with infiltration of the nodes with lymphocytes, plasma cells, eosinophils and histiocytic cells and maintenance of the general structural architecture. Many of the cases have been initially labelled as showing only reactive lymphoid changes. There is a great variability in the pathology, from lymphoma through atypical hyerplasia to a benign polymorphous infiltrate (Marsh *et al.* 1981).

Diagnosis may be suspected from the fairly characteristic clinical features but can only be made on immunochemical

analysis of serum and urine proteins. Both serum and urine show an abnormal protein band in the beta to beta-gamma region of the electrophoretic separation, the mobility being identical in both serum and urine samples. The abnormal protein reacts with antisera to the Fc region of the IgG globulin and does not react with antisera to κ or λ light chains. It does not have the characteristic thermal solubility properties of a Bence Jones protein. More sophisticated analysis of the abnormal protein shows it to have a sedimentation coefficient between 3.5 and 4s, and there appears to be an unusual preponderance of $\gamma 3$ heavy chain subclass molecules. Recent studies of plasma cells from patients with this disease in short-term tissue culture (Ein *et al.* 1969) have shown active synthesis of γ heavy chains and a total failure of production of light chains. This lack of light chain synthesis must be considered a basic feature of the defect in this condition.

ALPHA HEAVY CHAIN DISEASE

Since IgA globulins are produced by plasma cells lining the gastrointestinal tract and organs of external secretion, it is not surprising that Alpha heavy chain disease is found in patients with intestinal lymphoma, and is usually associated with severe malabsorption. The first report of this condition (Seligmann *et al.* 1968) was in a young adult with a 'Mediterranean lymphoma' who had an γA heavy chain protein in the serum, urine and jejunal juice. Since the initial description, cases have been described in populations of diverse geographical and ethnic origins, but the majority of cases are seen in patients of African and Sephardic Jewish origin.

The course of the disease is rapidly progressive with profound malabsorption, diarrhoea, weight loss and cachexia. Histologically there is a predominantly plasmacytic infiltration of the wall and lamina propria of the small intestine, but there appears to be little lymphoid involvement outside the intestinal tract. Jejunal biopsy (Doe *et al.*, 1972) shows a mononuclear infiltrate in the lamina propria with distortion and distension of the villous architecture and flattening of the crypts. The surface epithelium is relatively normal. The infiltrate contains recognizable mature plasma cells admixed with less mature cells which appear cytologically intermediate between lymphocytes and plasma cells.

Diagnosis again rests with the immunochemical characterization of the abnormal protein. This is complicated, however, by the fact that relatively small amounts of the free γA heavy chains are produced, and the serum abnormality may pass unrecognized except by careful immunoelectrophoresis, or immunoselection electrophoresis. Large quantities of the protein may, however, be detected in the jejunal juice. The abnormal protein is of beta or beta-gamma electrophoretic mobility, and reacts with antisera to γA heavy chains, there being no reaction with antisera to κ or λ light chains. Recent reports suggest that this may be more widespread than originally thought, and all cases of primary small intestinal lymphoma should be examined for the presence of alpha heavy chain disease protein (Seligmann *et al.* 1971).

MU HEAVY CHAIN DISEASE

The most recent of the heavy chain diseases to be described is that of the μ heavy chain (Forte *et al.* 1970). The three cases of long duration chronic lymphocytic leukaemia, which form the basis of this report, all had a rapidly migrating protein in the serum which reacted as a γM heavy chain on immuno-electrophoresis. The features that make these cases differ from chronic lymphocytic leukaemia are the presence of large numbers of vacuolated plasma cells in the bone marrow in addition to small lymphocytes, Bence Jones protein in the urine and the μ heavy chain protein in the serum. This entity differs from the other heavy chain diseases, however, in the fact that the abnormal serum component does not appear as a monoclonal band on zone electrophoresis and does not appear in the urine. It has also been shown (Zucker Franklin and Franklin 1970) that both μ and κ protein are produced by the same cell line, there being, apparently, a failure in assembly of the intact molecule due to a structural deletion in the Fd fragment of the μ heavy chain.

MACROGLOBULINAEMIA

Waldenström's initial description of essential macroglobulinaemia in 1944 has been modified somewhat over the intervening years. The condition may be defined as a progressive systemic proliferative disorder of the lymphoreticular system in which the cellular proliferation shows features of lymphoid and plasmacytoid development, and the serum contains a monoclonal IgM. The majority of patients are over 50 years of age, but there is no significant sex differential despite earlier reports to the contrary. Anorexia, malaise,

weight loss and recurrent infections are common symptoms; anaemia, a haemorrhagic diathesis, lymphadenopathy, hepato-splenomegaly and increased total serum protein with hyper-viscosity are common findings.

The *bone marrow* is hypercellular. The infiltrate consists of morphologically mature plasma cells and lymphocytes and of cells which appear intermediate between lymphocytes and plasma cells. These lymphoid cells have an eccentric nucleus with diffuse nuclear chromatin akin to the lymphocyte nucleus, and an intensely basophilic cytoplasm akin to that of the plasma cell. Dutcher and Fahey (1959) stressed the presence of intranuclear PAS-positive inclusions and this has become a much quoted diagnostic criterion. Harrison (1972) has, however, stressed that this is an elusive feature which cannot be relied upon. Lymph nodes are only moderately enlarged. The general architecture of the nodes is preserved despite an intense infiltration of lymphocytes and occasional plasmacytoid cells. The peripheral sinus is intact but there is pericapsular infiltration. Some follicular development is retained although the follicles tend to be small and rounded with scant reticulin framework. Mitotic figures are surprisingly infrequent. A characteristic feature is the intense eosinophilic staining of the plasma and lymph. Although numerous authors stress the high concentration of mast cells in the lymph node in this condition, this is an inconstant feature and cannot be relied upon to distinguish a macroglobulinaemic from a reactive node, although the relative numbers of mast cells are considerably higher than seen in malignant lymphoma. Liver involvement occurs in the majority of cases. There is an essentially lymphocytic infiltration of the portal tracts, with no increase in portal fibrosis. Several instances of lung involvement have been reported; the features being those of dense cellular infiltration almost obliterating the normal structure of the bronchi and peribronchial tissues. Remnants of mucous glands are scanty. The cellular infiltrate has the features of that seen in the lymph nodes with lymphocytes and plasma cells in almost equal numbers.

MONOCLONAL GAMMOPATHY IN MALIGNANT LYMPHOMA

Lymphomas are occasionally associated with monoclonal gammopathy (Krauss and Sokal 1966). This may be due to production of immunoglobulin by essentially stromal plasma-cytoid cells (Ward *et al.* 1971) but in the case of histiocytic lymphomas has been shown by immunocytological and ultrastructural techniques to be associated with immunoglobulin production by neoplastic B cells (Stein *et al.* 1974; Taylor 1974).

TREATMENT AND PROGNOSIS

Over the past 15–20 years it has been recognized that it is possible to improve the clinical status and increase survival time in patients with myelomatosis by the use of certain cytotoxic agents (Durie and Salmon 1982 for review). Melphalan and cyclophosphamide have commonly been employed both in low dose continuous or high dose intermittent regimes, the latter to reduce the incidence of prolonged myelosuppression. The therapeutic results with both of these drugs are virtually the same (Medical Research Council 1971 and 1980). Intermittent melphalan with prednisolone may further improve the response (Costa *et al.* 1973). Multi-drug combination chemotherapy is also proving successful (Azam and Delamore 1974; Alexanian *et al.* 1977) and studies of the role of biological response modifiers, e.g. levamisole, interferons, are also underway. Now, about 60% of patients respond slowly to chemotherapy, 20% of patients show no response and 20% show a rapid response. It appears that slow responders usually fare better than rapid responders. Responding patients improve clinically and show a fall in paraprotein level, sometimes with improvement in level of the uninvolved immunoglobulin classes. Bone lesions may also show some radiological resolution. It is thought that in most patients tumour regression reaches a plateau at which point no further regression occurs (Warner *et al.* 1974). Whilst chemotherapy has improved clinical status and survival, 50% of patients are dead within 2 years—relapse often being associated with tumour dedifferentiation and production of mutant proteins or immunoglobulin fragments. Unfavourable prognostic factors in myeloma are anaemia, impaired renal function, large cell mass (as estimated from paraprotein levels), extensive bone lesions, hypercalcaemia and failure to respond to initial therapy (Parker and Malpas 1979).

The importance of supportive therapy cannot be overemphasized—blood transfusion for anaemia, antibiotics for intercurrent infections, plasmapheresis for hyperviscosity, steroids and rehydration for hypercalcaemia, all have a vital role to play. Relief of pain is mandatory either by adequate analgesia or by treatment of local painful lesions by radiotherapy.

Treatment schedules should be monitored by periodic measurement of serum and urine monoclonal protein, escape from control being signalled by an increase in concentration of either protein abnormality.

Macroglobulinaemia may also respond to treatment with an alkylating agent (chlorambucil or melphalan) combined with prednisolone (Waldenström 1965). Symptomatic improvement is gratifying though individual responses vary. Plasmapheresis is important where there are symptoms reflecting hyperviscosity.

REFERENCES

ALEXANIAN R., SALMON S., BONNET J., GEHAN, E., HAUT A. & WEICK J. (1977) Combination therapy for multiple myeloma. *Cancer* **40**, 2878–82.

AZAM L. & DELAMORE I.W. (1974) Combination therapy for myelomatosis. *Brit. Med. J.* **3**, 560–64.

AZAR H.A. & POTTER M. (1973) *Multiple Myeloma and Related Disorders.* Harper and Row, Hagerstown.

BALLIEUX R.E., IMHOF J.W., MUL N.A.J., ZEGERS B.J.M. & STOOP J.W. (1968) Pathology of immunoglobulins: some aspects of monoclonal gammopathy. *Clin. Chim. Acta* **22**, 7–13.

BENCE JONES H. (1847) Papers in chemical pathology. *Lancet* **ii**, 88–92.

BLOCH K.J., LEE L., MILLS J.A. & HABER E. (1973) Gamma heavy chain diseases—an expanding clinical and laboratory spectrum. *Amer. J. Med.* **55**, 61–70.

COSTA G., ENGLE R.L., SCHILLING A., CARBONE P., KOCHAWA S., NACHMAN R.L. & GLIDEWELL O. (1973) Melphalan and prednisone: an effective combination for the treatment of multiple myeloma. *Amer. J. Med.* **54**, 589–99.

DALRYMPLE J. (1846) On the microscopic character of mollities ossium. *Dublin J. Med. Sci.* **11**, 85.

DOE W.F., HENRY K., HOBBS J.R., AVERY JONES F., DENT C.E. & BOOTH C.C. (1972) Five cases of alpha chain disease. *Gut* **13**, 947–57.

DUTCHER T.F. & FAHEY J.L. (1959) Histopathology of the macroglobulinaemia of Waldenstrom. *J. Nat. Cancer Inst.* **22**, 887–917.

DURIE B.G.M. & SALMON S.E. (1982) Current status and future treatment of multiple myeloma. *Clin. Haematol.* **11**, 181–210.

EIN D., BUELL D.N. & FAHEY J.L. (1969) Biosynthetic and structural studies of a heavy chain disease protein. *J. Clin. Invest.* **48**, 785–93.

FAHEY J.L., CARBONE P.P., ROWE D.S. & BACHMANN R. (1968) Plasma cell myeloma with D myeloma protein (IgD myeloma). *Amer. J. Med.* **45**, 373–80.

FATEH MOGHADEM A., WURZ H., OESER R.M. & KNEDEL M. (1968) Doppelparaproteinamie. *Deutsch. Med. Wschr.* **93**, 1695–1702.

FORTE F.A., PRELLI F., YOUNOT W.J., JERRY L.M., KOCHAWA S., FRANKLIN E.C. & KUNKEL H.G. (1970) Heavy chain disease of the μ (γM) type: report of the first case. *Blood* **36**, 137–44.

FRANKLIN E.C., LOWENSTEIN J., BIGELOW B. & MELTZER M. (1964)

Heavy chain disease: a new disorder of serum gamma globulins. Report of the first case. *Amer. J. Med.* **37**, 332–50.

FRIMAN C., TORNROTH T. & WEGELIUS O. (1970) IgD myeloma associated with multiple extramedullary amyloid containing tumours and amyloid casts in the renal tubules. *Ann. Clin. Res.* **2**, 161–6.

GROSS M., McDONALD H. & WATERHOUSE K. (1968) Anuria following urography with Meglumine diatrizoate (Renografin) in multiple myeloma. *Radiology* **90**, 780–81.

HARRISON C.V. (1972) The morphology of the lymph node in the macroglobulinaemia of Waldenström. *J. Clin. Path.* **25**, 12–16.

HOBBS J.R. (1969) Immunochemical classes of myelomatosis. Including data from a therapeutic trial conducted by the Medical Research Council working party. *Brit. J. Haemat.* **16**, 599–606.

HOBBS J.R. (1971) Immunocytemia o' mice an' men. *Brit. Med. J.* **2**, 67–72.

HORN M.F., KNAPP M.S., PAGE F.T. & WALKER W.H.C. (1969) Adult Fanconi syndrome and multiple myelomatosis. *J. Clin. Path.* **22**, 414–16.

JOHANSON S.G. & BENNICH H. (1967) Immunological studies of an atypical (myeloma) immunoglobulin. *Immunology* **13**, 381–94.

KAHLER O. (1889) Zur symptomatologies des multiplen Meyloms. Beobachtung von Albumosurie. *Prager. Med. Wschr.* **14**, 33–5.

KRAUSS S. & SOKAL J.E. (1966) Paraproteinaemia in the lymphomas. *Amer. J. Med.* **40**, 400–13.

LOEFFLER H., KNOPP A. & KRECKE H.J. (1967) Cases of multiple myeloma (plasmacytoma) 'without paraprotein'. *German Med. Monthly* **12**, 226–9.

MacINTYRE W. (1850) Case of mollities and fragilitas ossium. *Med. Chim. Soc. Tr.* **33**, 211–32.

MALDONADO J.E., BAYRD E.D. & BROWN A.L. (1965) The flaming cell in multiple myeloma. A light and electron microscopy study. *Amer. J. Clin. Path.* **44**, 605–12.

MARSH W.C., WORTHMAN J.W. & SPIEGELBERG H.L. (1981) The pathology of gamma heavy chain disease. *Cancer* **47**, 2878–82.

MEDICAL RESEARCH COUNCIL (1971) Myelomatosis: comparison of melphalan and cyclophosphamide therapy. *Brit. Med. J.* **1**, 640–1.

MEDICAL RESEARCH COUNCIL (1973) Report of the first myelomatosis trial: I. Analysis of the presenting features of prognostic importance. *Brit. J. Haematol.* **24**, 123–39.

MEDICAL RESEARCH COUNCIL (1980) Report of the second myelomatosis trial after 5 years of follow-up. *Brit. J. Cancer.* **42**, 813–22.

MILLER D.G. & KORNGOLD L. (1966) Monoclonal immunoglobulins in cancer. *Med. Clin. N. Amer.* **50**, 667–74.

PARKER D. & MALPAS J.S. (1979) Multiple myeloma. *J. Royal Coll. Phys.* **13**, 146–53.

PETO R. (1971) Urea, albumin and response rates. *Brit. Med. J.* **2**, 324.

PRESTON F.E. & WARD A.M. (1974) Acute renal failure in myelomatosis from intravascular coagulation. *Brit. Med. J.* **1**, 604–5.

RIVER G.L., TEWKSBURY D.A. & FUDENBERG H.H. (1972) 'Non secretory' multiple myeloma. *Blood* **40**, 204–6.

RUDDERS R.A., YAKULIS V. & HELLER P. (1973) Double myeloma. Production of both IgG type lambda and IgA type lambda myeloma proteins by a single cell line. *Amer. J. Med.* **55**, 215–21.

RUSTIZKY J. VON (1873) Multiples Myelom. *Dt. Z. Chir.* **3**, 162–72.

SALMON S.E. (Ed.) (1982) Myeloma and related disorders. *Clinics in Haematol.* Vol. II, No. 1.

SELIGMANN M., DANON F., HUREZ D., MIHAESCO E. & PREUD 'HOMME J.L. (1968) Alpha chain disease: a new immunoglobulin abnormality. *Science* **162**, 1396–7.

SELIGMANN M., MIHAESCO E. & FRANGIONE B. (1971) Alpha chain disease. *Ann. N.Y. Acad. Sci.* **190**, 487–500.

SNAPPER I. & KAHN A. (1975) Myelomatosis. In *Lymphoproliferative Diseases* (Ed Molander D.W.). Thomas, Springfield.

STEIN H., KAISERLING E. & LENNERT K. (1974) Evidence for B-cell origin of reticulum cells sarcoma. *Virschows Arch. Path. Anat.* **364**, 51–67.

STICH M.H., SWELLER A.I. & MORRISON M. (1955) The 'grape cell' of multiple myeloma. *Amer. J. Clin. Path.* **25**, 601–2.

TAYLOR C.R. (1974) The nature of Reed–Sternberg cells and other malignant reticulum cells. *Lancet* ii, 802–7.

WALDENSTRÖM J. (1944) Incipient myelomatosis or essential hyperglobulinaemia with fibrinogenopenia—a new syndrome? *Acta. Med. Scand.* **117**, 216–47.

WALDENSTRÖM J. (1965) Macroglobulinaemia. *Adv. Metab. Dis.* **2**, 115–58.

WARD A.M., SHORTLAND J.E. & DARKE C.S. (1971) Lymphosarcoma of the lung with monoclonal (IgM) gammapathy. A clinicopathologic, histochemical, immunologic and ultrastructural study. *Cancer* **27**, 1009–28.

WARNER N.L., POTTER M. & METCALF D. (Eds.) (1974) Multiple myeloma and related immunoglobulin producing neoplasms. UICC Technical Report Series Volume 13, Chapter 7, pp. 73–7.

ZAWADZKI Z.R., BONEDEK T.G., EIN D. & EASTON J.M. (1969) Rheumatoid arthritis terminating in heavy chain disease. *Ann. Intern. Med.* **70**, 335–47.

ZUCKER FRANKLIN D. & FRANKLIN E.C. (1970) Ultrastructural and immunofluorescence studies of the cells associated with μ chain disease. *Blood* **37**, 257–71.

The histological examination of the spleen is a problem which presents itself less often to the pathologist than the examination of lymph nodes. Spleens are removed because of splenomegaly, often in the presence of an obscure haemolytic anaemia, because of splenic rupture, often in the presence of acute splenic enlargement, as a diagnostic staging procedure in lymphoma and as a matter of surgical convenience during gastrectomy. The histology of the spleen at necropsy frequently presents problems.

The spleen should be measured, weighed and then cut in its long axis; in the absence of a gross lesion it should be cut into slices 0.5–1 cm thick and 6–12 blocks taken; preferably from regions where the white pulp is prominent. A lymph node is usually present in the hilum; this should be examined histologically. The weight of the spleen varies very widely with body weight, with the manner of dying and notably with the degree of terminal venous congestion. A spleen weighing over 250 g is probably abnormal and one weighing over 300 g almost certainly abnormal.

A discussion of the histopathology of the spleen falls naturally into an analysis of the general tissue reactions involved, followed by a discussion of specific lesions. Reference should be made to Stuart's excellent discussion on this subject (Macpherson *et al.* 1973); to the classic review by Klemperer (1936) and to articles by Rappaport (1970), Lukes (1970) and Robb-Smith (1970).

THE TISSUE RESPONSES OF THE SPLEEN

The histopathology of the spleen represents the sum of the focal pathological lesions and the general tissue response. The latter can be considered under the following headings:

1 Hypertrophy of the white pulp (Fig. 11.1). Normally the ratio of white to red pulp is between 1:3 and 1:6. The white pulp may enlarge often with the development of active germinal centres similar to those of lymph nodes. This is accompanied by the appearance of foci of lymphocytes and plasma cells in the red pulp and represents a humoral immune response. Lukes (1970) discriminates between different types of activation. In graft rejection, infectious, mononucleosis, *Herpes simplex*, and after irradiation or bone marrow damage, the white pulp contains lymphocytes and large basophilic stem cells; in acute sepsis, measles, pertussis, typhoid and a number of chronic conditions like idiopathic thrombocytopenic purpura, acquired haemolytic anaemia and rheumatoid disease, there is a prominent follicular reaction with perivascular plasma cells. There is a prominent follicular reaction in the spleens of patients who have been on haemodialysis.

2 Reduction of the white pulp. In patients dying of severe generalized shock and toxaemia the white pulp may be grossly reduced; similar appearances may be induced in animals by massive doses of corticosteroids. Similarly, in patients dying after prolonged chemotherapy for malignant lymphoma there is often complete disappearance of the white pulp of the spleen (Fig. 11.2). Inactive white pulp, composed only of small lymphocytes, is found in the foetus, the unstimulated, the senescent, and in patients with agammaglobulinaemia. An infiltrate of plasmacytoid cells without hypertrophy is found in dysproteinaemias such as macroglobulinaemia.

3 Hypertrophy of splenic macrophages. In prolonged systemic infections the spleen comes to contain numerous large swollen macrophages rich in acid phosphatase and often iron pigment. This process is essentially a process of macrophage maturation induced mainly by phagocytosis, similar to that occurring during the maturation of monocytes into macrophages. Hypertrophy of macrophages is often accompanied by hypertrophy of splenic sinus endothelial cells.

4 Congestion of pulp cords. The extravascular compartment of the red pulp may become stuffed with red blood cells. This is accompanied secondarily by a moderate degree of hypertrophy of splenic macrophages and sinus endothelial cells with a high iron content. This occurs while there is severe erythrocytic abnormality, e.g. in spherocytic anaemia, and in severe venous congestion (Fig. 11.3).

5 Variation in the polymorph content of the spleen. The

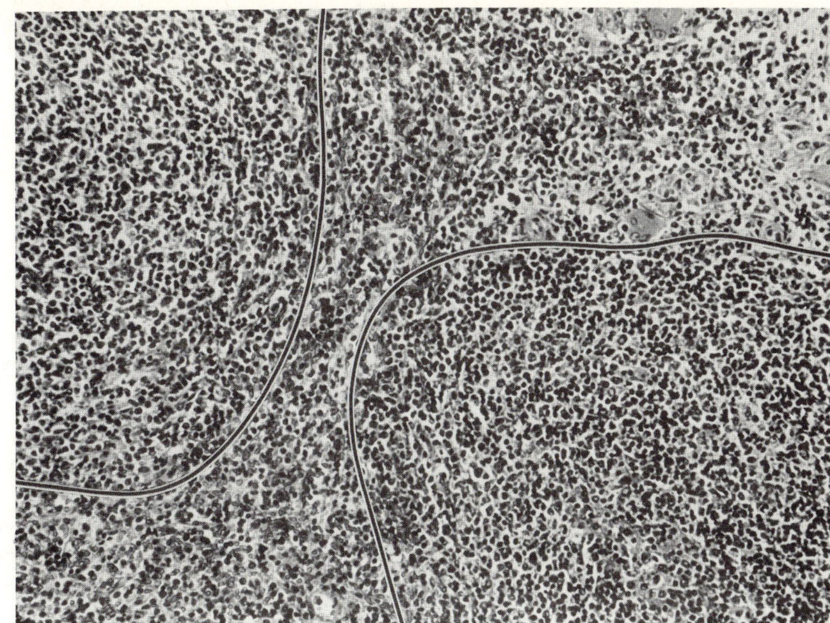

Fig. 11.1. Spleen from patient with Hodgkin's disease who did not have lymphomatous lesions in the spleen. The red pulp is compressed between hypertrophic nodules of white pulp (outlined). ×150.

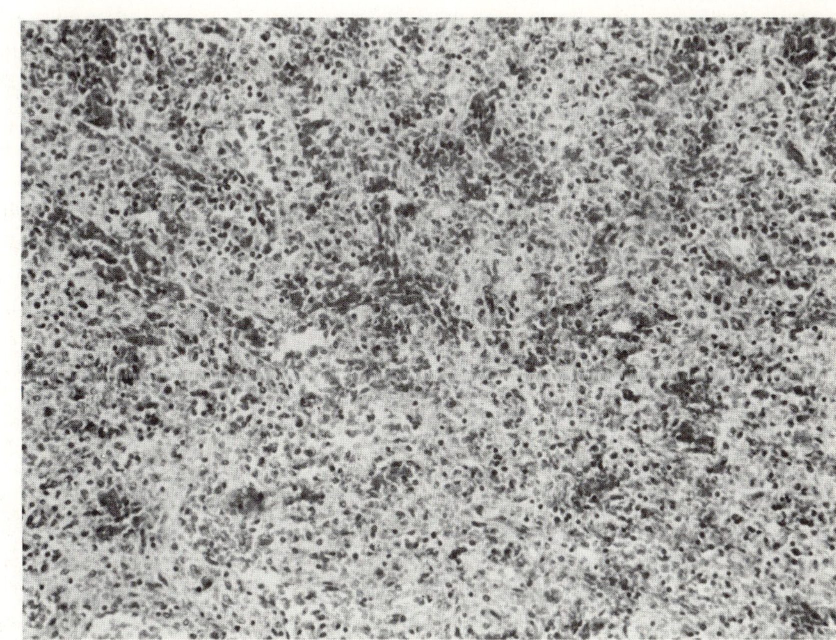

Fig. 11.2. Spleen from patient dying after extensive anti-cancer chemotherapy including steroid therapy. There is total atrophy of the white pulp. ×150.

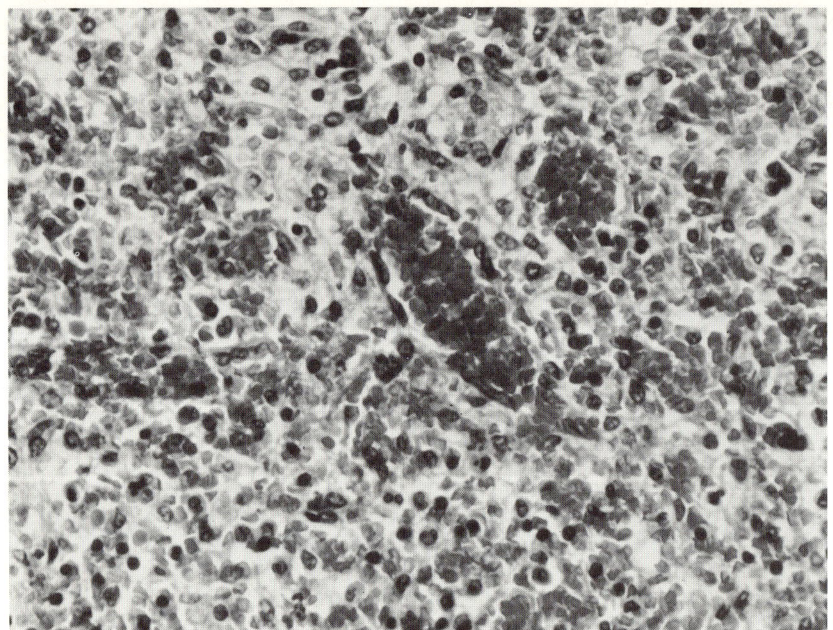

Fig. 11.3. Spleen from patient dying of congestive cardiac failure showing venous congestion; the sinusoids are distended with blood but there is no chronic interstitial fibrosis. ×375.

commonest example of this is the depletion of eosinophils, which occurs in the spleens of people dying of protracted disease; the spleen of someone killed suddenly in an accident normally contains numerous eosinophils.

Less commonly in patients dying of severe sepsis, the spleen will be stuffed with large numbers of neutrophil polymorphs. Commonly in severe infections this change is accompanied by white pulp hypertrophy.

Splenic lesions may be classified as follows:

1 Splenic rupture.
2 Circulatory disorders.
   (*a*) Portal hypertension.
   (*b*) Chronic venous congestion.
   (*c*) Infarction.
3 Degenerative disorders—Amyloidosis.
4 Infective and inflammatory disorders.
   (*a*) Acute pyogenic systemic infections—the 'septic' spleen.
   (*b*) Subacute systemic infections, notably subacute bacterial endocarditis. Rheumatoid disease.
   (*c*) Focal granulomatous lesions.
5 Lipidoses—Diabetes mellitus, Gaucher's disease, Niemann–Pick disease.
6 Blood disorders.
   (*a*) Idiopathic thrombocytopenic purpura.
   (*b*) Haemolytic anaemia.
   (*c*) Leukaemia.
   (*d*) Myelofibrosis.
7 Tumours.
   (*a*) Lymphoma, including malignant histiocytosis.
   (*b*) Secondary carcinomatosis.
   (*c*) Angiomata.
   (*d*) Cysts.
8 The spleen in hypersplenism.
9 Splenic atrophy.

1 Rupture

This is a common reason for splenectomy. A normal spleen does not rupture spontaneously but requires considerable external trauma. An enlarged spleen on the other hand requires little trauma to cause rupture and may indeed rupture spontaneously (Stites and Ultmann 1966). There may or may not be massive intraperitoneal haemorrhage; the peritoneal cavity may therefore be seeded with nodules of splenic tissue (Szabo 1961).

2 Circulatory disorders

a PORTAL HYPERTENSION

In portal hypertension, due to hepatic cirrhosis or less commonly to portal venous thrombosis with cavernous transformation of the portal vein, there is commonly gross splenic enlargement. This has been described in detail by McMichael (1934). The spleen is firm and the cut surface dark red with scattered brown spots which represent scars at the site of small haemorrhages. Histologically the white pulp is atrophic; the red pulp shows congestion though not so marked as in many other conditions and an increase in deposition of fine collagen (reticulin) fibres. Scattered throughout the spleen are small scars consisting of fibrous tissue containing iron and sometimes calcium—the site of organization of small haemorrhages. It is striking that after porto-caval anastomosis, there is little reduction in the size of the spleen (Macpherson *et al.* 1973). The pathological changes in the spleen in portal hypertension can be summarized as those of venous congestion, generalized reactive fine fibrosis, focal haemorrhage and focal reactive fibrosis.

b CHRONIC VENOUS CONGESTION

In generalized chronic venous congestion, due for instance to long-standing cardiac failure the changes are similar but less well-marked (see Fig. 11.3). The spleen is only slightly enlarged (200–300 g) firm and dark red; histologically the sinuses are congested with blood and there is slight fibrosis and often atrophy of the white pulp.

c INFARCTION

Infarction of areas of the spleen or even of almost the whole spleen may be due either to emboli from mural thrombi on the left side of the heart (as after myocardial infarction); or to local thrombosis. Local thrombosis may be due to such generalized arterial lesions as polyarteritis nodosa, or a local inflammatory lesion (Macpherson *et al.* 1973). Local thrombosis may also occur in the abnormal spleens of leukaemia, lymphoma, sickle cell anaemia and malaria. Infarcts may be single or several wedge-shaped necrotic areas which heal by peripheral fibrosis, leaving a yellow inert centre, or as in polyarteritis nodosa there may be multiple, small, usually central infarcts. Healed infarcts are usually evident on the splenic surface by the presence of a white fibrotic 'sugar iced' area.

3 Degenerative changes

The commonest degenerative change is hyaline change seen in splenic arterioles (Fig. 11.4). The arteriolar wall is deeply eosinophilic, thickened and structureless. Such a change is due to the insudation of plasmatic contents including fibrin; elsewhere in the body it would indicate hypertension but in this site is a normal phenomenon over the age of 30 years. Trabeculae of hyaline material are less commonly seen in the white pulp of the normal spleen (Fig. 11.5). The normal spleen contains a moderate diffusely scattered amount of Sudanophil lipid. Focal lipid globules in the white pulp have no particular significance (Wiland and Smith 1956).

Amyloid disease frequently affects the spleen, producing a moderate enlargement, usually up to 500 g. As indicated in Stirling's review (1975) amyloidosis occurs in patients with chronically elevated immunoglobulins due to chronic infection or multiple myeloma, and involves the deposition of a carbohydrate-protein complex containing immunoglobulin fragments. The material is laid down initially in a subendothelial position, either focally in the white pulp or diffusely.

4 Infective and inflammatory conditions

a ACUTE GENERALIZED

In severe acute generalized infections, especially in children, the spleen is moderately enlarged (up to 500 g in an adult), pale, soft and diffluent. The white pulp may be enlarged with prominent reactive germinal centres and the red pulp contains numerous polymorphs and plasma cells. In overwhelming infections the lymphoid tissue may be markedly depleted due to prolonged high output of gluco-corticoids, which cause degeneration of lymphocytes.

b SUBACUTE OR CHRONIC REACTIONS

In more chronic infections the above changes are seen to a lesser degree and are accompanied by increased numbers and size of macrophages in the red pulp.

In typhoid fever there is a diffuse mononuclear cell infiltrate, and in infectious mononucleosis there is a prominent diffuse infiltrate with large lymphocytes. Splenic rupture may occur in either condition. In rheumatoid disease the white pulp is very prominent with large germinal centres.

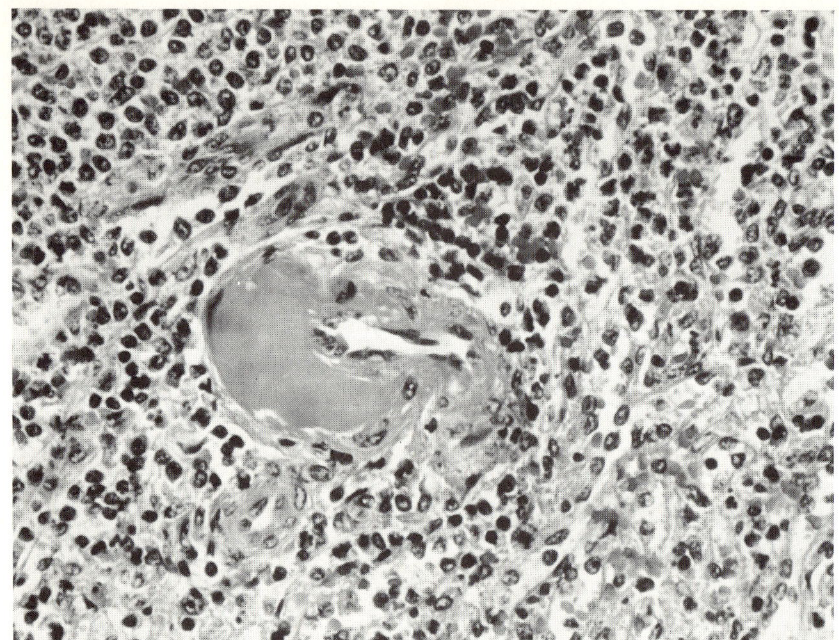

Fig. 11.4. Hyaline sclerosis of a splenic arteriole, occurring normally over the age of 30 years. ×375.

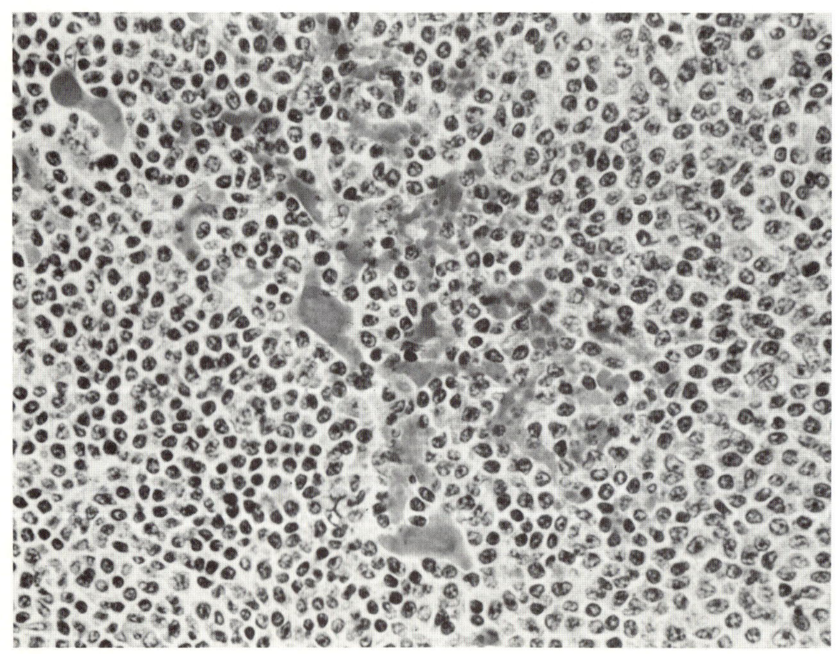

Fig. 11.5. Interstitial trabeculae of hyaline occurring in white pulp of a normal spleen. This material often gives 'amyloid' stains and contains collagen. ×375.

c FOCAL GRANULOMATOUS LESIONS

Focal granulomatous lesions are found in the spleen in a wide variety of systemic disorders—tuberculosis, atypical mycobacterial infections, brucellosis, syphilis and pneumocystis infection. The granulomas range from merely small aggregates of lymphocytes and macrophages to fully formed caseating giant cell granulomas with fibrosis. The nature of the granuloma may point to the diagnosis but often does not. In 20 patients with multiple splenic granulomas, reviewed by Kuo and Rosai (1974), organisms were isolated from only 3—atypical mycobacteria, *Histoplasma capsulatum*, and *Sporotrichum schenkii*. Small granulomas are frequently found, often containing lipid, in spleens removed as a staging procedure in lymphoma but are not of course diagnostic thereof (Kadin *et al.* 1970). The spleen is commonly affected in miliary tuberculosis.

5 Lipidoses

In untreated diabetes mellitus, while the spleen is not grossly enlarged, an excess of cholesterol and sometimes Sudanophilic lipid may be found in macrophages. In Gaucher's disease the spleen is often grossly enlarged, up to 6 kg, and shows diffuse infiltration of the red pulp with large (up to 80 μm), often multinucleate macrophages clear and hyaline in appearance due to the presence of kerasin; the cytoplasm shows a finely fibrillar appearance. The appearances in Niemann–Pick disease are similar, but the macrophages tend to be smaller and usually mononuclear.

6 Blood disorders

a IDIOPATHIC THROMBOCYTOPENIC PURPURA

The spleen in this condition is of normal size or only slightly enlarged. The germinal centres are rather prominent and active and there may be evidence of phagocytosis of platelet masses by macrophages (Firkin *et al.* 1969). The latter cells are large and have foamy, finely granular cytoplasm, containing much phospholipid (Saltzstein 1961). Evidence of other causes of thrombocytopenia is absent.

b HAEMOLYTIC ANAEMIA

Here the spleen is moderately enlarged (300–600 g) though sometimes much larger, particularly in the acquired haemolytic anaemias. The cords are intensely congested with red cells and there is marked phagocytosis by the enlarged red pulp macrophages which come to contain an excess of iron.

In addition to this general picture there is marked focal pooling of blood around the white pulp in sickle cell anaemia, with episodes of infarction and fibrosis. The spleen may ultimately become small, shrunken and fibrotic. In the acquired haemolytic anaemias the white pulp germinal centres are prominent presumably because of an immunological response. In haemolytic anaemia with haemoglobinuria there is only slight splenomegaly, with some congestion of the medulla but little evidence of excess erythrophagocytosis or haemosiderin deposition.

c LEUKAEMIA

Splenic enlargement is found in all forms of leukaemia reaching an extreme degree in the chronic leukaemias notably chronic myeloid leukaemia. In lymphocytic leukaemia the cellular infiltrate is confined at least initially to the white pulp while in myeloid leukaemia there is greater cellular pleomorphism, at least a few immature myeloid cells may be seen and the infiltrate at least initially is confined to the red pulp, with compression atrophy of the white pulp (Fig. 11.6). In hairy-cell leukaemia enlargement may be moderate or gross (up to 4000 g). The leukaemic infiltrate is diffuse, and primarily involves the red pulp with widening of the splenic cords and engorgement of the sinuses; the leukaemic cells often have pointed or indented nuclei and abundant pale cytoplasm containing tartrate-resistant acid phosphatase, demonstrable in smear preparations. Visible only with EM are numerous cytoplasmic processes (Burke *et al.* 1974; Ahmann *et al.* 1966; Kostick and Rappaport 1965). There may be considerable hypersplenism. The changes in monocytic leukaemia are not extensively documented but appear to be similar to those in myeloid leukaemia (Rappaport 1970).

d MYELOFIBROSIS

When the marrow is replaced by fibrous tissue myeloid metaplasia is found in the spleen, i.e. all of the constituents of normal haemopoietic marrow can be recognized. Of these the easiest to identify are megakaryocytes. There may be in addition excessive red cell breakdown and a few atypical histiocytic cells.

Similar changes may be found when haemopoietic marrow is replaced by, e.g. secondary carcinoma or, rarely, without evident cause.

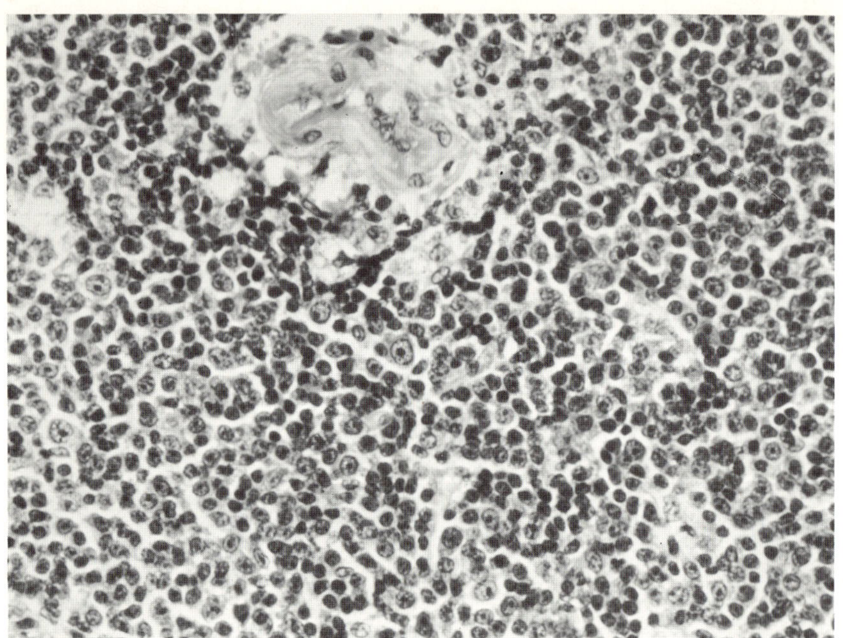

Fig. 11.6. White pulp of spleen from a patient with chronic lymphatic leukaemia in an acute phase. Large blast cells are scattered throughout the lymphoid tissue. ×375.

7 Tumours

a LYMPHOMA

The spleen is often affected in malignant lymphoma usually secondarily, very rarely as the isolated primary site of disease. In terminal untreated lymphoma the spleen may be very large (2–3,000 g) showing either nodular or diffuse infiltration with grey to white neoplasm.

In early Hodgkin's disease, as seen in staging splenectomy specimens, there is commonly hyperplasia of the white pulp with predominant germinal centre formation (see Fig. 11.1). Often no abnormal cells can be seen. The earliest deposits are usually seen in the white pulp in a paravascular position. The walls of veins may be invaded. There may be small lipid granulomata or a sarcoid reaction and in up to 50% of cases overt Hodgkin's lesions are present (Harrison 1975; Farrer-Brown *et al.* 1971).

In non-Hodgkin's lymphoma the earliest lesions are similarly usually in the white pulp. Early lesions may be difficult to distinguish from reactive hyperplasia. In nodular lymphomas there may be multiple, fairly large lesions restricted to white pulp but these ultimately become confluent to form masses 2 cm or more in diameter, indistinguishable from a diffuse lymphoma. Histiocytic lymphoma tends to be less restricted to white pulp than lymphocytic lymphoma. Angiosarcoma and malignant fibrous histiocytoma of spleen are rare and highly malignant (Wick *et al.* 1982). Diffuse splenic infiltration occurs characteristically in malignant histiocytosis.

Primary lymphoma of the spleen is rare. Ahmann *et al.* (1966) described 49 patients in whom the lesion appeared to start in the spleen. Of these 8 had tumour in the spleen only and another 9 had tumour in the spleen and splenic hilar node only. Hodgkin's disease was less common than other lymphomas, and lesions varied from homogenous infiltration through small miliary and multiple larger nodules, to single nodules. Nodular or follicular lymphomas, occurring primarily in the spleen, have a good prognosis after splenectomy (Hickling 1960, 1964).

b SECONDARY CARCINOMATOSIS

While the spleen is not a characteristic site for secondary carcinoma (Fig. 11.7), scattered carcinoma cells may be found in about 5% of patients dying of carcinomatosis and nodules of tumour in about 1%. The periarterial lymphatics may be distended with carcinoma cells (Kostick and Rappaport 1965).

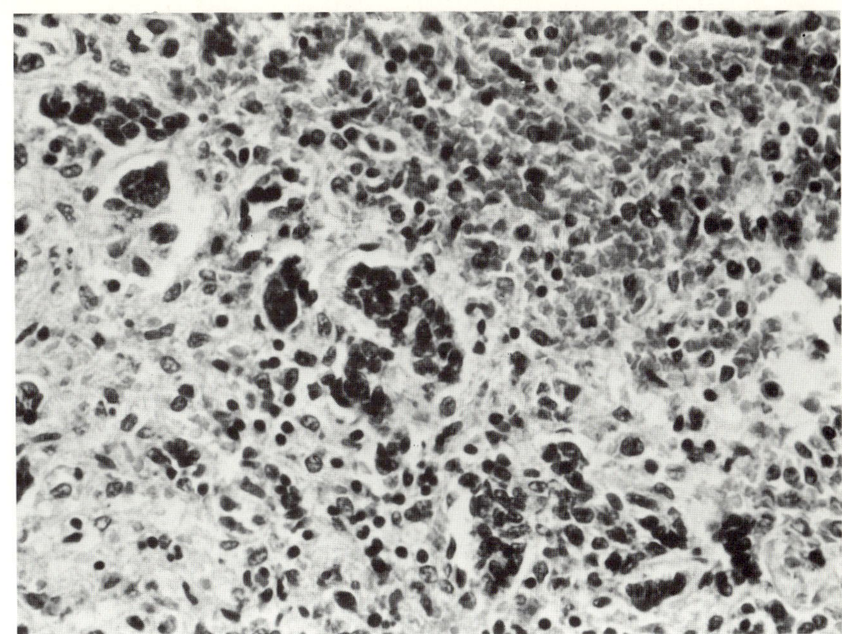

Fig. 11.7. Red pulp of spleen from patient dying of disseminated anaplastic small cell carcinoma of bronchial origin. Clumps of cancer cells distend the sinusoids. × 375.

c CAPILLARY OR CAVERNOUS HAEMANGIOMATA

In the spleen these may be single or multiple or even involve the whole spleen. Occasionally they result in massive haemorrhage.

d CYSTS

Cysts of the spleen are rare. They may be (a) parasitic, usually due to *Taenia echinococcus*; (b) dermoid, sometimes with hair follicles and sebaceous glands; (c) degenerative, following the liquefaction necrosis of infarcts or thrombosed angiomata (reviewed by Macpherson 1980).

8 The spleen in hypersplenism

The term hypersplenism means functional hyperactivity of the spleen and is commonly applied to a clinical syndrome where there is massive splenomegaly and anaemia. The haematological findings include reticulocytosis, neutropenia and thrombocytopenia. There are not usually immature red or white blood cells in the circulation and the bone marrow shows no gross abnormality. The physiologic aspects have been reviewed by Richmond (1980).

Many of these patients have a malignant lymphoma, a lipoidosis (notably Gaucher's disease) or evident persistent chronic infection—e.g. tuberculosis, brucellosis, kala-azar or malaria. The spleens from these patients show, in addition to the primary lesion, a hyperplasia of red pulp macrophages with erythrophagocytosis and increase in iron deposition. Hypersplenism may also occur in rheumatoid disease, where again there is some hyperplasia of red pulp macrophages but the prominent feature is the germinal centre hyperplasia. Hypersplenism occurs occasionally in diffuse carcinomatosis with splenic involvement.

Hypersplenism also occurs in the absence of demonstrable primary lesions, usually in tropical countries (reviewed by Geary *et al.* 1980). The pathology of the spleen in tropical hypersplenism in New Guinea has been described by Pitney *et al.* (1968). The spleens concerned were grossly enlarged (mean weight 3200 g) and showed inconspicuous white pulp; the red pulp showed distension of venous sinuses with swollen endothelial cells showing active phagocytosis. Red pulp macrophages were prominent showing evidence of phagocytosis of cell debris and iron, and moderate fibrosis (see Fig. 11.8). There was some evidence of myeloid transformation. Kirk (1957) described the pathology of the spleen in kala-azar. There is initially a proliferation of macrophages parasitized by the leishmania, followed by stasis of blood and excessive non-selective phagocytosis. This leads to fibrosis and dila-

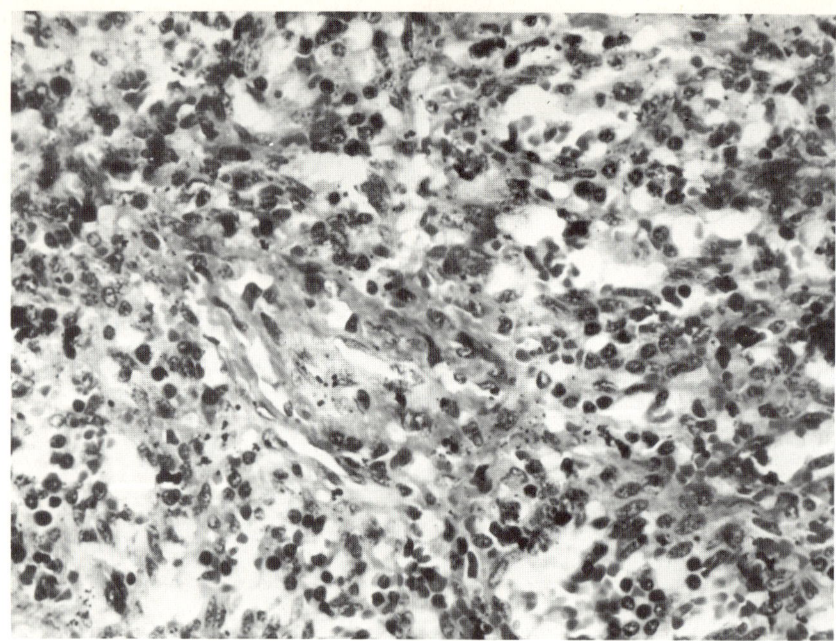

Fig. 11.8. Spleen from patient with idiopathic tropical splenomegaly showing interstitial fibrosis and numerous granules of iron-containing pigment. × 375.

tation of sinusoids. The splenomegaly common in Egypt may well be due to a similar process initiated by schistosomal infection, while the very common splenomegaly of malaria is explicable on a similar train of events initiated by the plasmodium of malaria.

Splenectomy normally corrects the cytopenia of hypersplenism but should not be undertaken lightly in view of the greater morbidity and mortality in such patients. In tropical splenomegaly long-term anti-malarial therapy is often appropriate in the first instance and in lymphomas, where modern cytotoxic chemotherapy or radiotherapy is commonly effective in shrinking the spleen, splenectomy is usually unnecessary except in certain low grade lymphomas and chronic lymphocytic leukaemia where it may be of palliative value (Holt and Witts 1966).

A similar syndrome occurs in temperate climates—nontropical idiopathic splenomegaly (primary hypersplenism) (Dacie *et al.* 1969). The spleens are grossly enlarged (mean 2400 g). About half show white pulp hyperplasia. There is usually dilatation of venous sinuses and increased macrophage activity in the red pulp with erythrophagocytosis. There are small lymphocytic foci but no myeloid metaplasia. Two of the ten patients in Dacie's group subsequently developed lymphosarcoma.

9 Splenic atrophy

Splenic atrophy is rare. As an exceptional occurrence the spleen may be congenitally absent or small, sometimes associated with marrow hypoplasia. Acquired atrophy may be due to autodestruction by numerous small infarcts in sickle cell anaemia or, rarely, in thrombocytopenic purpura. A diffuse atrophy may uncommonly occur in coeliac disease and other malabsorption states and even less often in alcoholism, hypopituitarism and hyperthyroidism (reviewed by Crosby 1963) and rarely without evident cause. The normal reserve of splenic function is great but when splenic mass sinks below about 20 g a failure of haemophagocytic functions results in the appearance of excessively thin red blood cells in peripheral films ('leptocytes') often containing abnormal inclusions, notably nuclear fragments (Howell–Jolly bodies) and denatured haemoglobin (Heinz bodies). Impaired splenic function may be detected in malabsorption states in life by impaired clearance of chromium labelled RBC and by reduction of splenic size as seen radiographically (McCarthy *et al.* 1966; Marsh and Stewart 1970). In a recent series of 14 patients with splenic atrophy diagnosed clinically, by red cell survival studies and radiographically, 8 had intestinal malabsorption and the remainder had a high incidence of autoimmune disease. There seems to be some correlation between auto-antibody formation and splenic atrophy (Wardrop *et al.* 1975).

Other possible consequences of impaired splenic function (Bullen and Losowsky 1979) include peripheral blood leucocytosis and thrombocytosis, the latter with possible consequences of thrombosis and/or haemorrhage.

Hyposplenism has been demonstrated in inflammatory bowel disease (Ryan *et al.* 1978) and there is some evidence that these patients may be prone to severe bacterial infection. It is recognised that infections, often with *Diplococcus pneumoniae* and *Haemophilus influenzae*, may occasionally follow removal of the spleen, sometimes many weeks or months later (Desser and Ultmann 1972). Patients having splenectomy for traumatic rupture rarely suffer such complications and those having the operation for idiopathic thrombocytopenic purpura, hereditary spherocytosis, local tumour or aplastic anaemia run only a small hazard. In contrast, the risks with thalassaemia major, portal hypertension and malignant lymphoma may be greater. Predisposing factors in the latter condition may be youth and immunosuppressive therapy. The risk of infection may be related to the falls in serum IgM observed after splenectomy, the failure to clear particulate antigens, or the fall in the level of the phagocytosis stimulating polypeptide tuftsin (Leader 1978). It is possible that long-term penicillin therapy or the administration of pneumococcal polysaccharide vaccine may help reduce the incidence of pneumococcal infections in such patients.

The complications of splenectomy done as part of the staging of Hodgkin's disease are discussed more fully in Chapters 4 and 13.

REFERENCES

AHMANN D.L., KIELY J.M., HARRISON E.G. & PAYNE W.S. (1966) Malignant lymphoma of the spleen. A review of 49 cases in which the diagnosis was made at splenectomy. *Cancer* **19**, 461–9.

BULLEN A.W. & LOSOWSKY M.S. (1979) Consequences of impaired splenic function. *Clin. Sci.* **57**, 129–37.

BURKE J.S., BYRNE G.E. & RAPPAPORT H. (1974) Hairy cell leukaemia. (Leukaemic reticulo–endotheliosis.) I. A clinical pathologic study of 21 patients. *Cancer* **33**, 1399–410.

CROSBY H.H. (1963) Hyposplenism: an enquiry into normal functions of the spleen. *Ann. Rev. Med.* **14**, 349–70.

DACIE J.V., BRAIN M.C., HARRISON C.V., LEWIS S.M. & WORLLEDGE S.M. (1969) Non-tropical idiopathic splenomegaly (primary hypersplenism): a review of ten cases and their relationship to malignant lymphoma. *Brit. J. Haemat.* **17**, 317–33.

DESSER R.K. & ULTMANN J.E. (1972) Risk of severe infection in patients with Hodgkin's disease or lymphoma after diagnostic laparotomy and splenectomy. *Ann. Intern. Med.* **77**, 143–46.

FARRER-BROWN G., BENNETT M.M., HARRISON C.V., MILLETT Y. & JELLIFFE A.M. (1971) The pathological findings following laparotomy in Hodgkin's disease. *Brit. J. Cancer* **25**, 449–57.

FIRKIN B.G., WRIGHT R., MILLER S. & STOKES E. (1969) Splenic macrophages in thrombocytopenia. *Blood* **33**, 240–45.

GEARY C.G., CLOUGH V. & McIVER J.E. (1980) The spleen: tropical splenomegaly. *Brit. J. Hosp. Med.* **24/5**, 417–21.

HARRISON C.V. (1975) Lymph Node Diseases. In *Recent Advances in Pathology*, pp. 73–96 (Eds Harrison C.V. & Weinbren K.). Churchill Livingstone, Edinburgh.

HICKLING R.A. (1960) Giant follicle lymphoma of the spleen; recovery after splenectomy. *Brit. Med. J.* **1**, 1464–7.

HICKLING R.A. (1964) Giant follicle lymphoma of the spleen. A condition closely related to lymphatic leukaemia but apparently curable by splenectomy. *Brit. Med. J.* **1**, 787–90.

HOLT J.M. & WITTS L.J. (1966) Splenectomy in leukaemia and the reticuloses. *Quart. J. Med.* **35**, 369–84.

KADIN M.E., DONALDSON S.S. & DORFMAN R.F. (1970) Isolated granulomas in Hodgkin's disease. *N. Eng. J. Med.* **283**, 859–61.

KIRK R. (1957) The pathogenesis of some tropical splenomegalies. *Ann. Trop. Med. Parasit. (Liverp.)* **51**, 225–34.

KLEMPERER P. (1936) The pathological anatomy of splenomegaly. *Amer. J. Clin. Path.* **6**, 99–159.

KOSTICK N.D. & RAPPAPORT H. (1965) Diagnostic significance of the histologic changes in the liver and spleen in leukaemia and malignant lymphoma. *Cancer* **18**, 1214–32.

KUO T. & ROSAI J. (1974) Granulomatous inflammation in splenectomy specimens. Clinico-pathologic study of 20 cases. *Arch. Path.* **98**, 261–8.

LEADER (1978) After splenectomy. *Brit. Med. J.* **2**, 1042.

LUKES R.J. (1970) The pathology of the white pulp of the spleen. In LENNERT K. & HARMS D. (eds.), *The Spleen*, pp. 130–8. Springer-Verlag, Berlin.

McCARTHY C.F., FRASER I.D., EVANS K.T. & READ A.E. (1966) Lymphoreticular dysfunction in idiopathic steatorrhoea. *Gut* **7**, 140–8.

McMICHAEL J. (1934) The pathology of hepatolienal fibrosis. *J. Path. Bact.* **39**, 481–502.

MacPHERSON A.I.S., RICHMOND J. & STUART A.E. (1973) *The Spleen*, pp. 83–151. Thomas, Springfield.

MacPHERSON A.I.S. (1980) The spleen cysts and tumours. *Brit. J. Hosp. Med.* **24/5**, 413–16.

MARSH G.W. & STEWART J.S. (1970) Splenic function in adult coeliac disease. *Brit. J. Haemat.* **19**, 445–57.

PITNEY W.R., PRYOR D.S. & TAIT-SMITH A. (1968) Morphological observations on livers and spleens of patients with tropical splenomegaly in New Guinea. *J. Path. Bact.* **95**, 417–22.

RAPPAPORT H. (1970) The pathologic anatomy of the splenic red pulp. In LENNERT K. & HARMS D. (eds.), *The Spleen*. Springer-Verlag, Berlin.

RICHMOND J. (1980) The spleen. Hypersplenism. *Brit. J. Hosp. Med.* **24/5**, 405–12.

Robb-Smith A.H.T. (1970) Pathological lesions in surgically removed spleens. *Brit. J. Hosp. Med.* **3**, 19–21.

Ryan F.P., Smart R.C., Holdsworth C.D. & Preston F.E. (1980) Hyposplenism in inflammatory bowel disease. *Gut* **19**, 50–5.

Saltzstein S.L. (1961) Phospholipid accumulation in histiocytes of splenic pulp associated with thrombocytopenic purpura. *Blood* **18**, 73–88.

Stirling G.A. (1975) Amyloidosis. In Harrison C.V. & Weinbren K. (eds.), *Recent Advances in Pathology*, pp. 249–72. Churchill Livingstone, Edinburgh.

Stites T.B. & Ultmann J.E. (1966) Spontaneous rupture of the spleen in chronic lymphatic leukaemia. *Cancer* **19**, 1587–90.

Szabo A. de K. (1961) Splenosis. The autotransplantation of splenic tissue. *Amer. J. Surg.* **101**, 208–14.

Wardrop C.A., Dagg J.H., Lee F.D., Singh H., Dyet J.F. & Moffat A. (1975) Immunological abnormalities in splenic atrophy. *Lancet* **2**, 4–7.

Wick M.R., Scheithauer B.W., Smith S.L. & Beart R.W. (1982) Primary non-lymphoreticular malignant neoplasms of the spleen. *Am. J. Surg. Pathol.* **6**, 229–42.

Wiland O.K. & Smith E.B. (1956) Morphology of the spleen in congenital haemolytic anaemia (hereditary spherocytosis). *Amer. J. Clin. Path.* **26**, 619–29.

As has been discussed in Chapter 1, the thymus is a lympho-reticular organ which undergoes physiological atrophy with age, or stress under the influence of corticosteroids. In children and young people dying suddenly the thymus may not have had time to atrophy, giving rise to the legend of 'status thymolymphaticus' and the view that the enlarged thymus was in some way the cause rather than the consequence of the sudden death. The thymus rarely fails to atrophy in adult life but atrophy is less complete than usual in thyrotoxicosis, Hashimoto's disease and Addison's disease. True thymic hyperplasia can be established by comparison of weight with a standard graph (Levine and Rosai 1978).

The role of the thymus in immune deficiency states has been discussed in Chapter 2 and is reviewed by Henry (1975). The pathology of the thymus in these conditions will be briefly summarized here. If the immunological defect is primarily a defect of T-lymphocyte function rather than production, such as occurs in the Wiskott–Aldrich syndrome, then the thymus may be normal in appearance. This will also be the case if the immune deficiency only affects B-lymphocytes (Bruton-type agammaglobulinaemia). However, since the thymus arises from two sources, embryological abnormalities could arise from failure of either the epithelial or lymphoid elements to develop. Thus in the Di George and Nezelof syndromes, the development of the thymus from the third pharyngeal pouch is defective and the thymus is either absent or severely defective. In the case of the Di George syndrome the parathyroids may also be absent, indicating a deficient development of the fourth pharyngeal pouch, and other congenital abnormalities may be present. In ataxia–telangiectasia the thymus may be hypoplastic due to defective formation of the mesenchymal elements.

In other cases the epithelial elements of the thymus may develop normally but a failure of lymphocyte production results in these cells being absent from the organ. Such is the case in reticular dysgenesis, Swiss-type agammaglobulinaemia, thymic alymphoplasia and thymic dysplasia.

Since the thymus has a role in immunological surveillance, defects in this may result in the onset of autoimmune disease and this may be associated with a thymoma or other thymic abnormalities, to be discussed later in the chapter. The thymus and particularly thymic neoplasia are also related to such conditions as myasthenia gravis. A further discussion of thymic pathology therefore must start with a consideration of thymic neoplasms.

THYMOMA

Tumours of the thymus form approximately 40% of swellings in the anterior mediastinum, exclusive of metastatic lesions (O'Gara et al. 1958). Early classifications failed to take account of the predominance of metastatic carcinoma in this area and it was not until the study of Symmers (1932) that the concept of a primary thymoma became established. Since then a number of other classifications have emerged, listed by Bernatz et al. (1961). These authors themselves describe the pathologic features of 138 cases incorporating both gross and microscopic findings.

CLINICAL ASPECTS

Of these 138 patients 64 (46%) had myasthenia gravis. In the myasthenic group the average age was 45 years, compared with 52 years for patients without myasthenia. In myasthenic patients undergoing thymectomy for non-neoplastic thymic enlargement, females predominate 2:1 whereas in the tumour group the sex distribution is equal. The average age of women in the former group is 28, considerably younger than in those myasthenics with a thymoma. Where no myasthenia is present, the lesion is most often discovered on a routine chest X-ray and the lesion is clinically symptomless. Symptoms of compression or local invasion may indicate malignancy and are usually of serious import particularly when pain is present (Seybold et al. 1950).

The clinical presentation in 54 cases of thymoma was studied by Batata et al. (1974). The tumour was asymptomatic in 22 patients and was detected only on routine chest X-ray.

The predominant symptoms in the remaining 32 patients were cough (14 patients), chest pain (14), dyspnoea (12), weight loss (16) and unexplained fever (8). Other symptoms included dysphagia, hoarseness, superior vena caval obstruction, enlarged cervical lymph nodes, pleural effusion, erythroid hypoplasia and hypogammaglobulinaemia. Four patients presented with myasthenia gravis and one developed this complaint after thymectomy. All of the 54 patients underwent surgical exploration. The tumour was in the anterior mediastinum in every case, 10 in the upper third, 27 in the middle third and 3 in the lower third. The radiological features of thymoma are discussed by Holmes Sellors *et al.* (1967) and by Kreel (1973).

Cases of familial thymoma do occur, as reported by Matani and Dritsas (1973), but these are rare. The tumour is also rare in children. Bearing in mind the embryological derivation of the thymus from the third pharyngeal pouch, ectopic thymic tissue may be found in the neck, where it may come into proximity with the parathyroids. Thymomas therefore may also be found in these situations.

GROSS PATHOLOGY

Most thymomas are well-circumscribed, although it may be evident at surgery that the tumour is, in fact, invasive. The cut surface shows a well-defined fibrous capsule with wide fibrous trabeculae extending into the interior of the tumour which is thus separated into greyish nodules. Significant cyst forma-

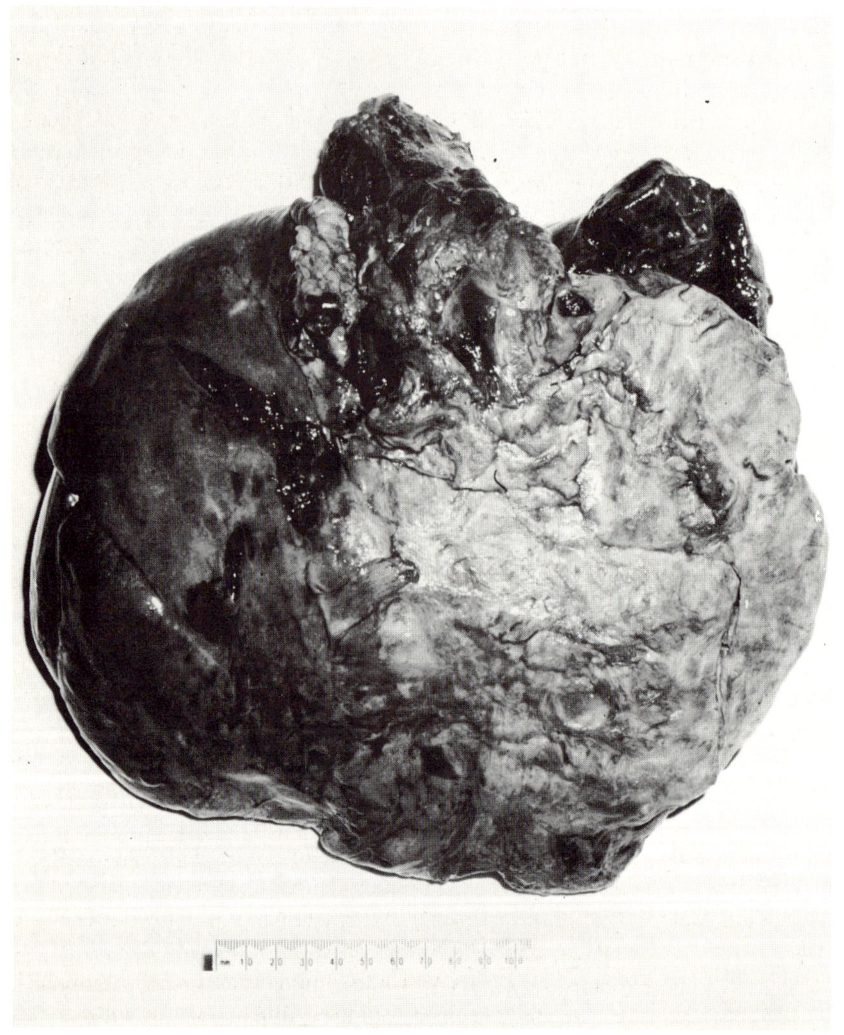

Fig. 12.1. Thymic tumour removed at postmortem from a man aged nineteen years. The lesion was an epithelial thymoma.

tion is seen in about one-sixth of the cases and calcification may occur in the walls of such cysts. While the larger tumours may have destroyed the original thymus, a thymic remnant is frequently present. In the series of Bernatz *et al.* (1961) the size varied from 15 cm to 3 cm in diameter and the weight from 915 g to 36 g. Occasionally tumours may be multiple. Some thymomas are not evidently trabeculated and are seen on cut surface as a diffuse sheet of homogeneous soft, grey tissue (Fig. 12.1).

HISTOLOGIC FEATURES

A comprehensive study of the histologic appearance of thymomas was undertaken by Lattes (1962). Most cases show a mixture of cells and the pattern may vary in different parts of the same tumour. The final classification of any individual tumour therefore tends to reflect the predominant pattern. Lattes (1962) subdivided a series of 103 cases as follows: (*a*) Lymphoid (42 cases); (*b*) Spindle cell (26 cases); (*c*) Epithelial (20 cases); (*d*) Granulomatous (7 cases); (*e*) Rosette (4 cases); (*f*) Seminoma (4 cases); (*g*) Epithelial+granulomatous (3 cases).

Most of the tumours in this group therefore contained a preponderance of lymphoid or epithelial cells. The frequency of the 'mixed' patterns led Bernatz *et al.* (1961) to include this as a separate category, dividing the tumours into the following categories:

Lymphoid	(30%)
Epithelial	(16%)
Mixed	(30%)
Spindle cell	(24%)

Legg and Brady (1965) have a similar classification using the term 'small-cell type' to refer to the lymphocytic and the term 'protoplasmic type' to refer to the epithelial types of other authors. This terminology is not commonly used. Thomson and Thackray (1957) recognize the variety of pattern which can be seen, and include all such variants in the 'epithelial' category, thus:

Epithelial (54 cases) This group was divided into sub-variants as follows: Differentiated (7 cases), Oval cell (7 cases), Spindle cell (7 cases), Lymphoepithelial (5 cases), Granulomatous (15 cases), Undifferentiated (20 cases)
    Lymphoid (10 cases)
    Teratomatous (2 cases)

This classification suffers from having a high proportion of undifferentiated tumours and by including 'granulomatous' thymoma. The latter is probably a manifestation of Hodgkin's disease and will be discussed later. It is probable that teratomatous lesions are not strictly of thymic origin and should not be considered among these tumours with the possible exception of the 'thymo-lipoma' (Shillitoe and Goodyear 1960) although even this may be a hamartomatous malformation rather than a true tumour.

Rosai and Levine (1976) suggest that all true thymomas arise from the epithelial cells of the thymus and are independent of the lymphocytic content of the tumour. Thus there would, for example, be no such entity as a 'predominantly lymphocytic thymoma' which should be considered as an epithelial tumour with a high content of lymphocytes. They point out that lymphomas of the thymus do occur, but usually in association with more generalized disease. 'Granulomatous' thymoma is considered to be a local manifestation of Hodgkin's disease and germ cell tumours of the mediastinum are placed in a separate category as being of doubtful thymic origin. Their classification of true thymomas, while commenting on the lymphocytic content, concentrates attention on the epithelial cells and the histological variations which may be found in relation to these.

A reasonable and simplified classification would seem to be as follows:

Predominantly lymphocytic
Mixed lymphocytic and epithelial (lymphoepithelioma)
Predominantly epithelial
Spindle cell (probably epithelial)
Germinal origin ('seminoma')

The continued classification into 'lymphocytic' and 'epithelial' types is justified by the ultrastructural studies of Toker (1968). The cells of epithelial thymomas show prominent desmosomes and intracellular fibrils and less often secretory granules. Ultrastructural examination is of real value in the diagnosis of thymomas (Fig. 12.2) since the presence of epithelial cells with well-developed desmosomes is essential for the diagnosis (Toker 1968). In their study of the ultrastructure of the normal thymus, thymic tumours and the thymus in myasthenia gravis, Bloodworth *et al.* (1975) describe six forms which the epithelial cell can take: syncytial, epithelioid, squamoid, spindle, fibrillary and secretory.

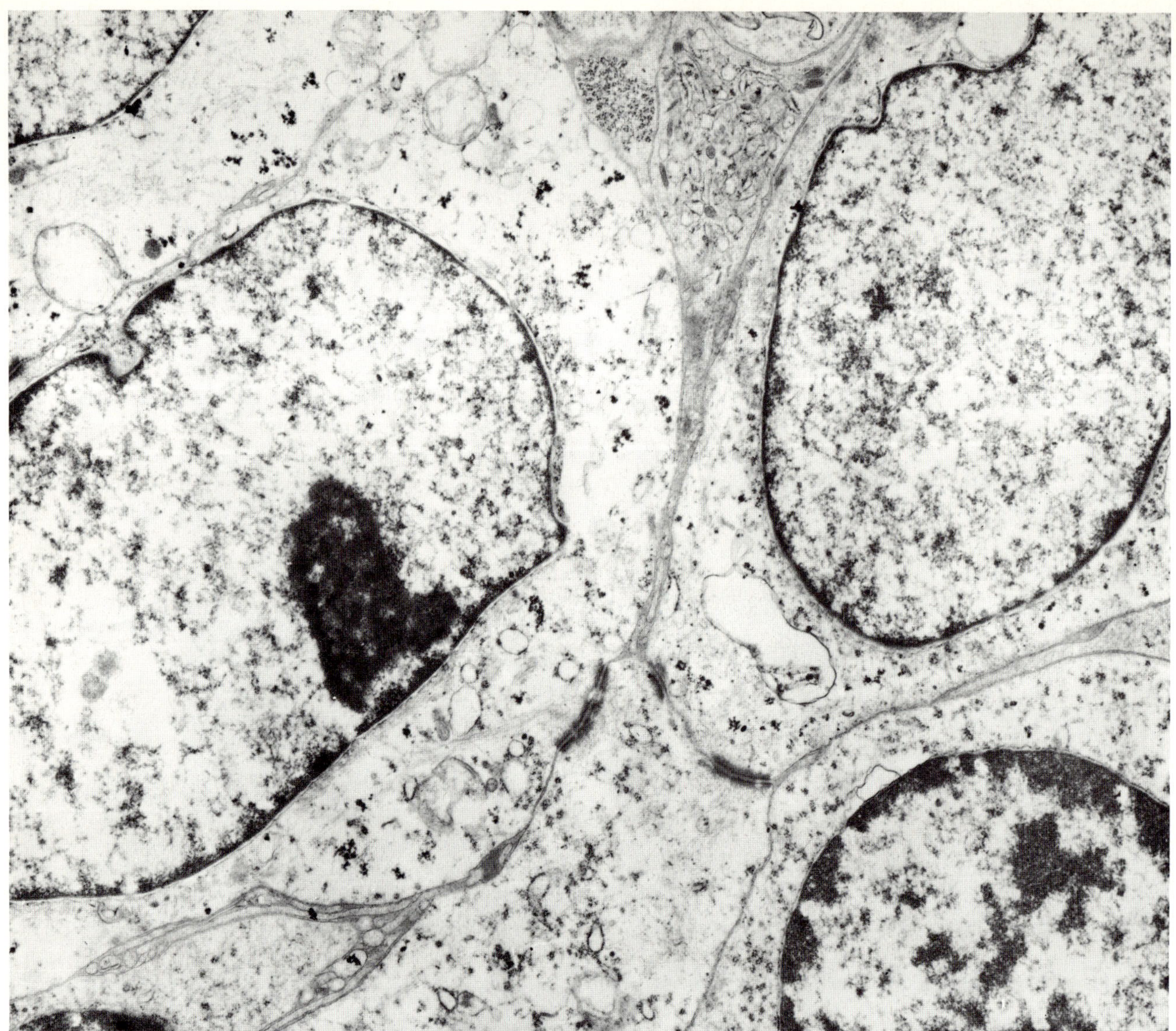

Fig. **12.2.** Electron micrograph of epithelial thymoma showing well developed desmosomes. ×6,100.

HISTOLOGICAL TYPES

Predominantly lymphocytic

Although the variant usually occurs in tumours showing gross fibrous trabeculation, little fibrosis is found within the tumour lobules. These consist of a diffuse sheet of small lymphocytes with no formation of follicles or germinal centres in most cases. A variable amount of reticulin can be demonstrated. No Hassall's corpuscles are seen. A few epithelial cells are invariably present, either singly or in small groups standing out against the smaller lymphocytes (Fig. 12.3). In the absence of epithelial cells, the diagnosis of a malignant lymphoma should be strongly considered.

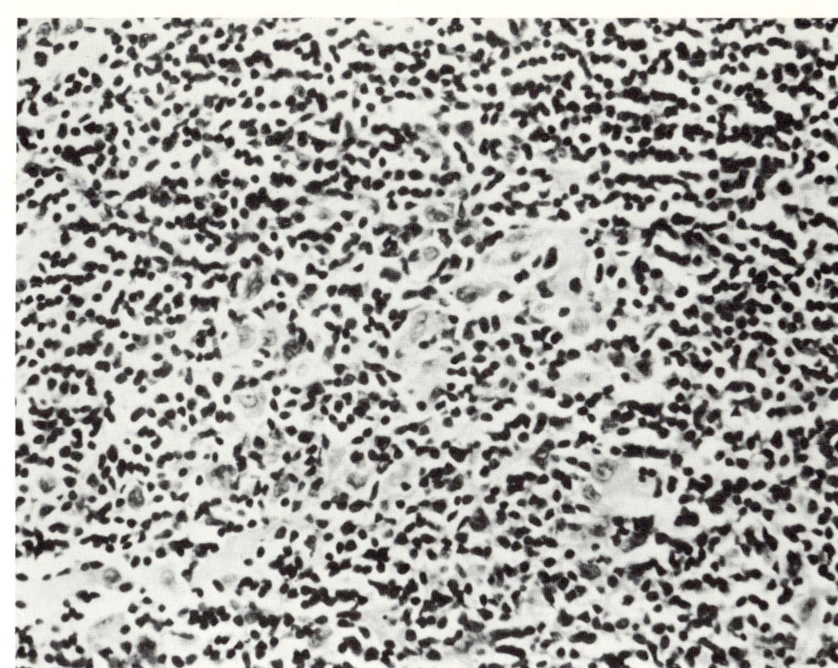

Fig. 12.3. Lymphocytic thymoma showing
diffuse replacement of normal thymic
structure by small lymphocytes with only a
few scanty residual epithelial cells. ×216.

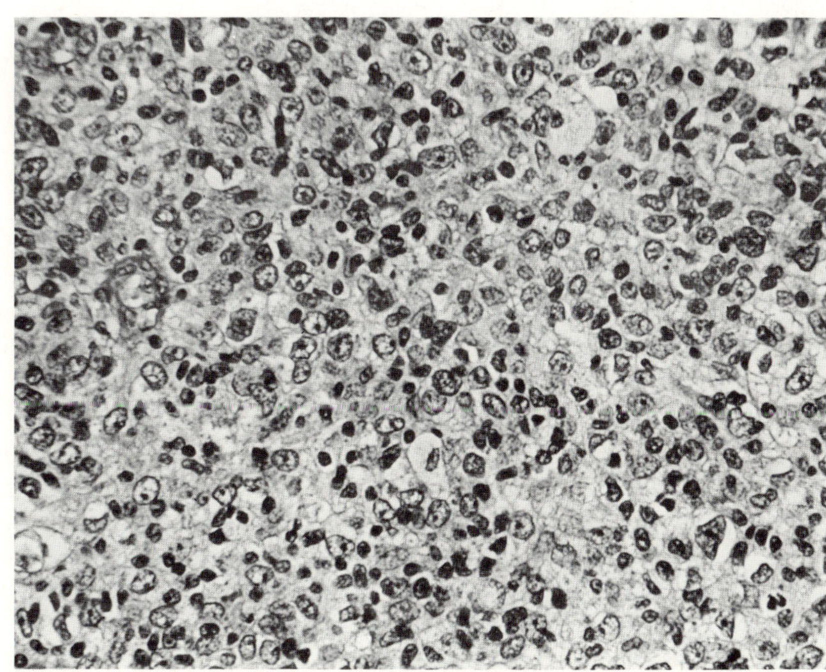

Fig. 12.4. Epithelial thymoma showing
diffuse replacement of thymus by large
epithelial cells with only a few
lymphocytes. ×216.

Predominantly epithelial

This type again occurs in association with fibrous trabeculae. The tumour nodules consist of a diffuse sheet of large pale cells with ill-defined cell boundaries giving the appearance of syncytial masses. There is no fibrosis or reticulin formation within the tumour. The individual cells have large nuclei and abundant cytoplasm which stains palely with eosin. Some variants show a 'clear-cell' pattern. Many of the cells contain PAS-positive granules; these cells may be of macrophage origin. The alignment of the cells in relation to each other causes them to adopt differing shapes from round to polyhedral and in addition to the syncytial appearance the tumour may show a whorled or fusiform pattern, or areas approaching a squamoid pattern. When well-formed whorls are present these may give the appearance of abortive formation of Hassall's corpuscles and in rare cases, these corpuscles can be definitely seen. Perivascular rosette formation may suggest a pseudoglandular pattern but this is probably not a separate histological type. Microcyst formation gives a cribriform pattern and as an extension of this Evans (1966) describes lymphangiomatous, adenomatoid or adamantinoma variants, although these are rare. Formation of larger cysts is common, such that these are grossly visible. Necrotic material containing cholesterol clefts may be seen in the cyst contents and calcification in the cyst wall. The epithelial cells may vary in size but there is usually no significant pleomorphism and the mitotic rate is normally low. Nucleoli are present. Occasionally cells containing large nuclei are sometimes seen, but no Reed–Sternberg cells. Scattered lymphocytes are always present and occasional lymphoid follicles with germinal cells are apparent (Fig. 12.4).

Lymphoepithelial

Here there is a variable admixture of lymphoid and epithelial cells but with both in significant proportions. Not only may the proportions of these two elements vary but also their relationship to one another. They may be intimately mixed, simulating a nasopharyngeal lymphoepithelioma although without the eosinophil content sometimes seen in these latter tumours. The lymphocytes and epithelial cells may be arranged in separate but contiguous islands or lymphocytic areas may be interposed between sheets of epithelial cells which compress the lymphocytes into cords. Occasionally, in a largely epithelial tumour, the lymphocytes may assume a perivascular distribution. On prolonged search lymphoid follicles with germinal centres may be seen and, rarely, Hassall's corpuscles are seen. The tumour is again lobulated and interspersed with fibrous trabeculae, which may be seen in tumour extending beyond the capsule, but the tumour tissue itself produces no collagen or reticulin. The morphologic details of the epithelial cells do not differ from the predominantly epithelial pattern, but cyst formation is rather less common. The ratio of lymphocytes to epithelial cells may vary between 0.27 and 4.10 and those with a greater proportion of epithelial cells tend to show features of malignancy. Most lymphocytes in a thymoma are T-lymphocytes (Cossman *et al.* 1978). Whether these are neoplastic in nature or are normal lymphocytes reacting against the tumour remains to be seen.

Spindle cell

In a significant number of cases the cells become fusiform and the whole tumour assumes a 'spindle cell' appearance simulating that of a sarcoma. This resemblance may be heightened when the cells are arranged in bundles or whorls. However, transitions are usually seen between obviously epithelial areas and spindle cells merging into one another. This, and a frequent admixture with lymphocytes indicates an epithelial origin of these tumours. This is confirmed by the ultrastructural study of Levine and Bensch (1972). A 68-year-old female had an asymptomatic mediastinal mass for 4 years. The resected tumour was well encapsulated and showed a spindle cell configuration. Electron microscopy showed a uniform population of interdigitating cells with large numbers of typical desmosomes and cytoplasmic filaments resembling the tonofilaments seen in the cells of Hassall's corpuscles, although no keratohyalin granules were demonstrated. Thus these tumours are certainly epithelial in nature, but should be considered separately because of their characteristic histological appearance and good prognosis. They are seldom associated with myasthenia gravis, but may be accompanied by a variety of other syndromes (Fig. 12.5).

ULTRASTRUCTURE OF THYMOMAS

The ultrastructure of thymic tumours has been studied by Toker (1968), Bloodworth *et al.* (1975) and by Rosai and Levine (1976). The cells composing a thymoma resemble those seen in a normal thymus. However, multiple blocks should be examined, since the ratio of cell types and the amount of stroma may vary in different areas of the same

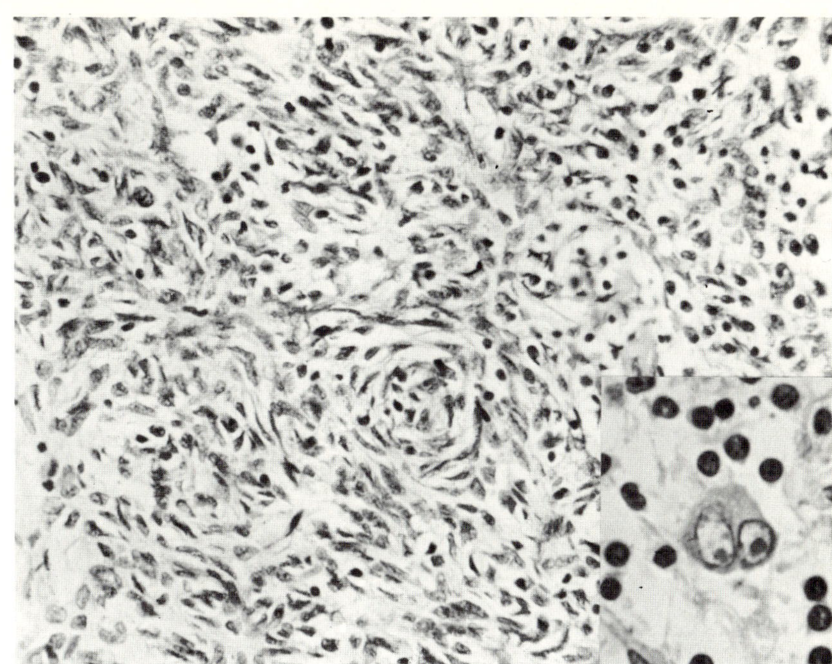

tumour. The epithelial cell of a thymoma is large, with elongated cell processes and containing tonofilaments (Levine *et al.* 1975). Some epithelial cells are polyhedral but desmosomes are seen in all cases. The epithelial nature of spindle cell thymomas is confirmed by Levine and Bensch (1972), the cells having some resemblance to those seen in Hassall's corpuscles. No dense-core granules are seen, but Bloodworth *et al.* (1975) report one case where the epithelial cells contained granules interpreted as being of a possible secretory nature. The lymphocyte morphology is variable and some show features of transformation. If the lymphocyte mitotic rate is high many degenerate lymphocytes may be seen. Llombart-Bosch (1975) reports a case where lymphocytes were present in both epithelial cells and macrophages. Snover *et al.* (1982) describe mixed, small cell, squamous carcinoma, basaloid carcinoma, mucoepidermoid carcinoma and sarcomatoid carcinoma as variants.

Seminoma ('germinoma')

In a few cases, some 4% of Lattes (1962) series, a tumour in the anterior mediastinum is histologically similar to a seminoma. The tumour may of course be metastatic from a seminoma of testis. This may be so small that the testis itself is not enlarged or on rare occasions may even regress, leaving a scar. However, if such an event can be excluded, there are some cases where the mediastinal tumour appears to be primary. The tumour consists of round cells with clear cytoplasm containing glycogen. The nuclei show coarse stippling of the chromatin pattern and a prominent nucleolus but mitotic figures are rare. These features combined with relative paucity of cytoplasmic organelles are particularly obvious at the ultrastructural level. Ultrastructural examination demonstrates convincingly that this is a distinct type of tumour (Levine 1973). The tumour is not lobulated as with the lymphoid or epithelial thymomas and presents a homogeneous grey-pink appearance on its cut surface, but histologically it may be separated into islands by thin trabeculae containing a little reticulin. Areas of granulomatous inflammation may occur. Lymphoid follicles are not a feature, but otherwise the resemblance to a seminoma is very striking. Although included by some as a thymoma (Iverson 1956; Lattes 1962) this is a distinct lesion, not associated with myasthenia or other autoimmune syndromes. Levine (1973) lists 61 such cases, again suggesting a thymic lesion and indicating a good response to irradiation rather than surgery. Pachter and Lattes (1964) found all such cases to be in males and Steinmetz and Hays (1961) report a case with metastasis to lungs, hilar lymph nodes, spleen and adrenal. There is some indication that these tumours may originate in an anterior mediastinal teratoma. Pugsley and Carleton (1953) report one case with both teratomatous and seminomatous elements, and similarly Woolner *et al.* (1955). It is therefore possible that a seminoma represents one facet of a malignant teratoma and may, in fact, be altogether separate from the thymomas. Electron microscopy is useful in this condition, the tumour having the ultrastructural characteristics of the true testicular seminoma.

In addition to the pure seminomatous tumour, malignant teratoma (Bloodworth *et al.* 1975) and embryonal carcinoma, choriocarcinoma and yolk-sac tumours have also been described (Rosai and Levine 1976) suggesting that these lesions arise from germ cell elements present in the thymic region.

TUMOURS WITH A MYOID COMPONENT

The occurrence of striated muscle cells in the medulla of the thymus has been known for some time, being re-emphasized by Henry (1966 and 1968) and Feltkamp-Vroom (1966). They may be found in the foetal, perinatal and adult thymus and although found in a variety of species are more common in the human organ. Their presence has considerable importance in considering the relationship of the thymus to myasthenia gravis (q.v.) but in morphologic terms two thymomas have been reported where a content of striated muscle fibres was established. Henry (1972) described a 68-year-old female with a cystic tumour in the thymus. This consisted of spindle cells and ovoid cells with scanty cytoplasm and occasional mitoses. In addition, large rounded cells were present, with plentiful, eosinophilic cytoplasm. Myofibrils were present in these latter cells on PTAH staining but although no cross-striations were observed, electron microscopy confirmed their nature as being of striated muscle origin. In a series of 56 tumours of the thymus, Friedman (1967) details one in a 51-year-old female as having the appearance of a myosarcoma.

CARCINOID TUMOUR

This, first described by Fell *et al.* (1966), is now regarded as a separate entity, possibly arising from Kultschitsky cells (Rosai and Higa 1972). Since then a number of cases have been reported (Wick 1980), some associated with multiple endocrine adenomatosis (Rosai *et al.* 1972). The histologic features are those of carcinoids elsewhere; the tumour cells are often arranged in ribbons or festoons with pseudo-acini, punctuate necrosis and calcification. Cushing's syndrome occurs in about one-third of cases (Kay and Willson 1970; Levine and Rosai 1978). Metastasis to regional lymph nodes, or even distantly to bone, occurs in 41% of cases, more commonly in patients with Cushing's syndrome (Levine and Rosai 1978).

GRANULOMATOUS THYMOMA (HODGKIN'S DISEASE OF THE THYMUS AND OTHER LYMPHOMAS)

A certain number of tumours have a histological appearance closely resembling Hodgkin's disease. These tumours have been designated as 'granulomatous' thymoma and accounted for 7 of the 107 cases of thymoma reported by Lattes (1962). They tend to occur in young women and at first the disease is localized to the mediastinum. Later the regional lymph nodes may become involved and a certain number of cases terminate with disseminated disease. Basically, the problem is to decide whether these tumours represent a localized manifestation of Hodgkin's disease or are specifically thymomas in their own right. The frequent association of thymic involvement with Hodgkin's disease led Thomson (1955) to speculate on the thymic origin of this condition, but the study of Marshall and Wood (1957) showed that in many cases of Hodgkin's disease the thymus was not involved. The histologic appearance is usually that of a rather fibrotic Hodgkin's disease with lymphocytes, plasma cells, eosinophils and large mononuclear cells with broad bands of fibrous tissue dividing the tumour into lobules. Reed–Sternberg cells are present (Fig. 12.6), although these may be somewhat atypical and contain PAS-positive granules, a feature not usually seen in the classical Reed–Sternberg cell. A thymic element is often present and may show squamoid cells or cysts lined by columnar cells, which later may be surrounded by foci of neoplasm. Hassall's corpuscles may be seen in the centres of the nodules associated with clusters of the atypical Reed–Sternberg cells. These features, described by Katz and Lattes (1969) are considered by these authors to represent a local manifestation of Hodgkin's disease modified by a response peculiar to the thymus. These authors detailed 24 cases of which 6 developed disseminated lesions indistinguishable from Hodgkin's disease. Since the classical varieties of thymoma seldom develop extrathoracic metastases this tendency to dissemination indicates a difference in the behaviour of granulomatous thymoma. This was emphasized by Nickels *et al.* (1973) who also pointed out that the mean age of patients with granulomatous thymoma (27 years) was lower than in those with other forms of the tumour (42 years). They felt that the histologic appearance was identical with nodular sclerosing Hodgkin's disease, in agreement with the view of Fechner (1969). Keller and Castleman (1974) studied 44 cases of Hodgkin's disease limited to the mediastinum. In 10 of these the disease involved only the thymus but in a further 11 both the thymus and mediastinal lymph nodes were affected. They too noted the histological similarity with nodular sclerosing Hodgkin's disease, including the presence of lacunar cells, in association with cysts lined by thymic epithelium. They revive the speculation of Thomson by suggesting that nodular sclerosing Hodgkin's disease has its origin in the thymus. The view of most authors (to which we subscribe) is that granulomatous thymoma is a variant of Hodgkin's disease. It is not usually associated with the other disorders which may accompany thymoma although one case of granulomatous thymoma with erythroid hypoplasia has been reported (Remigio 1971). The prognosis of Hodgkin's disease of the thymus is probably marginally better than that of Hodgkin's disease of similar histological type at other sites. Lymphoblastic lymphoma (see Chapter 5) may arise in the thymus, usually in young people, and is often accompanied by leukaemia. Histiocytic lymphoma is uncommon and hard to distinguish from carcinoma except by EM examination (Levine and Rosai 1978).

Criteria of malignancy in thymomas

The usual histologic criteria of malignancy are difficult to apply in thymomas and most authors use the terms 'benign' and 'malignant' with great caution. Again, while some histological classifications use an assessment of differentiation, the criteria for this are not clear-cut. Some tumours with 'benign' cellular features and a low mitotic rate may recur rapidly after excision while others, seemingly more aggressive, do well. The microscopic appearance, therefore is a poor guide to behaviour, although it can be stated in general terms that the epithelial variety is more malignant than the other histological groups. Thymomas do have a tendency to local infiltration and even tumours which seem well-encapsulated at surgery show invasion of the capsule histologically and it may be evident that excision is not complete. In any assessment of prognosis the usual practice in most series is to divide the thymomas into 'invasive' and 'non-invasive' types, rather than 'malignant' and 'benign'. Wilkins and Castleman (1979) suggest a system of histological staging:

Stage I   Intact capsule or growth within capsule
Stage II   Pericapsular growth into mediastinal fat tissue or adjacent pleura or pericardium
Stage III Invasive growth into the surrounding organs, intrathoracic metastasis or both.

Levine and Rosai (1978) point out that there is a good but not absolute correlation between cytologic atypia and invasion in thymomas. In general the non-invasive tumours have a better prognosis than the invasive ones, but on histological analysis the features of malignancy, apart from invasion, form no basis for predicting the subsequent behaviour of the tumour. Jain and Frable (1974) point out that in 'malignant' thymomas necrosis is more common, the lobular pattern is less well-marked and there is no calcification. 'Benign' tumours are characterized by well-marked nodular pattern, calcification and an absence of necrosis. The relative proportion of invasive tumours differs considerably in various series. Castleman (1955) quotes a figure of 25%, Bernatz *et al.* (1973) 36% and Batata *et al.* (1974) 66%. However, Effler and McCormack (1956) consider that all thymomas may have a malignant potential. Of their 19 cases, 16 (89%) showed some evidence of local spread or metastases. There is a tendency for granulomatous thymoma to show local spread and to develop a diffuse systemic involvement but if this type of tumour is considered as a form of Hodgkin's disease it should be excluded from the analysis of outcome. When this has been done, it is clear that distant metastasis of a thymoma is an exceedingly rare occurrence. Guillan *et al.* (1971) report only 11 such cases up to 1971. The case of Rachmaninoff and Fentress (1964) showed metastasis to the brain and that of Mottet (1964) to the pleura and lungs. Penn and Hope-Stone (1972) report two further cases, one metastasizing to the lungs and one to bone. However, the rarity of distant metastases should not be allowed to minimize the aggressive nature of the local invasion in some cases, to involve the lung, pleura, pericardium and great veins. Many of the encapsulated tumours may retain a portion of normal adjacent thymus but in widely invasive thymomas all vestiges of the the original thymus may be obliterated.

The treatment of 54 cases of thymoma was reviewed by Batata *et al.* (1974). The ages ranged from 6 to 74 years (average 48 years) with an equal sex ratio. The tumour was benign and non-invasive in 18 cases, and malignant in 36 cases, 10 of these showing invasion of the capsule while the remaining 26 showed no capsule at all. All of the cases were explored surgically, and all of the 18 encapsulated tumours were completely removed. This was also possible in 11 of the invasive tumours. Partial resection was performed in 8 cases. In 17, no resection was possible and tissue was taken for biopsy purposes only. 11 of the patients with invasive tumours had resection and external irradiation and in 2 of these chemotherapy was added. 17 patients with unresectable tumours had external irradiation and 4 received chemotherapy. Of the patients with non-invasive tumours, one died postoperatively and one after 3 years from anaemia. The remainder were alive and well at the time of review (83% 5-year survival). Of the 36 patients with invasive tumours 54% were alive at 5 years, although more than half of these survivors had recurrent disease. In invasive cases it appears that better results are obtained when surgery is supplemented by radiotherapy of not less than 4,000 rads in 4 weeks. Poor prognosis is associated with pleural effusion, superior vena caval obstruction, tracheal invasion or distant metastases.

These figures reflect the findings of a study by Kilman and Klassen (1971). In their cases of non-invasive tumour, 84% were alive and well at 5 years with a mean survival of 5.1 years whereas the 5-year survival of invasive cases was 33% (mean survival 2.8 years). In addition to the evidence of gross invasion, the histologic pattern does reflect the prognosis to some extent. Bernatz *et al.* (1973) point out that the spindle cell variant is more slowly growing and tends to have a better prognosis that the epithelial forms.

The place of radiotherapy in the management of malignant thymoma has been discussed by Penn and Hope-Stone (1972). They recommend a combination of surgery with postoperative radiotherapy as did Keynes (1949 and 1955). Although preoperative radiotherapy may be given to patients with myasthenia this has been discouraged by other authors (Henson *et al.* 1965). Surgery is usually performed first, to establish the histologic diagnosis and degree of invasion. If resection is not possible, palliative radiotherapy offers some relief. In the series of Penn and Hope-Stone, 18 cases were studied and followed for at least 3 years. 4 had myasthenia gravis. All of the seven cases given radical therapy were alive

at 3 years and 3 of the 4 cases followed for 10 years. Since the response of late recurrences to radiotherapy is diappointing these authors recommend postoperative radiotherapy in malignant thymoma even when the tumour appears to have been completely removed surgically.

Holmes Sellors *et al.* (1967) studied 88 cases where thymectomy had been performed, 38 of whom had myasthenia. The majority of the latter were epithelial or lymphoepithelial on histology. Surgery was complemented by pre- or postoperative radiotherapy in some cases. They felt that although many of the tumours were extremely radiosensitive, this was not a curative procedure, since in patients explored after irradiation, viable tumour was often found. These authors correlated the results of thymectomy with the histologic pattern of the tumour. In 25 cases of epithelial thymoma, 19 had myasthenia; 16 patients were alive with 9 deaths; 16 cases of lymphoepithelial thymoma were seen, 14 with myasthenia with survival in 13 cases. In 16 cases of oval and spindle cell tumours, 3 with myasthenia, 12 were alive and well. Out of 50 non-myasthenic tumours, 27 had radiotherapy in addition to surgery, early death occurred in 2 cases and late death in 12. On balance, radiotherapy seems to be a useful addition to surgery.

Wilkins and Castleman (1979) no longer consider that the presence of myasthenia gravis *per se* carries an adverse prognosis for thymectomy, due to improvements in postoperative management. Where total excision of the thymic tumour is possible they quote a cumulative 10-year survival of 68%.

THE THYMUS IN MYASTHENIA GRAVIS

The association of thymoma with myasthenia gravis was first reported by Weigert in 1901 and since then many such cases have been reported. Approximately 10% of patients with myasthenia have a thymoma. The incidence of myasthenia in patients with thymoma varies in different series. Lattes (1962) quotes a figure of 28% and Katz (1953) one of 75% while other reports quote a proportion of cases between these figures (Iverson 1956; Bernatz *et al.* 1961; Effler and McCormack 1956). In patients with myasthenia and a thymoma, the tumour is malignant in 10% of cases (Morgan and Dudley 1955). The histology of the tumours is usually the epithelial or lymphoepithelial (mixed) pattern. A spindle cell tumour does occur with myasthenia but is rare (Gillespie 1941; Bernatz *et al.* 1973). In 10% of cases of myasthenia the thymus is histologically normal, but the remaining 80% show a thymic abnormality, variously known as thymic hyperplasia or, preferably, dysplasia. The histology of these thymuses shows the presence of well-formed lymphoid follicles in the medulla with formation of germinal centres and increased numbers of plasma cells (Alpert 1971; Ringertz 1951; Levine and Rosai 1978). There is normally a circulation of lymphocytes through the thymus (Sainte-Marie and Leblond 1964), but the vascular endothelium is not normally of lymph node type. In patients with myasthenia gravis not only are lymphoid follicles seen in the thymus but the endothelium of the associated postcapillary venules is also similar to that seen in lymph nodes (Söderstrom *et al.* 1970). In 41 myasthenic patients reported by Bradfield (1973), 19 showed thymic lymphoid follicles with germinal centres and in 15 of these the endothelium of the postcapillary venules was of the high type. In a study involving both histochemical and electron microscopic techniques Tamaoki *et al.* (1971) showed that the thymic lymphoid follicles were identical in structure with those in peripheral lymphoid tissues and were not related to thymic epithelial cells (Fig. 12.7).

Lymphoid follicles may also be found in the thymic remnant adjacent to a thymoma (Alpert 1971; Goldstein 1971). The frequency of this was investigated by Watanabe (1971). In 10 cases where thymic tissue was attached to a thymoma, germinal centres were found in 7, of which 5 had myasthenia. A further case reported showed germinal centre formation in the tumour itself. This raises the question as to whether it is the thymoma itself or the changes in adjacent thymus which are associated with the myasthenia. Two of Watanabe's cases had myasthenia with a thymoma where no germinal centres were present in the adjacent thymus. Watanabe also speculates on the possibility of the thymoma being the result of the autoimmune process rather than its cause. Indeed, the lymphoid follicles with germinal centres found in myasthenia may themselves be the result of autoimmunity—a 'thymitis'. Habu *et al.* (1971) studied the incidence of thymic lymphoid follicles in myasthenia. In 37 cases of myasthenia they were found in 83.8% of the thymuses, but this figure rose to 100% if only the severe cases were considered. The high incidence was characteristic of every age group. Although myasthenia was found more commonly in women (30:7), the incidence of lymphoid follicles was almost identical in the two sexes (83.3:85.7%). The incidence of lymphoid follicles in hyperthyroidism and a group of autoimmune disorders is also raised, but not to the level seen in myasthenia. In addition to the increased incidence seen in myasthenia, the density of the follicles is greater than in other groups.

Lymphoid follicles with germinal centres may also be seen in the normal thymus. In 71 cases of accidental death Habu *et al.* (1971) found an incidence of 16.9%, and 5 of 15 control thymuses studied by Bradfield (1973) also showed lymphoid follicles. However, these tend to be less in density than in

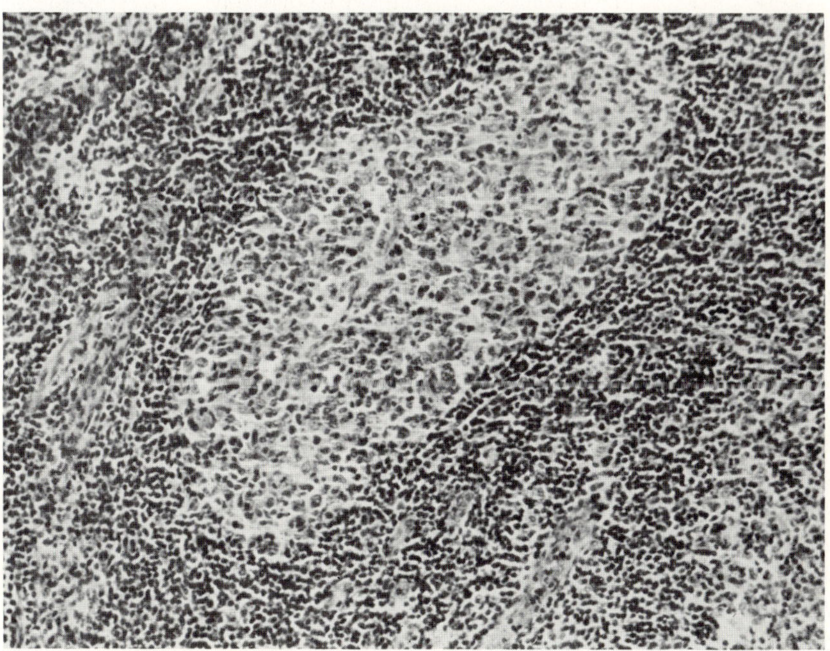

Fig. 12.7. Thymus in myasthenia gravis showing a germinal centre. × 108.

myasthenia and to involve younger persons, in the first two decades of life. The occurrence of these follicles in normal thymuses suggests that the 'blood–thymus barrier' is not absolute. Circulating antigens do not enter the thymic parenchyma or initiate the formation of secondary follicles as in the peripheral lymphoid system. However, if the barrier is artificially broken by intrathymic injection of antigen, typical lymphoid follicles with germinal centres are formed (Marshall and White 1961).

Autoimmune thymitis can be produced in the experimental animal by the injection of thymic tissue in Freund's adjuvant (Irvine 1970; Goldstein 1971). In addition to histological changes in the lymph, predominantly lymphocytic infiltration around Hassall's corpuscles, antibodies against striated muscle and defects in neuromuscular transmission are also produced. Therefore, although the association of myasthenia gravis with both thymoma and thymic lymphoid follicles is well-established, the exact mode of action has not yet been elucidated. In NZB mice, who develop a variety of autoimmune disorders in association with thymic lymphoid follicles, neonatal thymectomy does not prevent the systemic lesions. In these mice Irvine (1970) suggests that the thymic lesions are themselves a manifestation of the autoimmune disease rather than its cause, and postulates that a virus infection may initiate the pathological changes.

THYMECTOMY IN MYASTHENIA GRAVIS

The first operation for removal of a thymoma in a case of myasthenia gravis was undertaken by Blalock in 1939. Since then it has become clear that this operation results in either remission or substantial improvement in a significant proportion of cases. Similar results are obtained from the excision of non-neoplastic thymuses even though they may be of normal size. Goldstein (1971) indicates that some 70–80% of patients may show beneficial results following thymectomy. Simpson (1958) studied 451 cases of myasthenia, 47 with a thymoma and 404 without. The best results are obtained in females without a thymoma and with a history of less than 5 years. If the history covers a period of 7 years or longer, improvement is still obtained, but this is less marked. In cases of thymoma, the myasthenia is of later onset and is more difficult to control medically. Improvement is still obtained following thymectomy but only one-third of the patients survive. In 29 female and 18 male cases of thymectomy there were 9 postoperative deaths and an average survival of 5.3 years. Irvine (1970), Batata (1974) and Namba *et al.* (1978) record cases where the onset of myasthenia has followed the removal of a thymoma. Since no thymic tissue has been found on re-exploration of some of these patients Namba *et al.* (1978) postulate that the disease is due to a pool of long-lived extrathymic T-lymphocytes. Gradual depletion of such a pool may explain why some patients show a slow recovery from the myasthenia after thymectomy. In those cases where there is no improvement Goldstein (1971) suggests that this may be due to remaining ectopic thymus, to incomplete removal of the thymus or tumour, or to irreversible changes in the neuromuscular end organs.

Although recent series (Buckingham *et al.* 1976) have shown good results from thymectomy, some authors have cast doubt on this. Ferguson (1962), in reviewing 145 cases, reports 7 deaths in 12 operated cases and considers the results of thymectomy unpredictable, considering the tendency of the disease to undergo remission and relapse. This view is echoed by Adams *et al.* (1962) who felt that while remission after surgery could be obtained, this was barely greater than the natural remission rate. However, Henson *et al.* (1965) report a favourable result in 36 cases, stable remission being achieved in 15 out of 30 patients without tumours, although less impressive results were obtained in the cases involving a thymoma. Other reported series of thymectomy in myasthenia gravis are those of Eaton and Clagett (1955); Schwab and Leland (1953) and Keynes (1946, 1955).

In the series of Holmes Sellors *et al.* (1967) 38 thymic tumours were removed in myasthenic patients. Most of these were histologically epithelial or lymphoepithelial and only 5 were oval or spindle celled. The purely epithelial thymoma tended to be more malignant than the other varieties, being involved in 8 of the 13 deaths in the series.

An informative review of the historical aspects of myasthenia gravis is given by Viets (1953).

ANTIBODY FORMATION IN THYMOMA AND THYMIC HYPERPLASIA

The majority of patients with myasthenia gravis show a circulating antibody against acetylcholine receptors of the neuromuscular junction, and circulating lymphocytes active against these receptors are also present in the peripheral blood (Lennon 1978). Experimental autoimmune myasthenia gravis can be produced using these receptors. In some 30–40% patients with myasthenia gravis a circulating antibody is found, active against myoid cells found in the normal thymus and against the 'I' band of skeletal muscle (Strauss and Kemp 1967; Goldstein 1971). The proportion of positive sera is greater in patients with thymoma and myasthenia. Thus, van der Geld and Strauss (1966) found that in 336 patients antibody was demonstrable in 99 patients at a titre of 1:60, the titres against thymic myoid cells and skeletal muscle being almost identical. In contrast, antibody was found at a titre of 1:60 in 19 out of 20 patients with myasthenia and thymoma. However, on further examination of this disparity, it may be found that the existence of the antibody is correlated with the occurrence of lymphoid follicles in the adjacent thymus rather than in the presence of the tumour itself. The antibody fixes complement but has no action against the neuromuscular end plate. Many sera from patients with other autoimmune disorders and even control sera may contain the antibody at titres up to 1:30 but only sera from myasthenic patients achieve a titre of 1:60 (Strauss 1968). The antibody may appear following the production of experimental autoimmune thymitis using Freund's adjuvant (Goldstein 1971). The role of the antibody in producing the defect in neuromuscular transmission is debatable. Goldstein and Hofmann (1969) postulate a hormone 'thymin' secreted by the normal thymus; blood levels may be increased in myasthenia gravis. Twomey *et al.* (1979) correlated improvement following thymectomy with lowered serum levels of thymic hormone. As previously noted in Chapter 1, thymic epithelial cells have secretory properties (Vetters and MacAdam 1973). Membrane bound, presumably secretory granules have been described in a thymoma (MacAdam and Vetters 1969) although this was not confirmed by Timperley and Ahmed (1970). Fukawa *et al.* (1978) studied T cell responses after thymectomy. In patients who improved rapidly the postoperative T cell level fell, in those who showed slow, or no improvement, the levels were unchanged, and in those who showed an exacerbation of the disease, T cell levels rose postoperatively. It may well be that in the development of myasthenia, both antibody and sensitized lymphocytes are involved.

THYMIC LESIONS IN OTHER AUTOIMMUNE DISORDERS

This subject has been reviewed by Barnes and Irvine (1973).

In most cases where thymic and autoimmune disease are associated, the thymus shows an increased evidence of lymphoid follicles rather than a thymoma. If hyperthyroidism is considered to be autoimmune in origin, then Habu *et al.* (1971) found thymic lymphoid follicles in 13 of 29 cases of autoimmune disease, compared with 3/59 other diseases and 12/71 cases of accidental death.

Hyperthyroidism

In the series of Habu *et al.* (1971) four of their six cases of hyperthyroidism showed thymic lymphoid follicles. Gunn *et al.* (1964) undertook thymic biopsy in patients undergoing thyroidectomy. In 50 cases of thyrotoxicosis, thymic lymphoid follicles were present in 34, compared with 2 in 45 cases of non-toxic goitre. The presence of thymic lymphoid follicles also correlated with the presence of lymphoid follicles in the thyroid itself, but not with circulating antithyroid antibodies. In a further study, Michie *et al.* (1967) found that total thymic size as judged radiologically, in cases of hyperthyroidism and Hashimoto's disease, was about twice that seen with nodular goitre.

Hashimoto's disease

20% of cases studied by Habu *et al.* (1971) showed thymic lymphoid follicles.

Systemic lupus erythematosus

Several cases of thymoma associated with systemic lupus erythematosus have been reported (Larsson 1963), and a number of patients with thymoma and myasthenia gravis or pure red cell aplasia have circulating anti-nuclear antibody. Habu *et al.* (1971) found thymic follicles in two of their four cases of SLE. Mackay *et al.* (1963) reporting a case of SLE treated by thymectomy stated that the thymus showed islands of epithelial and spindle cells with scattered lymphocytes and few plasma cells. No lymphoid follicles or germinal centres were seen. No clinical response was observed following the thymectomy.

Rheumatoid arthritis

In a case of rheumatoid arthritis studied by Burnet and Mackay (1962) the thymus showed conspicuous epithelial activity intermingled with small lymphocytes with germinal centre formation surrounded by a narrow rim of lymphocytes.

Two of the three cases of this condition studied by Habu *et al.* (1971) showed thymic lymphoid follicles. In one reported case, thymectomy had a beneficial effect (Karaklis *et al.* (1964). The thymus contained large numbers of plasmablasts and a few mature plasma cells, indicating intense immuno-logical activity, these cells being a possible source for the abnormal antibody. No lymphoid follicles were seen. A similar case was reported by Wilmers and Russell (1963). An excellent animal model of spontaneous autoimmune haemoly-tic anaemia exists in the NZB strain of mice; the thymuses of these animals have a high incidence of thymic lymphoid follicles with germinal centre formation (Burnet and Mackay 1962).

THYMOMA ASSOCIATED WITH PURE RED CELL APLASIA

In certain cases of anaemia due to pure red cell aplasia, the patient is discovered to have a thymoma. Mondhiry *et al.* (1971) estimates this proportion to be as high as 40%, and thus it is of some importance to investigate such patients for the presence of a tumour in the anterior mediastinum. Opinion differs as to the first reports of this association. Hirst and Robertson (1967) quote Matras and Priesel in 1928, Schmid *et al.* (1965) quote Polayes and Lederer in 1930 and Chalmers (1955) quotes Opsahl in 1939. The condition is rare but sufficient instances had been reported by 1967 to allow Hirst and Robertson to review 56 cases in the literature and add two of their own.

The anaemia is normochromic and normocytic and the peripheral blood shows an almost total absence of reticulo-cytes. The marrow may show a normal degree of cellularity but erythropoietic activity is absent. The content of eosino-phils, monocytes and lymphocytes may be slightly increased. Schmid *et al.* (1965) drew attention to the sex distribution in these cases which shows a 2:1 female predominance while this ratio is reversed in cases of aplastic anaemia without thymoma. Hirst and Robertson (1967) report that 7 of the 56 recorded cases also had myasthenia gravis. The tumour is usually small and non-invasive, although Hirst does detail one case of a malignant tumour and another which achieved a diameter of 18 cm. The tumour itself, however, is usually symptomless.

The histology of the tumour varies in different series, but there does appear to be a greater tendency for the spindle cell variety to occur than is the case with myasthenia gravis. Both of the cases reported by Chalmers and Boheimer (1954) were lymphoepitheliomas, whereas the spindle cell variety accounted for 17 of the 19 cases of Schmid *et al.* (1965) where histology was available. There may be a mixture of spindle cells and lymphocytes (Ross *et al.* 1954; Jacobs *et al.* 1959). The latter authors also report a case of the lymphocytic variety as do Weinbaum and Thompson (1955). Thus in their review of 56 cases, Hirst and Robertson (1967) quote 4 cases of spindle cell thymoma, 33 of the spindle and lymphocytic variety and 9 lymphoepitheliomas in those cases where histology could be assessed. Only one case of granulomatous thymoma with this condition has been reported (Remigio 1971).

Removal of a thymoma with pure red cell aplasia was first undertaken by Humphreys and Southworth in 1945. Their case showed remission of the haematological abnormality with a reticulocyte response, but since then the results of surgery have been varied. Chalmers and Boheimer (1954) reported successful removal of a thymoma, but in two cases of Clarkson and Prockop (1958) there was no improvement of the anaemia. The latter authors report that up to 1958, of 11 cases undergoing surgery, 2 showed a cure of the anaemia, 2, partial remission and 7, no effect. Nevertheless, Zeok *et al.* (1979) consider that 25–30% patients are improved by thymectomy; therefore, it is probable that where a thymoma is found, removal is indicated.

The cause of the anaemia has come under investigation by several authors. Both Jepson and Lowenstein (1966) and Mondhiry *et al.* (1971) found that the serum contained a factor depressing erythropoiesis. Field *et al.* (1968) also demonstrated a stem cell suppressing factor in the serum, which disappeared when erythropoiesis recovered following irradiation of the thymic tumour. Erythropoietin levels were not raised and the authors speculated whether the serum factor could be an antibody against erythropoietin. Inhibition of erythropoietin and of nucleoprotein synthesis by marrow cells by a serum factor was demonstrated by Hamilton and Conley (1969) and this was identified as a gammaglobulin by Jepson *et al.* (1968). Barnes (1966) found that of 9 patients with refractory anaemia and thymoma all had positive antinuclear antibody present in the serum, although no striated muscle antibodies could be demonstrated. In contrast none of 35 patients with a similar anaemia but without thymoma showed an antinuclear antibody. Although his patient did not have a thymoma, the findings of Krantz *et al.*

(1969) in a case of red-cell aplasia are of some interest. When the patient's marrow was incubated *in vitro* an increase in haem synthesis was observed, further accentuated by addition of erythropoietin. The plasma contained an antibody of IgG type active against erythroblast nuclei and inhibiting haem synthesis; both of these effects were abolished by treatment with cyclophosphamide. It may therefore be the case that in thymoma the pure red cell aplasia is brought about by the action of an antibody against the nuclei of red-cell precursors in the marrow, and that the condition should properly be classified as an autoimmune disease. The subject is reviewed by Krantz (1976).

THYMOMA ASSOCIATED WITH OTHER HAEMATOLOGICAL ABNORMALITIES

In addition to pure red-cell aplasia thymoma may be associated with other haematological abnormalities. A patient presenting with red-cell aplasia may develop a deficiency of polymorph leucocytes and platelets as the disease progresses, with a final state of aplastic anaemia involving all marrow elements. However, pancytopenia may be present in the initial stages (Burrows and Carroll 1971) and may be associated with hypogammaglobulinaemia (Rogers *et al.* 1968) or Hashimoto's disease (Dawson 1972). There is one report of thymoma presenting with thrombocytopenic purpura and a marrow megakaryocytopenia (Sundström *et al.* 1972), this case having also a positive Coombs' test, indicating an autoimmune process. Sundström (1972) has also reported a case of thymoma presenting with erythrocytosis.

THYMOMA ASSOCIATED WITH ABNORMALITIES OF THE PLASMA PROTEINS

Lehar and Heard (1970) report a case of agammaglobulinaemia and thymoma and cite 20 such cases in the literature, sometimes associated with red-cell aplasia or myasthenia gravis. Hypogammaglobulinaemia and thymoma are also reported by Brasher *et al.* (1972). A case of multiple myeloma is described by Lindstrom *et al.* (1968) in a patient known to have had a thymoma of several years' duration. Pure red-cell aplasia developed as a terminal event. The occurrence of immunoglobulin abnormalities may be surprising if the

thymus produces only T cells which theoretically should not produce immunoglobulin. However, the thymus does have a co-operative role in antibody production in response to some antigenic stimuli (Miller 1962). Plasma cells can be demonstrated in the human thymus (Henry 1967) and culture of thymus from foetal lambs previously infected with *Toxoplasma gondii* showed continuing release of antibody into the culture fluid (Beverly and Archer, unpublished observations). In view of the interaction between T- and B-lymphocytes which is necessary for good antibody production, a thymoma which produces a destruction of thymic tissue and consequent deficiency of T-lymphocytes may in fact result in a failure to produce immunoglobulins.

THYMOMA AND MUSCLE ABNORMALITIES

In cases of myasthenia gravis due to thymoma or to thymic hyperplasia, the skeletal muscles may contain focal infiltrations of lymphocytes and plasma cells known as 'lymphorrhages' first described by Buzzard (1905). The muscle fibres in the region of the infiltrate are normal. These are inconstant findings and their relation to the autoimmune process is not clear. However, other cases have been reported in which there is a more direct inflammation of the muscle itself, and involvement of the myocardium. 4 such cases have been reported (Waller *et al.* 1957; Langston *et al.* 1959; Rundle and Sparks 1963; Burke *et al.* 1969). All of the patients were female with ages ranging from 45 to 60 years. One had myasthenia gravis and one skin lesions similar to erythema nodosum. In each case a lymphoepithelial thymoma was present. Each case showed identical changes in the heart and skeletal muscles, a giant cell inflammation with areas of muscle loss, granulation tissue formation and a mixed inflammatory exudate. In view of the capacity of certain viruses to produce giant cell inflammation, a viral infection cannot be ruled out in these cases, but the association is sufficiently striking that the presence of a thymoma should be sought when giant cell myositis is present.

10 published cases of thymoma associated with myopathy have been reviewed by Kater and van Toorn (1969).

THYMOMA AND CUSHING'S SYNDROME

The rare association of these two conditions has been reported, firstly by Leyton *et al.* (1931) and then by Hubble

(1949). In 1959, Scholz and Bahn reviewed 12 cases in the literature and added 1 of their own. Castleman (1955) reports that in each case the histology of the thymoma showed epithelial cells with virtually no lymphocytes. 2 cases showed a spindle cell pattern, 5 showed evidence of malignancy and 1 had metastatic spread to hilar and supraclavicular lymph nodes. All cases showed bilateral adrenal hyperplasia with no adrenal tumour. The presumption is that the tumour was undertaking inappropriate secretion of ACTH. The ultrastructure of one such tumour was described by Kay and Willson (1970). The tumour cells contained small membrane bound secretory granules. When this association is encountered, the possibility of an oat cell carcinoma of bronchus metastasizing to the anterior mediastinum should be considered.

THYMOMA AND PEMPHIGUS

Krain (1974) reported 8 cases of thymoma associated with pemphigus. 5 of these had, in addition, myasthenia gravis and one, pure red cell aplasia and a positive LE cell test. This association is of interest in view of recent theories concerning the immunological aetiology of pemphigus.

THYMOMA AND NON-THYMIC MALIGNANCY

There is some suggestion that the presence of a thymoma is associated with an increased incidence of non-thymic malignancy. Soudjian *et al.* (1968) found that in 146 cases of thymoma followed for 20 years, 31 (21%) developed a malignant lesion of non-thymic tissue. Only 8% of 177 patients with a parathyroid adenoma had such lesions. Reviewing 1,030 reported cases, the same authors found a 20% incidence of non-thymic malignancy if the case was followed for 5 years or more. This may indicate that the immunological disturbances consequent on the development of a thymoma may predispose to malignancy in other sites.

REFERENCES

ADAMS R.D., DENNY-BROWN D. & PEARSON C.M. (1962) *Diseases of Muscle. A study in Pathology.* 2nd ed. Hoeber, New York.

ALPERT L.I. (1971) A historic reappraisal of the thymus in myasthenia gravis. A correlative study of thymic pathology and response to thymectomy. *Arch. Path.* 91, 55–61.

BARNES E.W. & IRVINE W.J. (1973) Clinical syndromes associated with thymic disorders. *Proc. Roy. Soc. Med.* 66, 151–4.

BARNES R.D. (1966) Refractory anaemia with thymoma. *Lancet* 2, 1464.

BATATA M.A., MARTINI N., HUVOS A.G., AGUILAR R.I. & BEATTIE E.J. (1974) Thymomas. Clinicopathologic features, therapy and prognosis. *Cancer* 34, 389–96.

BERNATZ P.E., HARRISON E.G. & CLAGGETT O.T. (1961) Thymoma —a clinico-pathologic study. *J. Thor. Cardiovasc. Surg.* 42, 424–44.

BERNATZ P.E., KOHNSARI S., HARRISON E.G. & TAYLOR W.F. (1973) Thymoma: factors influencing prognosis. *Surg. Clin. N. Amer.* 53, 885–92.

BEVERLY J.K.A. & ARCHER J.F. Unpublished observations.

BLALOCK A., MASON M.F., MORGAN H.J. & RIVEN S.S. (1939) Myasthenia gravis and tumours of the thymic region. *Ann. Surg.* 110, 544–60.

BLOODWORTH J.M.B., HIRATSUKA H., HICKEY B.C. & WU J. (1975) Ultrastructure of the human thymus, thymic tumours and myasthenia gravis. *Pathol. Ann.* 10, 329–91.

BRADFIELD J.W.B. (1973) Altered venules in the stimulated human thymus as evidence of lymphocyte recirculation. *Clin. Exp. Immunol.* 13, 243–52.

BRASHER G.W., HOWARD P.H. & BRINDLEY G.V. (1972) Thymoma and hypogammaglobulinaemia (Good's syndrome). *Surg. Clin. N. Amer.* 52, 429–38.

BUCKINGHAM J.M., HOWARD F.M., BERNATZ P.E., PAYNE W.S., HARRISON E.G., O'BRIEN P.C. & WEILAND L.H. (1976) The value of thymectomy in myasthenia gravis. *Ann. Surg.* 184, 453–8.

BURKE, J.S., MEDLINE N.M. & KATZ A. (1969) Giant-cell myocarditis and myositis associated with thymoma and myasthenia gravis. *Arch. Path. (Chicago)* 88, 359–66.

BURNET F.M. & MACKAY I.R. (1962) Lymphoepithelial structures and autoimmune disease. *Lancet* 2, 1030–33.

BURROWS S. & CARROLL R. (1971) Thymoma associated with pancytopenia. *Arch. Path.* 92, 465–8.

BUZZARD E.F. (1905) The clinical history and postmorten examination of five cases of myasthenia gravis. *Brain* 28, 438–83.

CASTLEMAN B. (1955) Tumours of the thymus gland. *Armed Forces Inst. Path. Fascicle.,* 19.

CHALMERS J.N.M. (1955) Anaemia in patients with thymic tumours. *Amer. J. Clin. Path.* 25, 790–1.

CHALMERS J.N.M. & BOHEIMER K. (1954) Pure red cell anaemia in patients with thymic tumours. *Brit. Med. J.* 2, 1514–18.

CLARKSON B. & PROCKOP D.J. (1958) A regenerative anaemia associated with benign thymoma. *N. Engl. J. Med.* 259, 253–8.

COSSMAN J., DEEGAN M.J. & SCHNITZER B. (1978) Thymoma. An immunologic and electron microscopic study. *Cancer* 41, 2183–91.

DAWSON M.A. (1972) Thymoma associated with pancytopenia and Hashimoto's thyroiditis. *Amer. J. Med.* 52, 406–10.

DEFENDI V. & ROOSA R.A. (1964) The role of the thymus in carcinogenesis. In Defendi V. & Metcalf D. (eds.), *The Thymus,* pp. 121–31. Wistar Institute Press, Philadelphia.

EATON L.M. & CLAGETT O.T. (1955) Symposium on myasthenia

gravis; present status of thymectomy in treatment of myasthenia gravis. *Amer. J. Med.* **19**, 703–17.

EFFLER D.B. & MCCORMACK L.J. (1956) Thymic neoplasms. *J. Thor. (Cardiovasc.) Surg.* **31**, 60–82.

EVANS R.W. (1966) *Histological appearances of tumours* (2nd Edn.), pp. 568–85. Churchill Livingstone, Edinburgh.

FECHNER R.E. (1969) Hodgkin's disease of the thymus. *Cancer* **23**, 16–23.

FELL S.C., SPRAYREGEN S. & BECKER N.W. (1966) Bilateral carcinoid tumours of the mediastinum. *Ann. Thor. Surg.* **2**, 429–34.

FELTKAMP-VROOM T. (1966) Myoid cells in hyman thymus. *Lancet* **1**, 1320–1.

FERGUSON F.R. (1962) A critical review of the clinical features of myasthenia gravis. *Proc. Roy. Soc. Med.* **55**, 49–52.

FIELD E.O., CAUGHI N.M., BLACKETT N.M. & SMITHERS D.W. (1968) Marrow suppressing factors in the blood in pure red-cell aplasia, thymoma and Hodgkin's disease. *Brit. J. Haem.* **15**, 101–10.

FRIEDMAN N.B. (1967) Tumours of the thymus. *J. Thor. Cardiovasc. Surg.* **53**, 163–82.

FUKAWA M., TORISU M., MIYAHARA T., HARASAKI H., KAI S., YAMAMOTO H., KONOMI K., NISHIMURA M. & TANAKA J. (1978) Immunological studies on myasthenia gravis. Operative indication and cell-mediated immunity. *Surgery* **83**, 293–302.

GILLESPIE B. (1941) Thymoma in myasthenia gravis. *Arch. Path.* **32**, 659–63.

GOLDSTEIN G. (1971) Myasthenia gravis and the thymus. *Ann. Rev. Med.* **22**, 119–24.

GOLDSTEIN G. & HOFMANN W.W. (1969) Endocrine function of the thymus affecting neuromuscular transmission. *Clin. Exp. Immunol.* **4**, 181–9.

GUILLAN R.A., ZELMAN S., SMALLEY R.L. & INGLESIAS P.A. (1971) Malignant thymoma associated with myasthenia gravis and evidence of extrathoracic metastases. An analysis of published cases and report of a case. *Cancer* **27**, 823–30.

GUNN A., MICHIE W. & IRVINE W.J. (1964) The thymus in thyroid disease. *Lancet* **2**, 776–8.

HABU S., KAMEYA T. & TAMAOKI N. (1971) Thymic lymphoid follicles in autoimmune diseases. I. Quantitative studies with special reference to myasthenia gravis. *Keio J. Med.* **20**, 45–56.

HAMILTON C.R. & CONLEY C.L. (1969) Pure red-cell aplasia and thymoma. *Johns Hopkins Med. J.* **125**, 262–9.

HENRY K. (1966) Mucin secretion and striated muscle in the human thymus. *Lancet* **1**, 183–5.

HENRY K. (1968) Striated muscle in human thymus. *Lancet* **1**, 638–9.

HENRY K. (1972) An unusual thymic tumour with a striated muscle (myoid) component (with a brief review of the literature on myoid cells). *Brit. J. Dis. Chest* **66**, 291–9.

HENRY K. (1975) The lymphocyte. In Harrison C.V. & Weinbren K. (eds.), *Recent Advances in Pathology* (9th Edn.), pp. 39–72. Churchill Livingstone, London.

HENRY L. (1967) Involution of the human thymus. *J. Path. Bact.* **93**, 661–71.

HENSON R.A., STERN G.M. & THOMPSON V.C. (1965) Thymectomy for myasthenia gravis. *Brain* **88**, 11–28.

HIRST E. & ROBERTSON T.I. (1967) The syndrome of thymoma and erythroblastopenic anaemia. *Medicine* **46**, 225–64.

HOLMES SELLORS T., THACKRAY A.C. & THOMPSON A.D. (1967) Tumours of the thymus. A review of 88 operation cases. *Thorax* **22**, 193–220.

HUBBLE D. (1949) Cushing's syndrome and thymic carcinoma. *Quart. J. Med.* **18**, 133–47.

HUMPHREYS G.H. & SOUTHWORTH H. (1945) Aplastic anaemia terminated by removal of a mediastinal tumour. *Amer. J. Med. Sci.* **210**, 501–10.

IRVINE W.J. (1970) The thymus in autoimmune disease. *Proc. Roy. Soc. Med.* **63**, 718–22.

IVERSON L. (1956) Thymoma; a reivew and reclassification. *Amer. J. Path.* **32**, 695–719.

JACOBS E.M., HUTTER R.V.P., POOL J.L. & LEY A.B. (1959) Benign thymoma and selective erythroid aplasia of bone marrow. *Cancer* **12**, 47–57.

JAIN V. & FRABLE W.J. (1974) Thymoma, an assessment of benign and malignant criteria. *J. Thor. Cardiovasc. Surg.* **67**, 310–21.

JEPSON J.H., GARDNER F.H., DEGNAN T. & VAS M. (1968) A gamma-globulin inhibitor of erythropoiesis in erythroblastopenic plasma from patients with thymoma. *Clin. Res.* **16**, 536.

JEPSON J.H. & LOWENSTEIN L. (1966) Inhibition of erythropoiesis by a factor present in the plasma of patients with erythroblastopenia. *Blood* **27**, 425–34.

KARAKLIS A., VALAES T., PANTELAKIS S.N. & DOXIADIS S.A. (1964) Thymectomy in an infant with autoimmine haemolytic anaemia. *Lancet* **2**, 778–80.

KATER L. & VAN TOORN D.W. (1969) Thymoma and myopathy. Report of a case of myopathy resembling muscular dystrophy and a granulomatous thymoma in an adult woman. *Arch. Neurol. (Chicago)* **20**, 461–7.

KATZ J.H. (1953) Medical progress: malignant thymoma in myasthenia gravis; report of an unusual case with brief discussion of role of thymus in disease. *New Engl. J. Med.* **248**, 1059–64.

KATZ A. & LATTES R. (1969) Granulomatous thymoma or Hodgkin's disease of the thymus. A clinical and histologic study and a re-evaluation. *Cancer* **23**, 1–15.

KAY S. & WILLSON M.A. (1970) Ultrastructural studies of an ACTH-secreting thymic tumor. *Cancer* **26**, 445–52.

KELLER A.R. & CASTLEMAN R. (1974) Hodgkin's disease of the thymus gland. *Cancer* **33**, 1615–23.

KEYNES G. (1946) The surgery of the thymus gland. *Brit. J. Surg.* **33**, 201–14.

KEYNES G. (1949) The results of thymectomy in myasthenia gravis. *Brit. Med. J.* **2**, 611–16.

KEYNES G. (1955) Investigations into thymic disease and tumour formation. *Brit. J. Surg.* **42**, 449–62.

KILMAN J.W. & KLASSEN K.P. (1971) Thymoma. *Amer. J. Surg.* **121**, 710–11.

KRAIN L.S. (1974) Association of pemphigus with thymoma or malignancy: a critical review. *Brit. J. Dermatol.* **90**, 397–405.

KRANTZ S.B. (1976) Diagnosis and treatment of pure red cell aplasia. *Med. Clin. N. Am.* **60**, 945–58.

Krantz S.B. & Kao V. (1969) Studies on red cell aplasia. II. Report of a second patient with antibody to erythroblast nuclei and a remission after immunosuppressive therapy. *Blood* **34**, 1–13.

Kreel L. (1973) Radiology of the thymus. *Proc. Roy. Soc. Med.* **66**, 157–8.

Langston J.D., Wagman G.F. & Dickenman R.C. (1959) Granulomatous myocarditis and myositis associated with thymoma. *Arch. Path.* **68**, 367–73.

Larsson O. (1963) Thymoma and S.L.E. in the same patient. *Lancet* **2**, 665–6.

Lattes R. (1962) Thymoma and other tumours of the thymus: An analysis of 107 cases. *Cancer* **15**, 1224–60.

Legg M.A. & Brady W.J. (1965) Pathology and clinical behaviour of thymomas. *Cancer* **18**, 1131–44.

Lehar T.J. & Heard J.L. (1970) Agammaglobulinaemia and thymoma associated with non-thymic cancer. *Cancer* **25**, 875–9.

Lennon V.A. (1978) The immunopathy of myasthenia gravis. *Hum. Pathol.* **9**, 541–51.

Levine G.D. (1973) Primary thymic seminoma—a neoplasm ultrastructurally similar to testicular seminoma and distinct from epithelial thymoma. *Cancer* **31**, 729–41.

Levine G.D. & Bensch K.G. (1972) Epithelial nature of spindle cell thymoma. An ultrastructural study. *Cancer* **30**, 500–11.

Levine G.D. & Rosai J. (1978) Thymic hyperplasia and neoplasia. A review of current concepts. *Hum. Pathol.* **9**, 495–515.

Levine G.D., Rosai J., Bearman R.M. & Pollack A. (1975) The fine structure of thymoma with emphasis on its differential diagnosis. *Amer. J. Pathol.* **81**, 49–86.

Leyton O., Turnbull H.M. & Bratton A.B. (1931) Primary cancer of the thymus with pluriglandular disturbance. *J. Path. Bact.* **34**, 635–60.

Lindstrom F.D., Williams R.C. & Brunning R.D. (1968) Thymoma associated with multiple myeloma. *Arch. Int. Med.* **122**, 526–31.

Llombart-Bosch, A. (1975) Epithelio-Reticular Thymoma with lymphocytic 'Emperipolesis'. An ultrastructural study. *Cancer* **36**, 1794–803.

Lundin P.M. & Schelin U. (1965) Ultrastructure of the rat thymus. *Acta. Path. Microbiol. Scand.* **65**, 379–94.

Macadam R.F. & Vetters J.M. (1969) Fine structural evidence for hormone secretion by a human thymic tumour. *J. Clin. Path.* **22**, 407–9.

MacKay I.R., Goldstein G. & McConchie I.M. (1963) Thymectomy in systemic lupus erythematosus. *Brit. Med. J.* **2**, 792–3.

Marshall A.H.E. & White R.G. (1961) The immunological reactivity of the thymus. *Brit. J. Exp. Path.* **42**, 379–85.

Marshall A.H.E. & Wood C. (1957) The involvement of the thymus in Hodgkin's disease. *J. Path. Bact.* **73**, 163–6.

Matani A. & Dritsas C. (1973) Familial occurrence of thymoma. *Arch. Path.* **95**, 90–1.

Matras A. & Priesel A. (1928) Ueber einige Gewasche des Thymus. *Bettr. z. Path. Anat. u.z. Allg. Path.* **80**, 270–306.

Michie W., Beck J.S., Mahaffy R.G., Honein E.F. & Fowler G.B. (1967) Quantitative radiological and histological studies of thymus in thyroid disease. *Lancet* **1**, 691–5.

Miller J.F.A.P. (1962) Effect of neonatal thymectomy on the immunological responsiveness of the mouse. *Proc. Roy. Soc. (B)* **156**, 415–28.

Miller J.F.A.P. (1967) The thymus in relation to neoplasia. In Crawford T. (ed.), *Modern Trends in Pathology* (2nd Edn.), pp. 140–75. Butterworths, London.

Mondhiry H.A., Zanjani E.D., Spivack M., Zalusky R. & Gordon A.S. (1971) Pure red cell aplasia and thymoma: loss of serum inhibitor of erythropoiesis following thymectomy. *Blood* **38**, 576–82.

Morgan W.L. & Dudley H.R. (1955) Malignant thymoma and myasthenia gravis. Report of case and review of literature. *N. Engl. J. Med.* **253**, 625–32.

Mottet N.K. (1964) Malignant thymoma. *Amer. J. Clin. Path.* **41**, 61–71.

Namba T., Brunner N.G. & Grob D. (1978) Myasthenia gravis in patients with thymoma. Reference to onset after thymectomy. *Medicine* **57**, 411–33.

Nickels J., Franssila K. & Hjelt L. (1973) Thymoma and Hodgkin's disease of the thymus. *Acta. Path. Microbiol. Scand. (A)* **81**, 1–5.

O'Gara R.W., Horn R.C. & Enterline H.T. (1958) Tumours of the anterior mediastinum. *Cancer* **11**, 562–90.

Opsahl R. (1939) Thymus-Karcinom og aplastisk anemi. *Nord. Med.* **2**, 1835–37.

Pachter M.R. & Lattes R. (1964) Germinal tumours of the mediastinum: a clinicopathological study of adult teratomas, teratocarcinomas, choriocarcinomas and seminomas. *Dis. Chest* **45**, 301–10.

Penn C.R.H. & Hope-Stone H.F. (1972) The role of radiotherapy in the management of malignant thymoma. *Brit. J. Surg.* **59**, 533–9.

Polayes S.M. & Lederer M. (1930) A recipient of many blood transfusions. *J. Amer. Med. Ass.* **95**, 407–9.

Pugsley W.S. & Carleton R.L. (1953) Germinal nature of teratoid tumours of the thymus. *Arch. Path.* **56**, 341–7.

Rachmaninoff N. & Fentress V. (1964) Thymoma with metastasis to the brain. *Amer. J. Clin. Path.* **41**, 618–25.

Remigio P.A. (1971) Granulomatous thymoma associated with erythroid hypoplasia. *Amer. J. Clin. Path.* **55**, 68–72.

Ringertz N. (1951) The pathology of the thymus and other organs in myasthenia gravis. *Acta Path. Microbiol. Scand.* **29**, 9–25.

Rogers B.H.G., Manligod J.R. & Blazek W.V. (1968) Thymoma associated with pancytopenia and hypogammaglobulinaemia. Report of a case and review of the literature. *Amer. J. Med.* **44**, 154–64.

Rosai J. & Higa E. (1972) Mediastinal endocrine neoplasm of probable thymic origin related to carcinoid tumour. Cliniopathologic study of 8 cases. *Cancer* **29**, 1061–74.

Rosai J., Higa E. & Davie J. (1972) Mediastinal endocrine neoplasm in patients with multiple endocrine adenomatosis; a previously unrecognised association. *Cancer* **29**, 1075–83.

Rosai J. & Levine G.D. (1976) Tumours of the thymus. *AFIP Atlas of Tumour Pathology*. Second series. Fascicle 13. Washington D.C.

Ross J.F., Finch S.C., Street R.B. & Streider J.W. (1954) The simultaneous occurrence of benign thymoma and refractory anaemia. *Blood* 9, 935–52.

RUNDLE L.G. & SPARKS F.P. (1963) Thymoma and dermato-myositis: a disease entity. *Arch. Path. (Chicago)* 75, 276–83.

SAINTE-MARIE G. & LEBLOND C.P. (1964) Cytologic features and cellular migration in the cortex and medulla of the thymus in the young adult rat. *Blood* 23, 275–99.

SCHMID J.R., KIELY J.M., HARRISON E.G., BAYRD E.D. & PEASE G.L. (1965) Thymoma associated with pure red cell agenesis. Review of literature and report of 4 cases. *Cancer* 18, 216–30.

SCHOLZ D.A. & BAHN R.C. (1959) Thymic tumours associated with Cushing's syndrome. Review of three cases. *Proc. Mayo Clin. Staff Meet.* 34, 433–41.

SCHWAB R.S. & LELAND C.C. (1953) Sex and age in myasthenia gravis as critical factors in incidence and remission. *J. Amer. Med. Ass.* 153, 1270–3.

SEYBOLD W.D., MCDONALD J.R., CLAGETT O.T. & GOOD C.A. (1950) Tumours of the thymus. *J. Thor. Surg.* 20, 195–215.

SHILLITOE A.J. & GOODYEAR J.E. (1960) Thymolipoma: a benign tumour of the thymus gland. *J. Clin. Path.* 13, 297–8.

SIMPSON J.A. (1958) An evaluation of the thymectomy in myasthenia gravis. *Brain* 81, 112–44.

SNOVER D.C., LEVINE G.D. & ROSAI J. (1982) Thymic carcinoma: Five distinctive histological variants. *Amer. J. Surg. Path.* 6, 451–70.

SÖDERSTROM N., AXELSSON J. & HAGELQVIST E. (1970) Post capillary venules of the lymph node type in the thymus in myasthenia. *Lab. Invest.* 23, 451–8.

SOUDJIAN J.V., SILVERSTEIN M.N. & TITUS J.L. (1968) Thymoma and cancer. *Cancer* 22, 1221–5.

STEINMETZ W.H. & HAYS R.A. (1961) Primary seminoma of the mediastinum. Report of a case with an unusual site of metastasis and review of the literature. *Amer. J. Roent.* 86, 669–72.

STRAUSS A.J.L. (1968) Myasthenia, autoimmunity and the thymus. *Advan. Intern. Med.* 14, 241–80.

STRAUSS A.J.L. & KEMP P.G. (1967) Serum autoantibodies in myasthenia gravis and thymoma: selective affinity for I-bands of striated muscle as a guide to identification of antigens. *J. Immunol.* 99, 945–53.

SUNDSTRÖM C. (1972) A case of thymoma associated with erythrocytosis. *Acta. Path. Microbiol. Scand.* 80, 235.

SUNDSTRÖM C., LUNDBERG D. & WERNER I. (1972) A case of thymoma in association with megakaryocytopenia. *Acta. Path. Microbiol. Scand. (A)* 80, 487–90.

SYMMERS D. (1932) Malignant tumours and tumour-like growths of the thymic region. *Ann. Surg.* 95, 544–72.

TAMAOKI N., HABU S. & KAMEYA T. (1971) Thymic lymphoid follicles in autoimmune diseases. II. Histological, histochemical and electron microscopic studies. *Keio J. Med.* 20, 57–68.

THOMSON A.D. (1955) The thymic origin of Hodgkin's disease. *Brit. J. Cancer* 9, 37–50.

THOMSON A.D. & THACKRAY A.C. (1957) The histology of tumours of the thymus. *Brit. J. Cancer* 11, 348–57.

TIMPERLEY W.R. & AHMED A. (1970) Histochemistry of the thymus and a thymoma. *Arch. Path. (Chicago)* 89, 405–9.

TOKER C. (1968) Thymoma: an ultrastructural study. *Cancer* 21, 1157–63.

TWOMEY J.J., LEWIS V.M., PATTON B.M., GOLDSTEIN G. & GOOD R.A. (1979). Myasthenia gravis. Thymectomy and serum thymic hormone activity. *Amer. J. Med.* 66, 639–43.

VAN DER GELD H.W.R. & STRAUSS A.J.L. (1966) Myasthenia gravis. Immunological relationship between striated muscle and thymus. *Lancet* 1, 57–60.

VETTERS J.M. & MACADAM R.F. (1973) Fine structural evidence of hormone secretion by the human thymus. *J. Clin. Path.* 26, 194–7.

VIETS H.R. (1953) A historical review of myasthenia gravis from 1672 to 1900. *J. Amer. Med. Ass.* 153, 1273–80.

WALLER J.V., SHAPIRO M. & PALTAUF R. (1957) Congestive heart failure in post-menopausal muscular dystrophy; myositis, myo-carditis and thymoma. *Amer. Heart J.* 53, 479–84.

WATANABE H. (1971) Thymoma and thymic germinal centre. *Keio J. Med.* 20, 69–75.

WEIGERT C. (1901) Pathologisch-anatomischer Beitrag zur Erb'schen Krankheit (Myasthenia gravis). *Neurol. Centralbl.* 20, 597–601.

WEINBAUM J.G. & THOMPSON R.F. (1955) Erythroblastic hypoplasia associated with thymic tumour and myasthenia gravis: report of case. *Amer. J. Clin. Path.* 25, 761–9.

WICK M.R. (1980) Carcinoid tumour of thymus. A report of 7 cases and review of the literature. *Mayo Clinic Proceedings* 55, 246–54.

WILKINS E.W. & CASTLEMAN B. (1979) Thymoma. A continuing survey at the Massachusetts General Hospital. *Annals, Thor. Surg.* 28, 252–6.

WILMERS M.J. & RUSSELL P.A. (1963) Autoimmune haemolytic anaemia in an infant treated by thymectomy. *Lancet* 2, 915–17.

WOOLNER L.B., JAMPLIS R.W. & KIRKLIN J.W. (1955) Seminoma (Germinoma) apparently primary in the anterior mediastinim. *N. Engl. J. Med.* 252, 653–7.

ZEOK J.V., TODD E.P., DILLON M., DE SIMEONE P. & UTLEY J.R. (1979) The role of thymectomy in red cell aplasia. *Ann. Thor. Surg.* 28, 257–60.

INVESTIGATION

The planned investigation of malignant lymphoma is aimed at providing an accurate assessment of extent of disease. Careful staging evaluation is essential to facilitate comparison of results from different centres and, more important to the patient, to give a guide to therapy and prognosis.

Until recently interest has centred on Hodgkin's disease and the improved results of planned treatment in this condition have confirmed the importance of staging. With non-Hodgkin's lymphomas the story is not yet as encouraging but there has been increasing interest in this group of conditions so that universally accepted histopathological and staging classifications may soon provide a good critical basis for defining treatment and prognosis.

The present internationally accepted staging classification is based on the Ann Arbor conference findings (Carbone *et al.* 1971). This modification of the Rye classification (Rosenberg 1966) was introduced with the realization that laparotomy and splenectomy could be of great help with accurate staging and with the appreciation that extranodal disease, if localized and related to an adjacent lymph node area, did not adversely affect survival. The patient is first staged clinically (CS) and then pathologically (PS) depending on assessment of further histological findings. A detailed description of the staging criteria is given in Chapter 4. The completed assessment can be summarized on a specially designed chart (Fig. 13.1). For example the staging of an asymptomatic patient with clinical involvement of one lymph node group who after laparotomy is shown to have involvement of spleen, but not of liver, bone marrow or abdominal lymph nodes could be summarized as CS IA PS $III_{S+H-M-N-}$. The symptomatic patient with generalized lymph node enlargement and clinical bone and spleen involvement who has positive hepatic, bone and bone marrow biopsies is summarized as CS IVB_{OS} PS IV_{H+O+M+}.

Extranodal lesions may either be localized (E lesions) or generalized (Stage IV disease). Thus the symptomatic patient with localized perihilar infiltration and ipsilateral hilar adenopathy on chest radiography with positive lung biopsy but negative pleural and laparotomy biopsy histology findings could be staged as CS II_EB_L PS $II_{EL+S-H-M-N-P-}$.

The Ann Arbor staging classification can be applied to non-Hodgkin's lymphomas but the centripetal and non-contiguous lymphatic distribution and increased incidence of extranodal disease must be kept in mind during investigation of these diseases.

Having stressed the importance of staging evaluation it is now intended to give a more detailed description of relevant investigations. Most of these are applicable to both Hodgkin's disease and non-Hodgkin's lymphoma but any differences will be discussed.

THE PATHOLOGICAL INVESTIGATION OF LYMPHORETICULAR DISEASE

The essential and usual problem presented to the pathologist is the examination of a lymph node. Ideally this should be received immediately, fresh and uncut from the operating theatre. The surgeon should be aware of the dangers of mutilation and compression of the node and should take not the nearest or most convenient node but the largest available node. The fresh node should be cut across its long axis with a fresh razor blade. One half should be put immediately into 10% buffered formalin. A thin slice (1 mm thick) should be removed from the other half and put into 3% buffered glutaraldehyde. The remaining fresh exposed surface should be pressed gently on four glass slides to make impression preparations. The damaged face should be trimmed and pieces quick frozen for immunofluorescence. Half of the residual material should be chopped in tissue culture fluid at $37°C$ for cell marker studies if the techniques are available and any residual material put into formalin. After 2 hours prefixation in formalin the definitive blocks for paraffin embedding should be taken with a fresh razor blade and after 15 minutes prefixation in glutaraldehyde the tissue for EM should be chopped into small blocks (0.5 mm diameter) for further fixation and embedding for EM.

WESTON PARK HOSPITAL

MALIGNANT LYMPHOMA

(Ann Arbor Classification)

Consultant.. Ward/O.P.........................

UNIT No. ....

NAME ....

FIRST NAME(S) ....

ADDRESS...

....

D.O.B. .... SEX ....

CONSTITUTIONAL SYMPTOMS

	+	—	?
Fever			
Night sweats			
Wt. loss 〉 10%			

HISTOLOGY

CLINICAL STAGING

PHYSICAL EXAM.

	+ R	L	— R	L	? R	L
Axilla						
Upper cerv.						
Lower cerv. s'clav.						
Iliacs.						
Ing. - fem.						
Spleen						
Liver						
Other (spec.)						

X-RAY

	+ R	L	— R	L	? R	L	Not done
Lung							
Pleura							
Hilar							
Mediast.							
Pericard.							
Lymphgr.							
IVP							
Bones							
Other (spec.)							

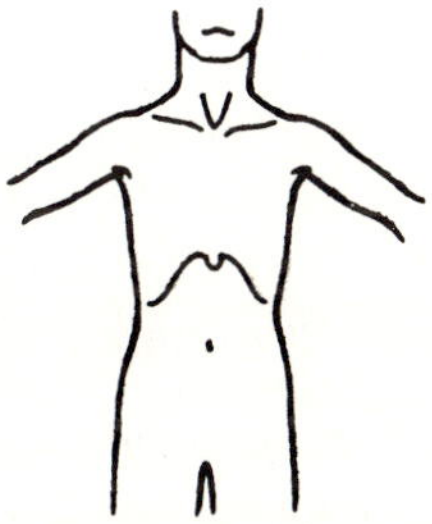

SCANS

	+	—	?	Not done
Bone				
Spleen				
Liver				
Gallium				
Other (spec.)				

CLINICAL STAGE

PATHOLOGICAL STAGING

	Not done	+	—	?	wt. gms
S — (Spleen)					
H — (liver, hepar)					
N — (paraaortic, nodes other nodes (spec.))					
M — (marrow)					
L — (lung)					
P — (pleura)					
O — (osseous)					

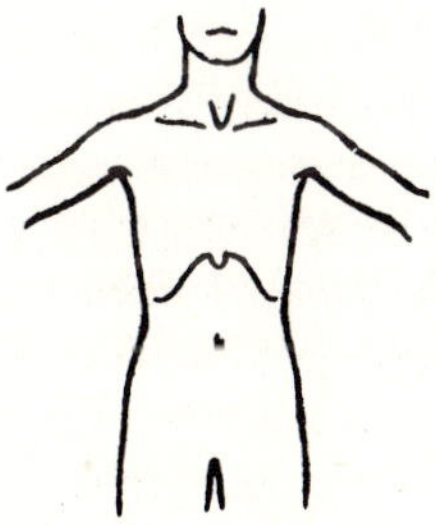

E — Localized extralymphatic involvement

PATHOLOGICAL STAGE

Fig. 13.1. Chart of the type used in Sheffield to summarize clinical and pathological findings in patients with malignant lymphoma. (Modified from the staging form used at the Stanford University Medical Center, USA.)

The standard stains to be used on all lymph node specimens should be haematoxylin and eosin, van Gieson—reticulin, periodic acid Schiff, and methyl green pyronin. Where the diagnosis is in doubt further sections should be cut deeper into the block.

It must be accepted that material referred to lymphoma centres has often not been prepared to these standards and it may occasionally be necessary in the patient's interest to request further biopsy. The accurate diagnosis of lymphoma is crucial in that potentially toxic but life-saving treatment is mandatory. Diagnosis must therefore be precise and absolute occasionally requiring review by several pathologists with special experience in lymphoreticular disease.

Splenectomy specimens should be sliced in their long axis. Where a gross lesion is not apparent it is wise to examine 6–12 sections from areas of spleen where the white pulp is notably prominent.

Bone marrow specimens should be decalcified using a schedule which preserves cytology, serially sectioned and one section in ten mounted (on one slide) for H & E staining ensuring adequate sampling. Single sections should be stained reticulin—van Gieson and for iron.

The interpretation of the difficult biopsy

Most lymph node biopsies are easy to interpret; some are difficult, and a very few are impossible even after consultation by several expert pathologists. In all save the most obvious cases a full clinical history should be available, obtained from a clinician who has personally seen the patient, and at least a peripheral blood film report. Where there is significant doubt as to whether a patient has lymphoma or not, a marrow report and the results of immunological investigations on serum proteins and, if possible, toxoplasma and infectious mononucleosis infection should be at hand.

The critical pathological question is—malignant or not?

The first point to be noted pathologically is the size of the node. A node over 5 cm in diameter is rarely (though occasionally!) a benign lesion. Next the node should be examined at the low power of the microscope; if the normal sinusoidal architecture is preserved and reticulin pattern preserved the lesion is probably benign. At a higher power the node should be surveyed systematically. Cellular infiltration of the capsule by lymphocytes or histiocytic cells suggests malignancy. Germinal centres which are uniform and have normal structure and peripheral reticulin pattern and contain dividing cells and tingible body macrophages are probably reactive. Centres which are grossly non-uniform where the reticulin pattern is breached and where large atypical cells spill out are likely to be malignant. The presence of numbers of polymorphs, and the presence of marked cuffing of postcapillary venules in paracortical areas, suggests inflammation. Finally the node should be surveyed at high power in search of atypical cells.

Where the node evidently contains neoplasm it may be difficult to determine whether it is primary or secondary. Anaplastic small cell carcinoma may be mistaken for small cell lymphoma and anaplastic large cell carcinoma for histiocytic lymphoma. Secondary neoplasms often distend sinusoids with destruction only at a late stage. Rapid EM examination even of paraffin embedded material re-embedded in araldite may clinch a diagnosis by demonstrating the presence of desmosomes in a carcinoma or melanosomes in melanoma while large cell carcinomas may show intracellular mucin.

The interpretation of splenectomy specimens rarely causes the same order of difficulty. Where neoplastic cells are present, they tend to be found first in the white pulp, particularly in the periarteriolar area, and around vessels.

HAEMATOLOGICAL INVESTIGATIONS

A full peripheral blood count with examination of a blood film is mandatory. Many forms of anaemia and white cell and platelet count abnormalities are described (Chapters 4 and 5) and with non-Hodgkin's lymphoma (particularly in the lymphocytic varieties) tumour cells may be seen in the blood.

The ESR may provide a guide as to prognosis and disease activity, and should be assessed serially.

Bone marrow biopsy is also essential. The incidence of bone marrow lesions in malignant lymphoma is only appreciated when thorough marrow examination is undertaken. Thus examination of a smear preparation will rarely lead to the identification of lymphoma cells. When a trephine biopsy is examined the incidence of positive identification rises and the more and the larger the specimens that are examined, the more often will a positive identification be made. A large bone biopsy is readily obtainable at staging laparotomy. The specimen received should be slowly decalcified and serially sectioned throughout. In some cases the identification of a lymphomatous deposit is easy—deposits showing the typical morphology of Hodgkin's disease or non-Hodgkin's lymphoma may be identified. The earliest such typical foci often lie in a paratrabecular position. Deposits can be identified in

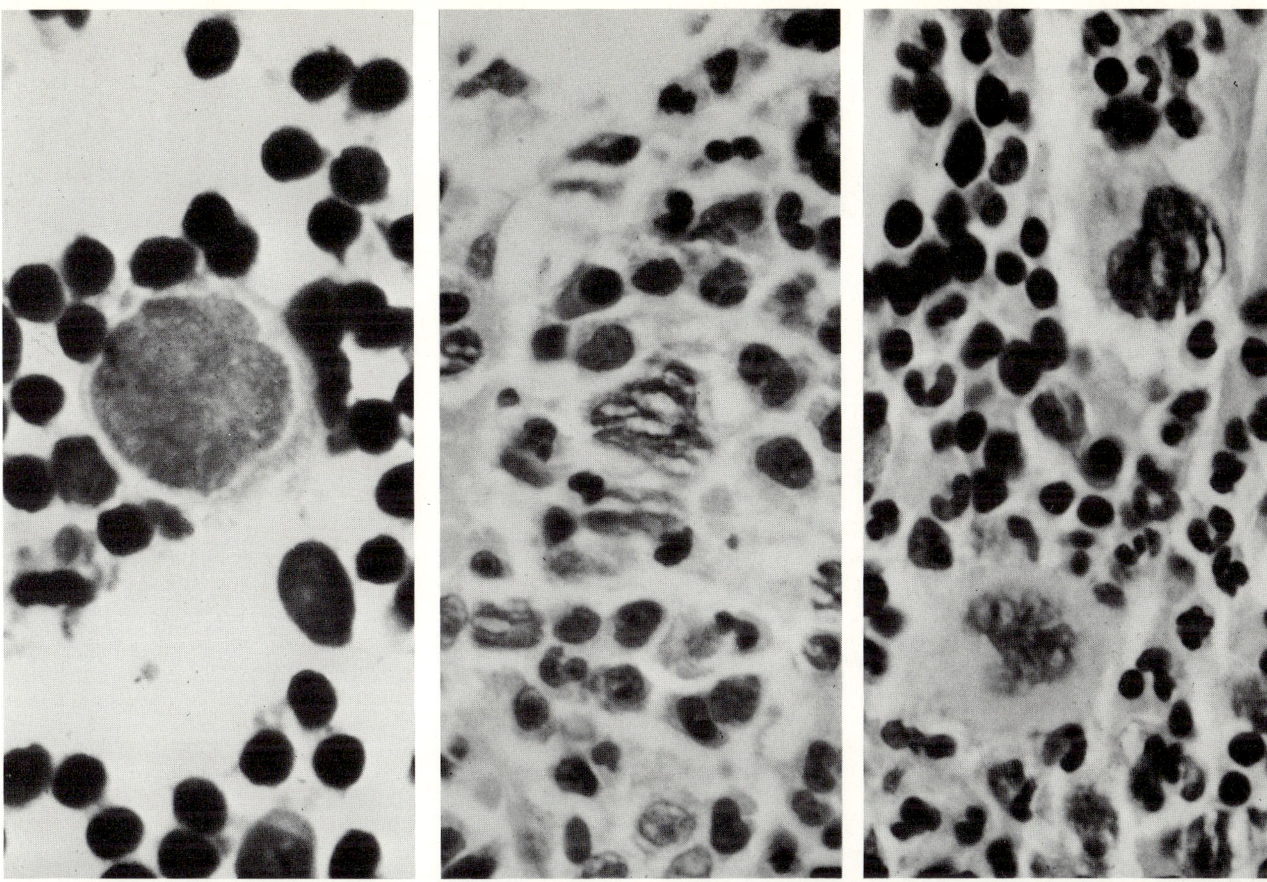

Fig. 13.2. (*left*) Bone marrow smear: A malignant histiocytic cell in Hodgkin's disease. × 1,400. Romanowsky stain.

Fig. 13.3. (*middle*) Bone marrow section: A malignant histiocytic cell in Hodgkin's disease. × 580.

Fig. 13.4. (*right*) Bone marrow section: A malignant histiocytic cell (*top*) and a megakaryocyte (*bottom*) in Hodgkin's disease. Differentiation between the two cell types can be very hard. The malignant histiocytic cell has less cytoplasm and a more densely staining nucleus. × 580.

some cases of Hodgkin's disease (Han *et al.* 1971; Webb *et al.* 1970) and more frequently in non-Hodgkin's lymphoma (Jones *et al.* 1972; Dick *et al.* 1974; McKenna *et al.* 1975). Apart from typical lymphomatous foci areas of histiocytic hyperplasia may be found in marrrow in both Hodgkin's disease and histiocytic lymphoma. Where those are widespread and diffuse they must be regarded as evidence of lymphoma in marrow even though they do not precisely correspond in pattern to the major lymphomatous deposit. Where they are scattered focal and minimal it is more difficult to interpret them. We do not regard them as constituting sufficient evidence of lymphoma in the marrow to change the patient's course of treatment. Focal aggregates of small lymphocytes are a feature of normal marrow and must not be

regarded as evidence of lymphoma. Oblique sections through megakaryocytes must not be mistaken for malignant 'Hodgkin' cells. Areas of fibrosis with atypical histiocytic cells in Hodgkin's disease, in the absence of Reed–Sternberg cells are regarded as evidence of Hodgkin's disease in the marrow. Where a single trephine biopsy is negative and there is strong clinical suspicion of dissemination, further trephine biopsy is indicated (Figs. 13.2–13.7).

Haemolysis (particularly of an autoimmune type) may be a feature of advanced Hodgkin's disease, but is more common in non-Hodgkin's lymphoma. An established method of estimating red cell survival involves the use of ^{51}Cr. When red cells are incubated with this isotope the chromium enters the cells and is bound to the haemoglobin molecule. The

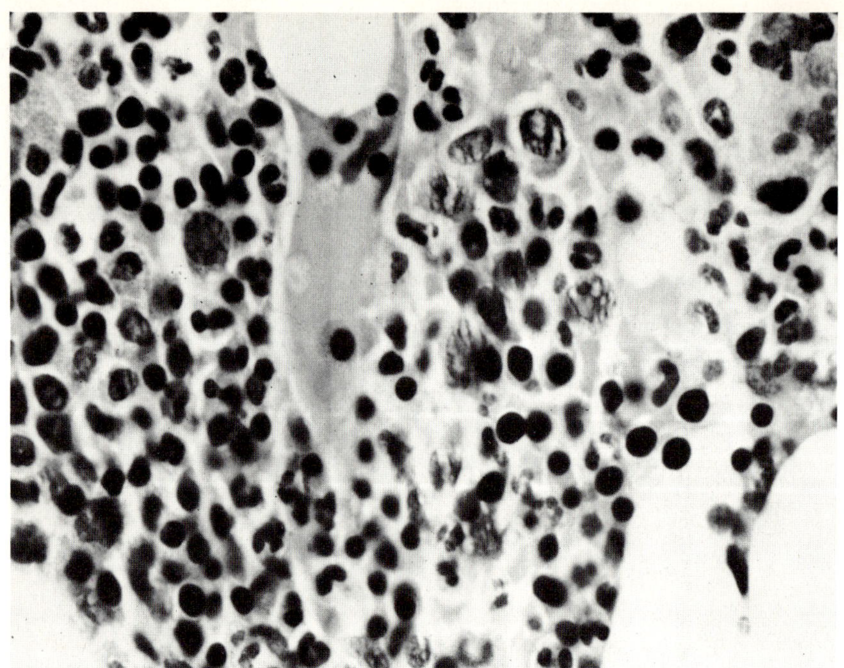

Fig. 13.5. Bone marrow section: Showing atypical histiocytic cell hyperplasia. Such appearances strongly suggest but are not quite diagnostic of lymphoma in the marrow. ×480.

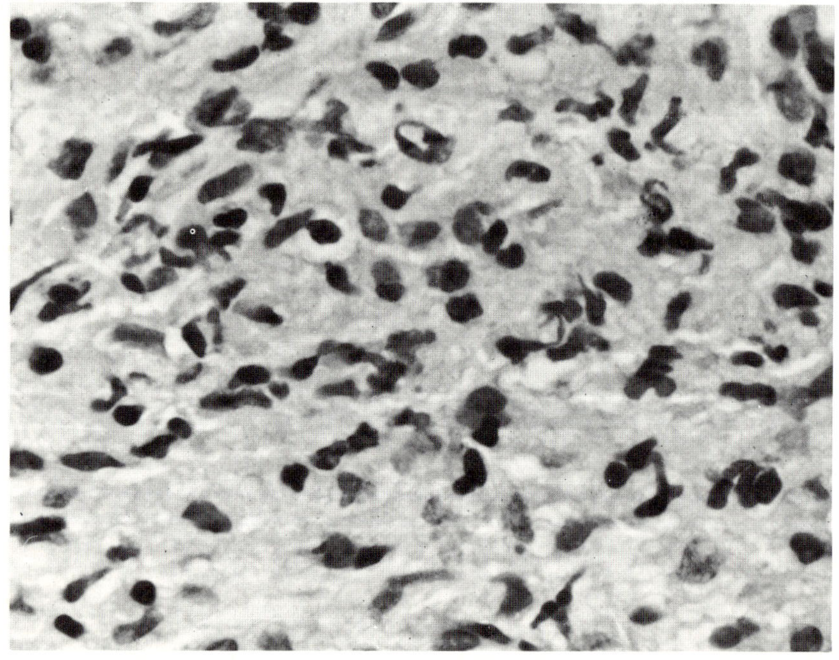

Fig. 13.6. Bone marrow section: Showing diffuse fibrosis and infiltration with atypical histiocytic cells in Hodgkin's disease. ×480.

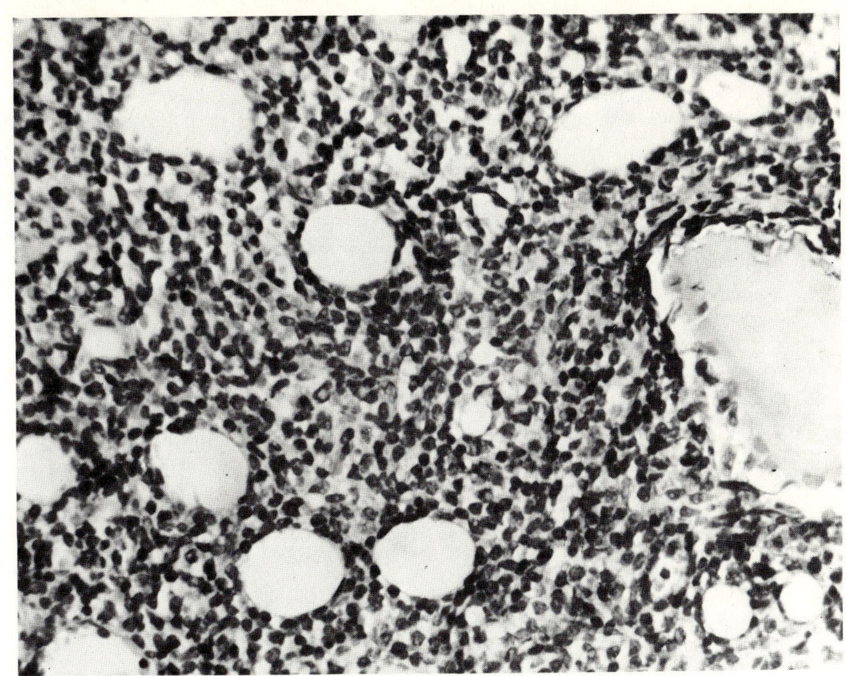

Fig. 13.7. Bone marrow section in
non-Hodgkin's lymphoma showing diffuse
infiltration with lymphoma cells. × 216.

labelled cells are re-injected into the patient and the rate of
disappearance of radioactivity in blood samples is followed
over the next 20 or 30 days. In the chromium test the red-cell
survival is usually expressed as the half-chromium time $T\frac{1}{2}Cr$
(normally about 25–32 days). This does not represent the true
half life of the red-cells, since there is a steady loss of
chromium from the cells by elution. However in standard
practice this test does give a useful idea of the red-cell life
span.

A more accurate estimate of red-cell life can be obtained by
using diisopropyl fluoro phosphate labelled with radioactive
phosphorus (DF ^{32}P) which is permanently attached to the
red cells without imparing their survival. However, since ^{32}P
is a β emitting isotope the preparation and counting of blood
samples is somewhat tedious.

Radioactive iron (^{59}Fe) can also be used to assess red-cell
life span. In the patient most of this appears in circulating
cells within 10 days and remains there until the end of the
red-cell life (about 110 days normally) when there is a
transient fall in activity. The survival data using ^{59}Fe tend to
be difficult to interpret but the information obtained from
plasma clearance and localization in organs may be of value in
assessing the disorders of iron utilization seen often in the
anaemia of malignant lymphoma.

Reticuloendothelial system phagocytic ability can be
assessed by measuring the clearance of ^{125}I labelled aggregated human serum albumin. In Hodgkin's disease clearance
is increased, advanced disease being associated with more
rapid and remission with slower clearance rates (Sheagren *et
al.* 1967).

BIOCHEMICAL INVESTIGATION

Blood samples should be taken for liver function tests (serum
bilirubin, alkaline phosphatase, liver enzymes, proteins); for
urea, calcium and electrolyte assessment (looking particularly
for renal abnormalities). Uric acid levels must be assessed
before and during treatment. Where it is available a multifactorial serum analysis gives a good general screen for biochemical abnormalities. Disease activity is often assessed by serial
measurements of levels of serum iron (depressed) and serum
copper (elevated). Ferritin, an iron storage protein, is elevated
in the serum in widespread malignant lymphoma and
elevation of this marker is also associated with poor prognosis
(Hancock *et al.* 1980). These serum ferritin abnormalities may
reflect the reticuloendothelial block of iron release in a chronic
disease or may represent a change in the immunological or

biochemical nature of the protein in lymphoma (Hancock *et al.* 1979).

It is often difficult to get an accurate clinical assessment of hepatic involvement. Hepatomegaly does not imply pathological involvement and conversely hepatic infiltration may be seen in the presence of a clinically normal liver with normal liver function tests and isotope scans. Carbone *et al.* (1971) suggest, that in the clinical staging evaluation, criteria for hepatic involvement should be (a) abnormal serum alkaline phosphatase with two or more other liver function test abnormalities; (b) an abnormal isotope liver scan with one or more abnormal liver function tests. A suitably sized hepatic biopsy taken at open operation is the most accurate way of assessing liver involvement.

IMMUNOLOGICAL INVESTIGATIONS
(see also Chapters 4 and 5)

These may be helpful in the investigation of lymphoma since it is likely that immune status is related to prognosis. Markedly depressed immunity, when it occurs, is nearly always a feature of disseminated disease.

In vivo investigations of cellular immunity include skin tests (recall antigens) or active sensitization with dinitrochlorobenzene (DNCB). *In vivo* tests include lymphocyte transformation, macrophage migration inhibition and E rosetting techniques. Humoral immunity may be assessed by measuring serum immunoglobulin levels, by estimating the proportion of B cells by immunofluorescent cell surface immunoglobulin labelling techniques or by assessing functional antibody formation, either by estimating natural antibodies or by test immunization. Classically the defect is of cellular immunity in Hodgkin's disease and of humoral immunity in non-Hodgkin's lymphoma; in practice however there may be overlap.

In non-Hodgkin's lymphoma particularly, monoclonal gammopathies are an occasional finding (see Chapter 10). Immunoglobulin quantitation and immunoelectrophoretic examination of blood and urine should be carried out in all cases.

ISOTOPE SCANNING

The visualization of radio isotope uptake in body tissues by means of either a rectilinear scanner or gammacamera may be of supportive help in the staging of lymphoma. Some authorities (Kaplan and Rosenberg 1975) consider that the yield and accuracy of such scans is too low to justify routine use in all cases. Perhaps they should be selectively used when indicated by clinical and other investigative findings.

Liver

Malignant lymphoma can involve the liver at an early stage and at autopsy over half of cases have such involvement. Clinical and biochemical findings are often inaccurate in the assessment of infiltration however and attempts have been made to increase this accuracy by hepatic scanning. Early studies with ^{131}I rose bengal gave apparently good results but more recently the use of ^{99m}Tc sulphur colloid (1–10 mCi) has allowed the better demonstration of space occupying lesions. The spleen is also visualized in this procedure. In lymphoma the liver scan supplements the clinical information of liver shape and size. Large discrete lymphoma deposits may show up as cold areas but the accuracy is not as great as that reported with other space occupying lesions. The liver may appear of normal size but show a diffuse patchy infiltration (Fig. 11.8) or multiple small filling defects. However, such findings are not a truly reliable sign of liver involvement. A strong suspicion of liver involvement, based on physical, radiographic, biochemical and scintigraphic findings, still requires biopsy confirmation.

Spleen

The spleen is often enlarged in lymphoma and therefore investigations into the nature of the splenic involvement have proved of great interest. The clinically enlarged spleen is not necessarily infiltrated by lymphoma (Kadin *et al.* 1971). It may be enlarged from congestion, reactive hyperplasia or granuloma formation. Several methods of spleen scanning are available which involve the labelling and denaturing of the patient's red cells. Improved visualization is obtained by using high activities of, for example, ^{99m}Tc sulphur colloid and such scans demonstrate size, shape and position of the spleen.

Rarely discrete deposits are seen but more commonly the abnormality is one of increased size (Fig. 13.8). The clinically and radiographically enlarged spleen, confirmed by scanning, is associated with pathological involvement in over 40% of cases but obviously histological examination is the only valid way of assessing splenic infiltration.

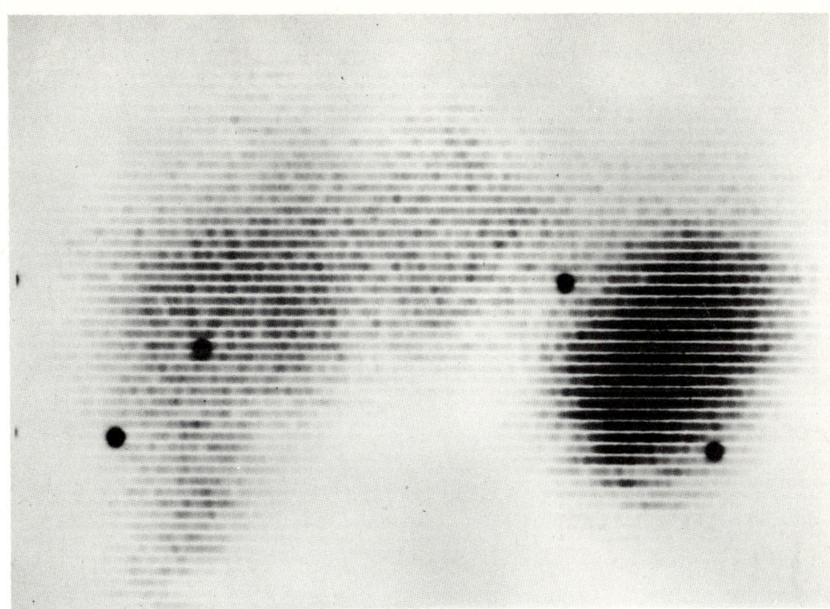

Fig. 13.8. ^{99m}Tc sulphur colloid scan showing diffuse patchy infiltration of the liver by Hodgkin's disease and enlargement of spleen.

Skeleton

Bony involvement is seen in up to a quarter of all patients with lymphoma. Lesions are more frequently osteolytic than sclerotic or mixed, and they may of course be multiple. Bone scans are of use in lymphoma where there is clinical or radiographic doubt as to whether a deposit is present. The appearances are however non-specific.

^{85}Sr has been one of the more frequently used radio isotopes but has a long half life and can only be given in low activities. Interest has centred recently on the use of ^{99m}Tc polyphosphate or pyrophosphate which can be given in smaller quantities and which have activities suitable also for the gammacamera.

Gallium scanning

Various tumour specific radionuclides have been assessed. The most useful at the moment is ^{67}Ga citrate which concentrates in tumours (including lymphoreticular tumours). This isotope also tends to accumulate in inflammatory tissue and hence some false positives are obtained. The main use of this, apart from hepatic and splenic visualization, seems to be in detecting mediastinal involvement (Fig. 13.9) and differentiating this from fibrosis (McCready 1973).

Kidneys

Renal involvement occurs rarely in Hodgkin's disease but is common in non-Hodgkin's lymphoma. Routine renography using ^{125}I or ^{131}I hippuran is not of particular value but in selected cases (for example, those with considerably elevated blood urea or in whom IVP has been unsuccessful) a useful assessment of renal function can be obtained. Such studies should of course be combined with biochemical (blood and urine) tests of renal function and if necessary with renal biopsy.

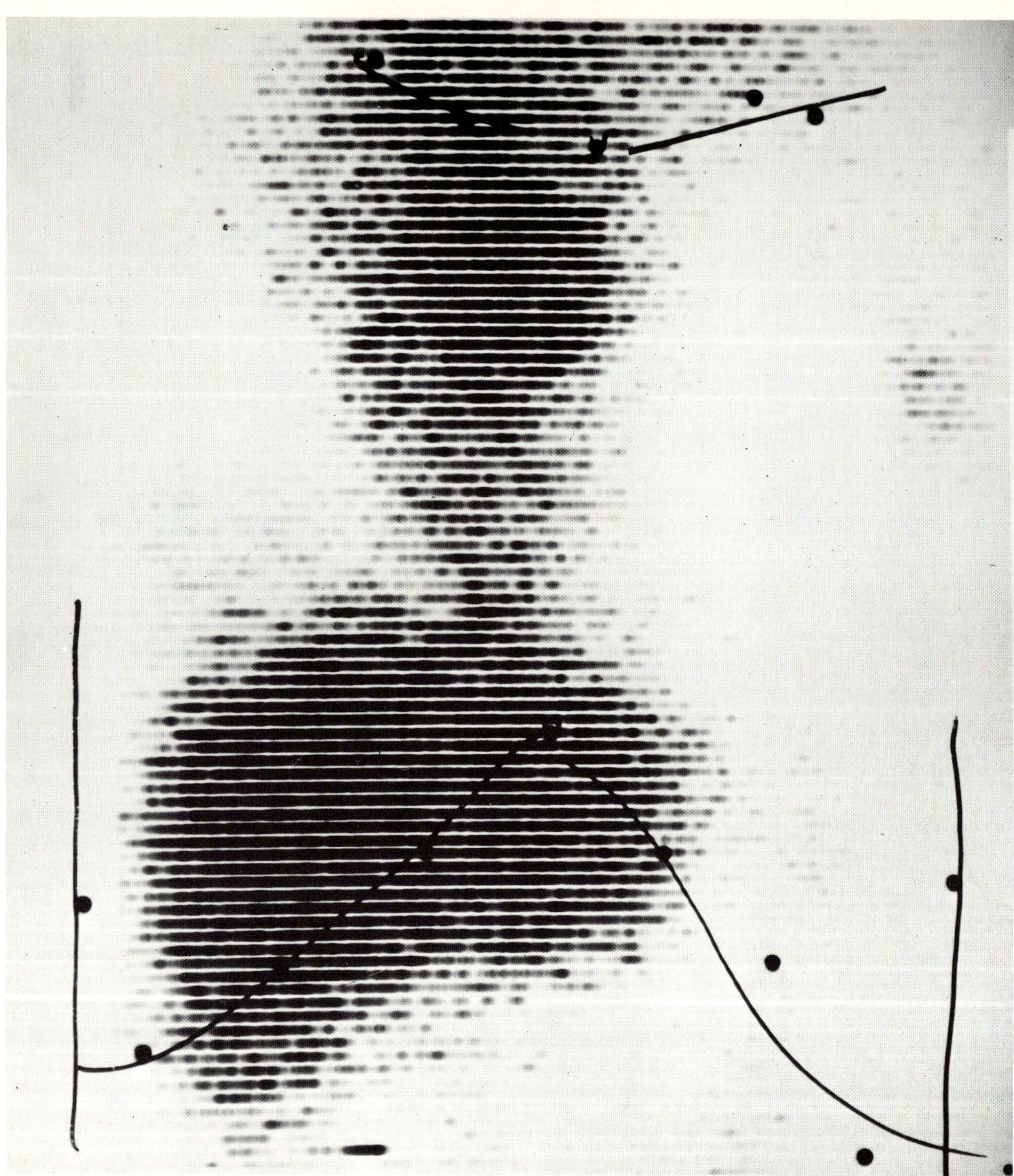

Fig. 13.9. ^{67}Ga citrate scan showing high uptake in mediastinal gland involved by Hodgkin's disease. Enlarged liver also shown.

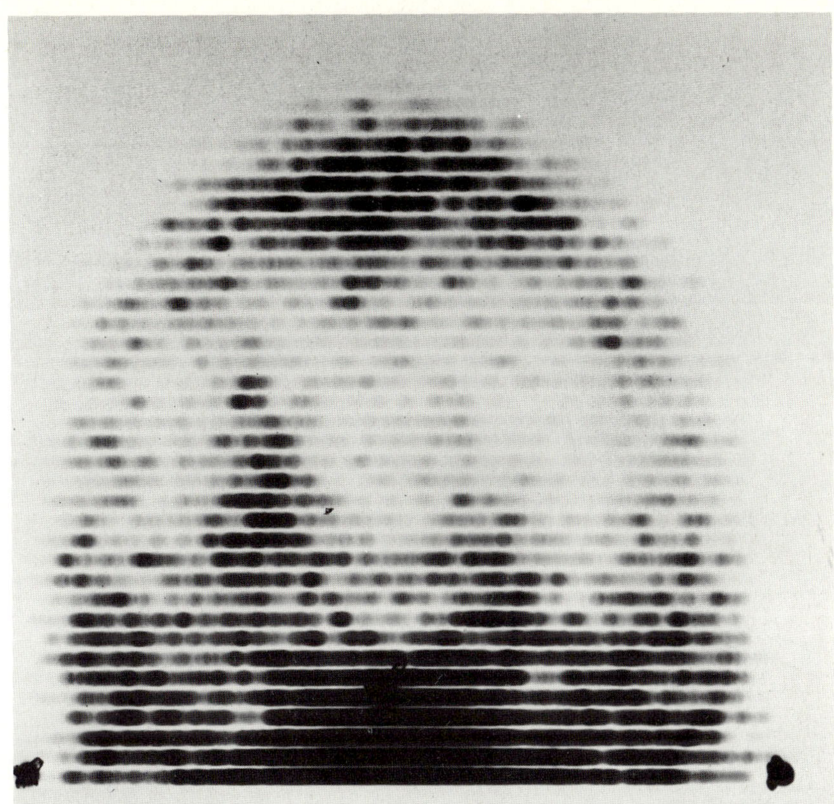

Fig. 13.10. ^{99m}Tc sulphur colloid brain scan showing deposit in the right frontal lobe of a patient with Hodgkin's disease presenting with major epilepsy.

Brain

A ^{99m}Tc brain scan may occasionally be of help in detecting cerebral lymphomatous deposits (Fig. 13.10).

RADIOLOGY

Many radiological investigations are of importance in the staging of lymphoma. Some, e.g. chest radiograph and lymphography, are mandatory in most patients, whereas others, e.g. skeletal survey, gastrointestinal studies, should be reserved for those patients in whom there is a good clinical indication.

Chest radiography

More than one quarter of patients with lymphoma have mediastinal involvement (Fig. 13.11) sometimes with hilar and paratracheal gland enlargement. Superior vena caval obstruction occurs occasionally. Mediastinal involvement is particularly common in the nodular sclerosing type of Hodgkin's disease.

The lung parenchyma is involved in about 10% of patients (usually in advanced or recurrent disease) either from local extension from thoracic lymph nodes or by lymphatic or haematogenous spread. The radiological appearance may therefore be one of infiltration (Fig. 13.12), discrete deposits (Fig. 13.13) (sometimes indistinguishable from bronchial neoplasm) or occasionally of miliary deposits (which require careful distinction from tuberculosis) or cavitation.

Pleural effusions, sometimes bilateral, are seen in up to one third of patients during the natural history of the diseases. Pericardial involvement from mediastinal gland masses may result in a pericardial effusion (Fig. 13.14). The cardiac shadow on chest radiograph should be serially reviewed to pick up this complication.

Post-irradiation fibrosis may be difficult to distinguish from mediastinal gland involvement. The use of tomography

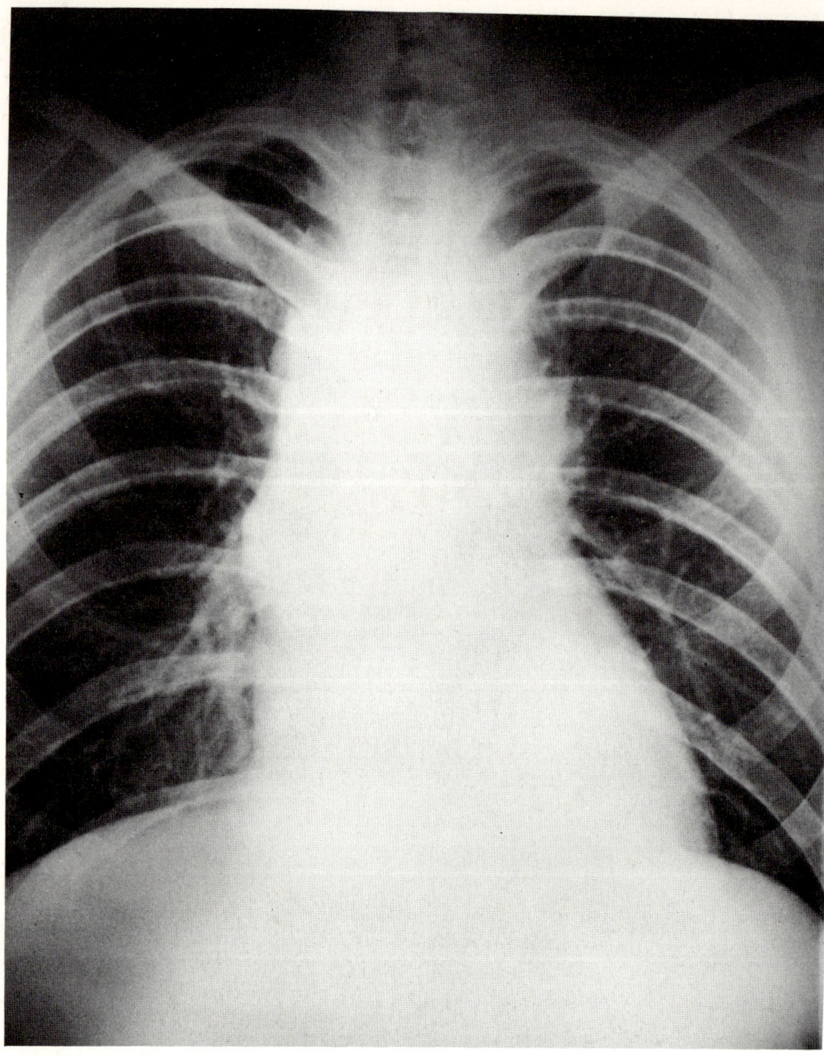

Fig. 13.11. Chest radiography showing enlarged mediastinal and hilar lymph nodes in patient with Hodgkin's disease.

and of ^{67}gallium citrate isotope scanning may help in resolving the problem.

Occasionally atypical infiltrations are seen and it is important in such cases to exclude opportunistic infections with bacteria (including *Mycobacterium tuberculosis*), candida, aspergillus, pneumocystis, cytomegalovirus and other rarer organisms.

Some difficulties are encountered in the staging of lung disease. Multiple nodules in one lobe, perihilar infiltration with ipsilateral lymphadenopathy and unilateral pleural effusion with hilar adenopathy are considered localized extralymphatic ('E') disease.

Lymphography

The place of bipedal lymphography in the staging of malignant lymphoma is now established (Viamonte 1971). This procedure has two basic aims, firstly to give information on the size and involvement of abdominal lymph nodes and secondly, in follow-up, as a marker of success of therapy or recurrence of disease. The procedure involves the isolation of lymphatic vessels on the dorsal surfaces of both feet. Identification of these vessels is aided by the injection of a marker dye into the skin above the toes. The lymphatic channel can then be cannulated after cut-down and contrast

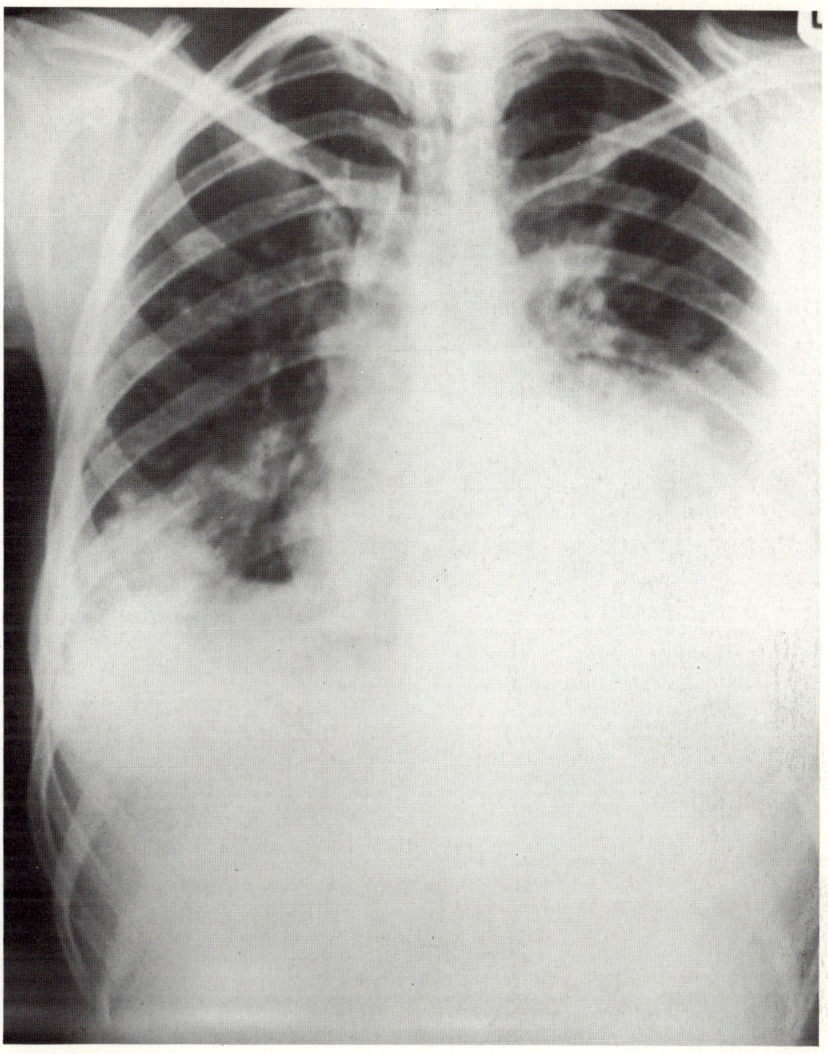

Fig. 13.12. Chest radiograph showing pulmonary parenchymal infiltrates in a patient with lymphocytic lymphoma.

(usually ultrafluid Lipiodol) is injected. The contrast is then visualized, by a series of radiographs, ascending the leg lymphatics and entering the lower abdominal nodes. A 24-hour series of films allows visualization of iliac and para-aortic nodes. It is important to bear in mind that Lipiodol is an oily medium and will eventually enter the lungs which act as a filter from the systemic venous circulation. A patient with low respiratory reserve (with lung, thrombo-embolic or cardiac disease) should be treated with special caution since the respiratory reserve may be lowered to dangerous or even fatal levels by Lipiodol in the lung. Severe respiratory impairment is therefore a contraindication to

lymphography. Therapeutic lung irradiation, which may paralyse lung capillaries, alters the filtering effect of the lungs and is therefore also a contraindication to lymphography.

Serious complications (mostly respiratory) occur in less than 1 in 100 cases in expert hands. Many patients experience a transient pyrexia following the procedure and anaphylaxis, sometimes severe, is an occasional complication of both marker dye and Lipiodol injection. As with other radiographic procedures using iodine containing contrast media thyroid function tests may be persistently disturbed (with elevation of the serum protein bound iodine level and depression of thyroidal radio iodine uptakes).

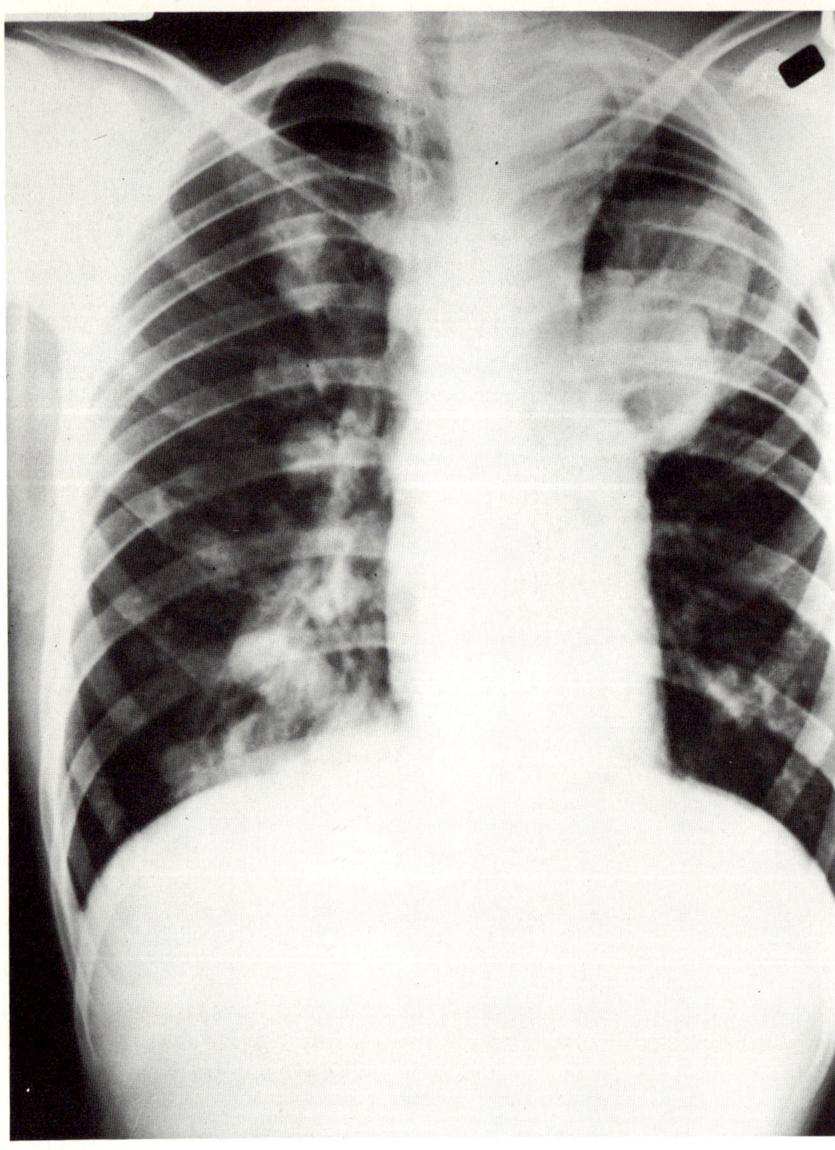

Fig. 13.13. Chest radiograph showing discrete deposits in both lungs in a patient with Hodgkin's disease.

The lymphographic changes in malignant lymphoma are non-specific. Normal lymph nodes show an almost homogeneous finely granular texture. Lymphoma involved nodes are enlarged but with retention of the marginal sinus; they show a reticular or 'foamy' appearance with or without filling defects (Fig. 13.15). Failed or delayed opacification of the abdominal nodes may indicate lymphatic obstruction by grossly involved nodes. In Hodgkin's disease of the lymphocyte depleted histology type, the nodes may occasionally be completely replaced by tumour and are therefore not visua-lized on lymphography. In non-Hodgkin's lymphoma there is a high incidence of mesenteric node involvement which is not detected by lymphography.

There is considerable overlap of the lymphographic appearance of malignant lymphoma with many diseases. Other tumours, sarcoidosis, specific and non-specific infections, autoimmune disease and macroglobulinaemia may give similar appearances. The findings of the lymphogram must therefore always be taken in conjunction with clinical judgement.

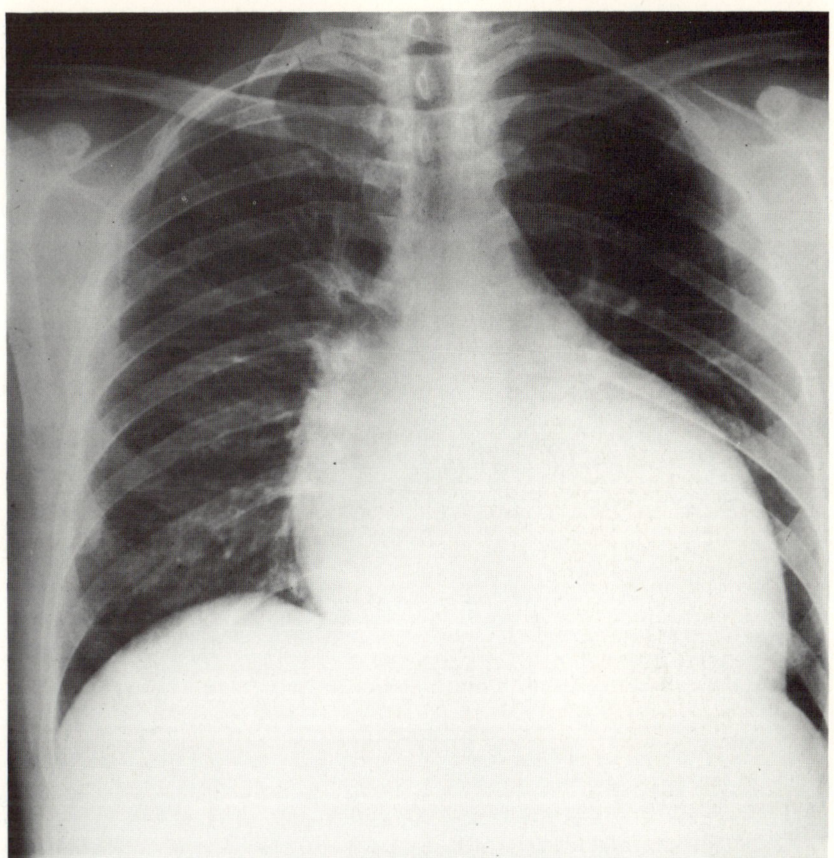

Fig. 13.14. Chest radiograph showing a pericardial effusion in a patient with Hodgkin's disease.

The importance of follow-up has been emphasized. The oily contrast remains in the nodes for up to 1 or 2 years and should be regularly visualized. The response to therapy can be assessed (Fig. 13.16a and b) and any abnormalities developing may give an early warning of recurrence of disease.

Undoubtedly many patients with malignant lymphoma are re-staged from clinical Stages I and II to Stage III by positive lymphographic findings.

The accuracy of such findings, as assessed by histological examination of radiographically involved nodes and by follow-up radiographic studies, is good, but the procedure should be regarded as complementary to other investigations including diagnostic laparotomy.

Renal radiography

Intravenous pyelography (IVP) may be of value as an accessory investigation to the lymphogram in demonstrating para-aortic node disease. The ureters may be displaced or obstructed. IVP (if necessary by high dose infusion) is mandatory in those patients with evidence of renal impairment. Renal involvement by malignant lymphoma may be seen as enlargement, often irregular, of one or both kidneys. Unilateral or bilateral hydronephrosis may indicate obstruction by retroperitoneal gland masses. The investigations should be assessed together with blood and urine tests of renal function, renogram and possibly renal biopsy. The radiographs of abdomen obtained during this procedure may of course give valuable information on the size of liver, spleen and kidneys (see Fig. 13.16).

Skeletal radiography

Bony deposits are found in up to 5% of patients with lymphoma (usually with late or recurrent disease) but most

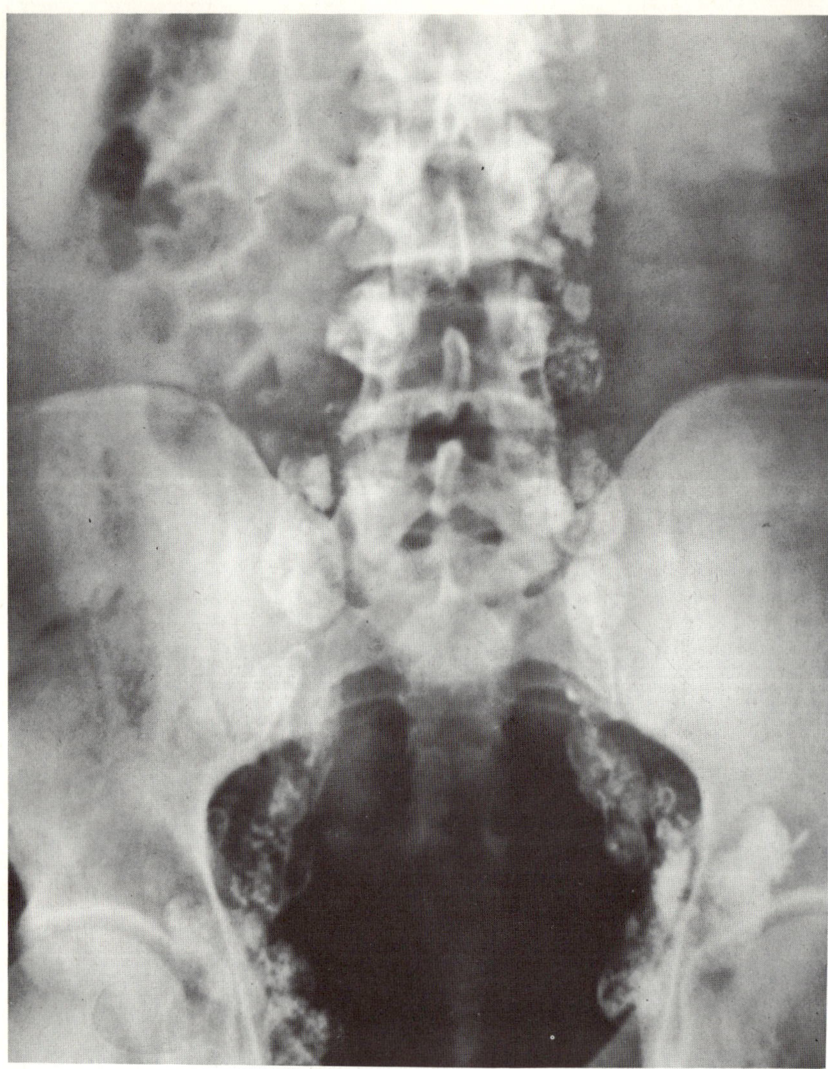

Fig. 13.15. Lymphogram showing enlarged foamy intra-abdominal lymph nodes in a patient with Hodgkin's disease.

authorities now consider that skeletal radiography (including surveys) should be reserved for those patients with clinical or biochemical indication of bone disease.

Deposits, whether from direct invasion or from haematogenous spread, can be single or multiple. They are more often osteolytic (Fig. 13.17) than osteosclerotic (Fig. 13.18) or mixed in type. The vertebral spine, ribs, pelvis and upper femora are most commonly involved but there are no radiographic features specific to lymphoma. Hypertrophic osteoarthropathy is a rare finding with intrathoracic lymphoma.

Gastrointestinal radiography

A barium swallow investigation may be useful in detecting posterior intrathoracic lymph node enlargement but the yield of positive findings is often considered too low for this to be considered as a routine investigation in malignant lymphoma.

Lymphomatous involvement (particularly by non-Hodgkin's lymphoma) may occur in stomach, small bowel and colon. Such lesions, demonstrated by barium studies, may be segmental or diffuse (Fig. 13.19); the gut appears rigid and the mucosal pattern is destroyed. Obstruction is occasionally

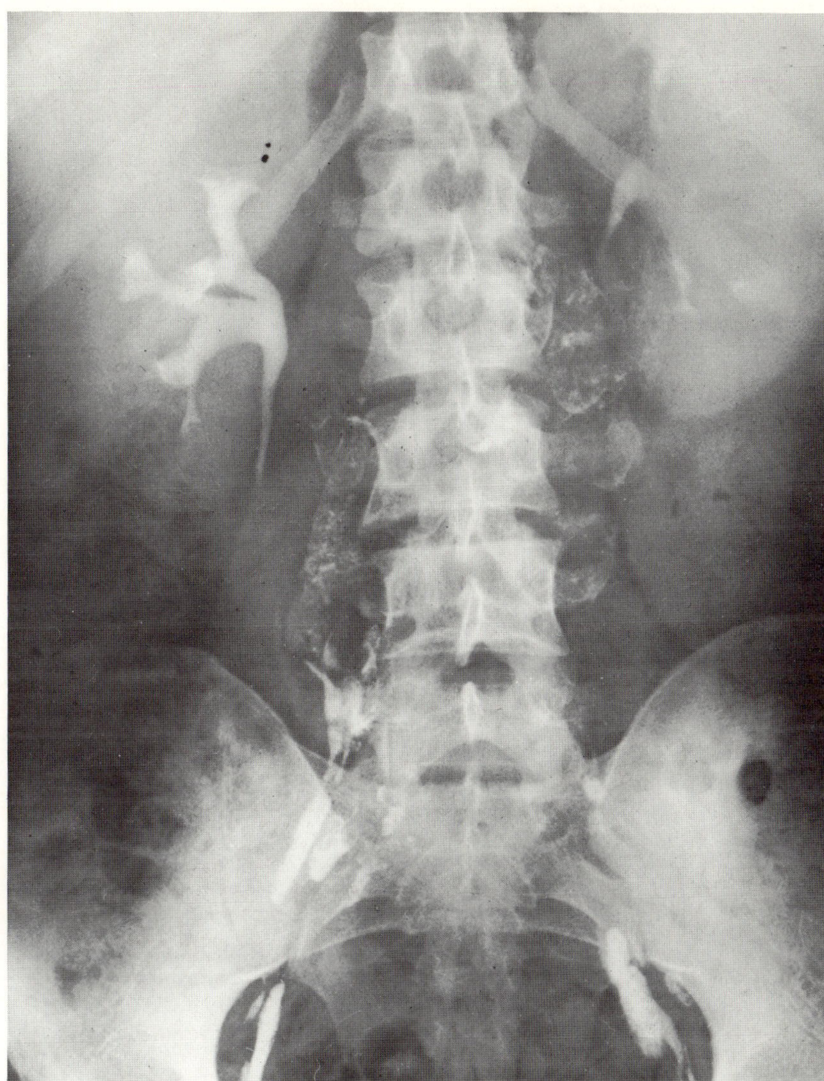

Fig. 13.16. (a) Abdominal radiograph of a patient with generalized Hodgkin's disease with abdominal radiograph lymphogram demonstrating para-aortic lymph node involvement and intravenous pyelogram showing displacement of ureters with infiltration and enlargement of the left kidney. Enlargement of the spleen is also seen.

seen. Conclusive evidence of bowel involvement is gained from laparotomy or occasionally from endoscopy.

Computerized tomography

Computerized axial tomography (CAT, CT scanning) is a non-invasive radiological technique which is of established value in the diagnosis of lesions in the brain and has also been recently applied to the whole body with equally good results. The technique may be of value in the staging of patients with malignant lymphoma (Blackledge *et al.* 1980) and particularly in detecting nodes in the upper abdomen where lymphography is of little value. CT scanning does not appear to help in the assessment of splenic involvement however and cannot replace diagnostic laparotomy in appropriate patients (Fig. 13.20a and b).

Ultrasonography

The diagnostic use of high frequency sound waves in the management of tumours is becoming important particularly in the non-invasive assessment of abdominal lesions. In

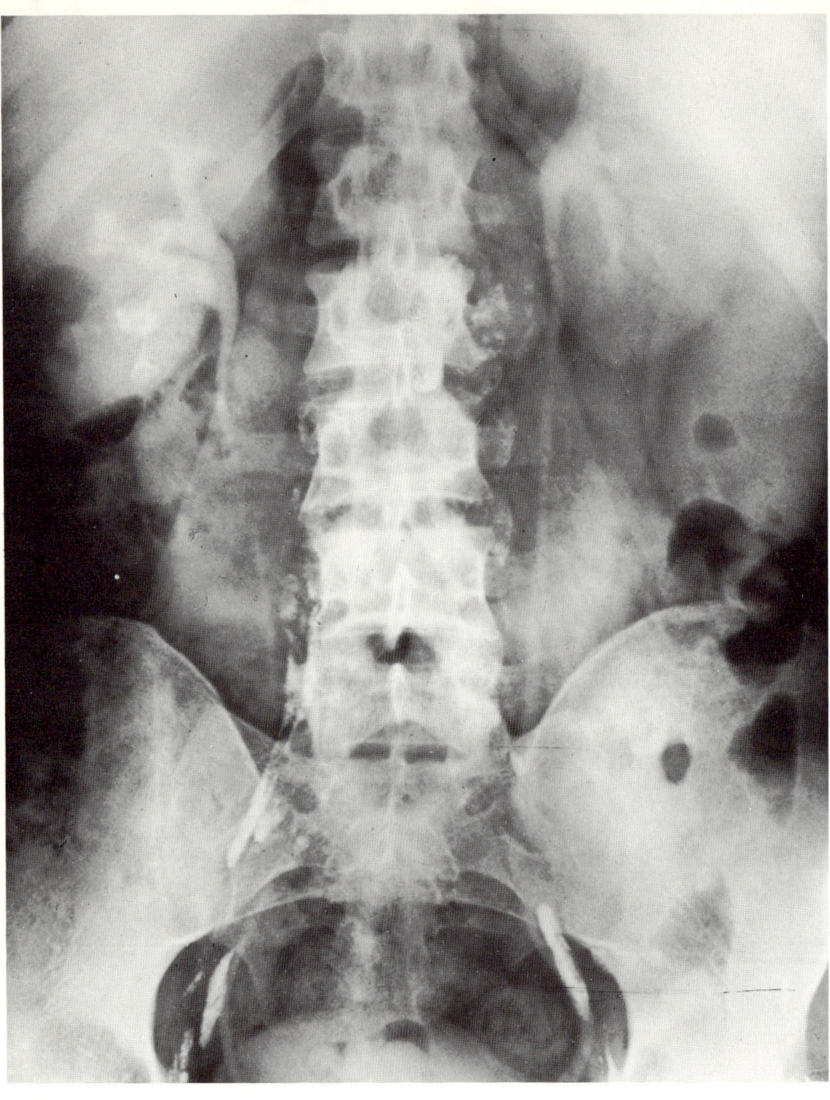

Fig. 13.16. (b) After cytotoxic chemotherapy there is regression of lymph node, left kidney and spleen enlargement.

malignant lymphoma helpful information can be gained on the size and involvement of structures such as the liver, spleen, kidneys and abdominal lymph nodes (Fig. 13.21).

LAPAROTOMY AND SPLENECTOMY

Over the past few years it has been recognized that intra-abdominal involvement with malignant lymphoma may accompany apparently isolated superficial lymphadenopathy remote from the abdomen. Certain categories are at high risk, particularly those with systemic symptoms and, in Hodgkin's disease, especially those with mixed cell and lymphocyte depleted histology. Neutrophil leucocytosis, eosinophilia and thrombocytosis may also indicate the presence of abdominal disease. In non-Hodgkin's lymphoma intra-abdominal involvement (of nodes, spleen, liver or bowel) is often found.

It is clear that the chances of error in assessing involvement of liver and spleen after clinical investigation are high. In Hodgkin's disease, for example, only about one half of clinically enlarged spleens are involved by disease the others showing congestion, hyperplasia or granuloma formation.

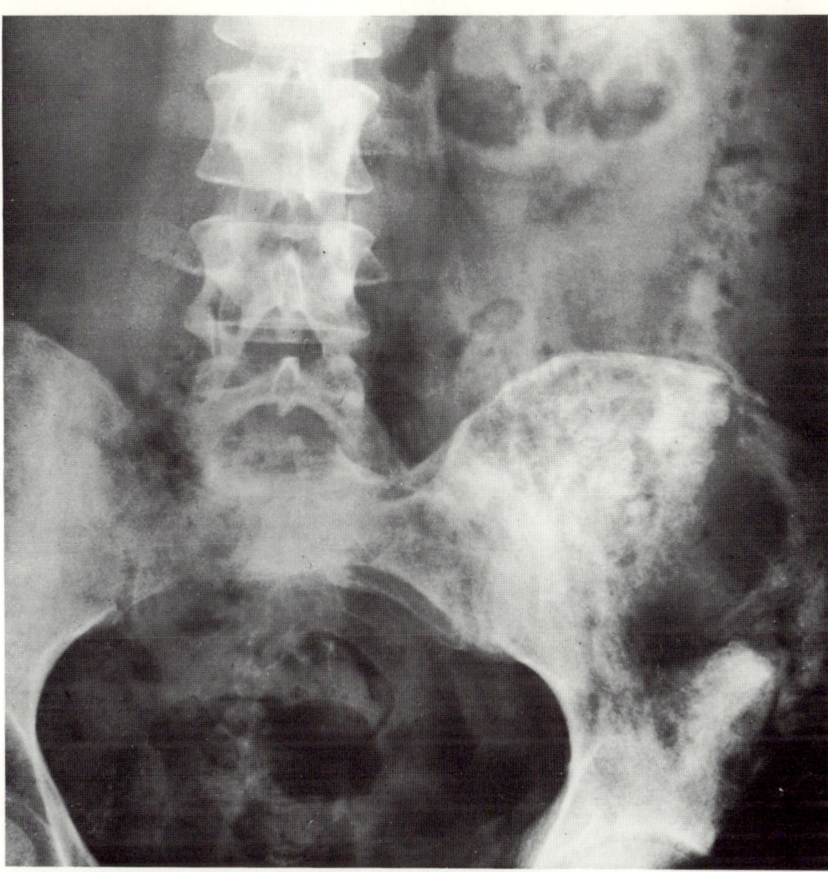

Fig. 13.17. Radiograph of the pelvis showing a large osteolytic deposit in the left ilium of a patient with Hodgkin's disease.

Conversely the clinically normal spleen shows pathological evidence of disease in one third of cases (Kadin *et al.* 1971).

It is for these reasons that diagnostic laparotomy with splenectomy and liver, lymph node and open bone marrow biopsy is now acknowledged to be an important part of the effective staging of many patients with Hodgkin's disease (Rosenberg 1971). The status of exploratory laparotomy in non-Hodgkin's lymphoma is as yet uncertain. Controlled trials are in progress but meanwhile operation is best left for those patients needing resection of intra-abdominal disease, e.g. bowel, spleen.

The advantages of splenectomy, apart from the obvious boon of total pathological inspection of the organ, are in the field of therapy. The drop in blood count that occurs with therapy may be lessened, and in those patients requiring abdominal irradiation the radiotherapy field can be reduced and better localized (particularly if the splenic pedicle is marked by radio-opaque clips), thus lessening the risk of radiation damage to the left kidney and left lung base. The occasional complication of hypersplenism is, of course, corrected by splenectomy.

The incision made at the time of operation must be large enough to allow mobilization and delivery of the spleen, a vertical midline approach usually being used. The abdominal cavity is carefully inspected, splenectomy performed and lymph nodes from several sites are sampled with reference to the pre-operative lymphographs. Obviously enlarged glands are removed, regardless of site, and radio-opaque clips are inserted at all sites of node biopsy and on the splenic pedicle; obvious hepatic nodules are biopsied or a wedge of tissue removed from the macroscopically normal liver. Bone biopsy from the iliac crest is an optional additional procedure. After closure sutures or skin clips are normally left in for 10–14 days.

Laparotomy and splenectomy is not without the morbidity and mortality of any major operation, though these are low in

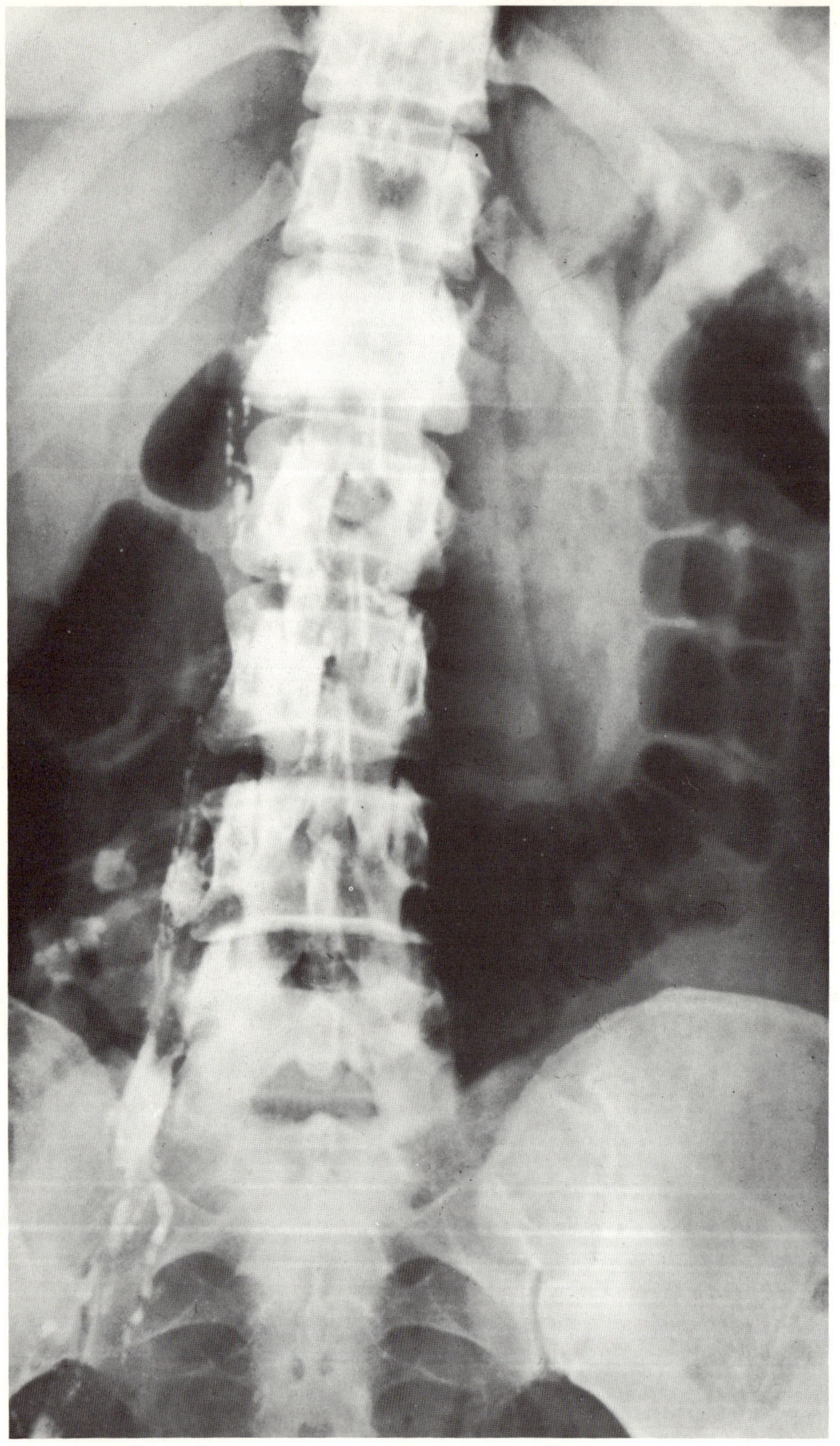

Fig. 13.18. Radiograph of the spine showing an osteosclerotic deposit in the first lumbar vertebra of a patient with Hodgkin's disease.

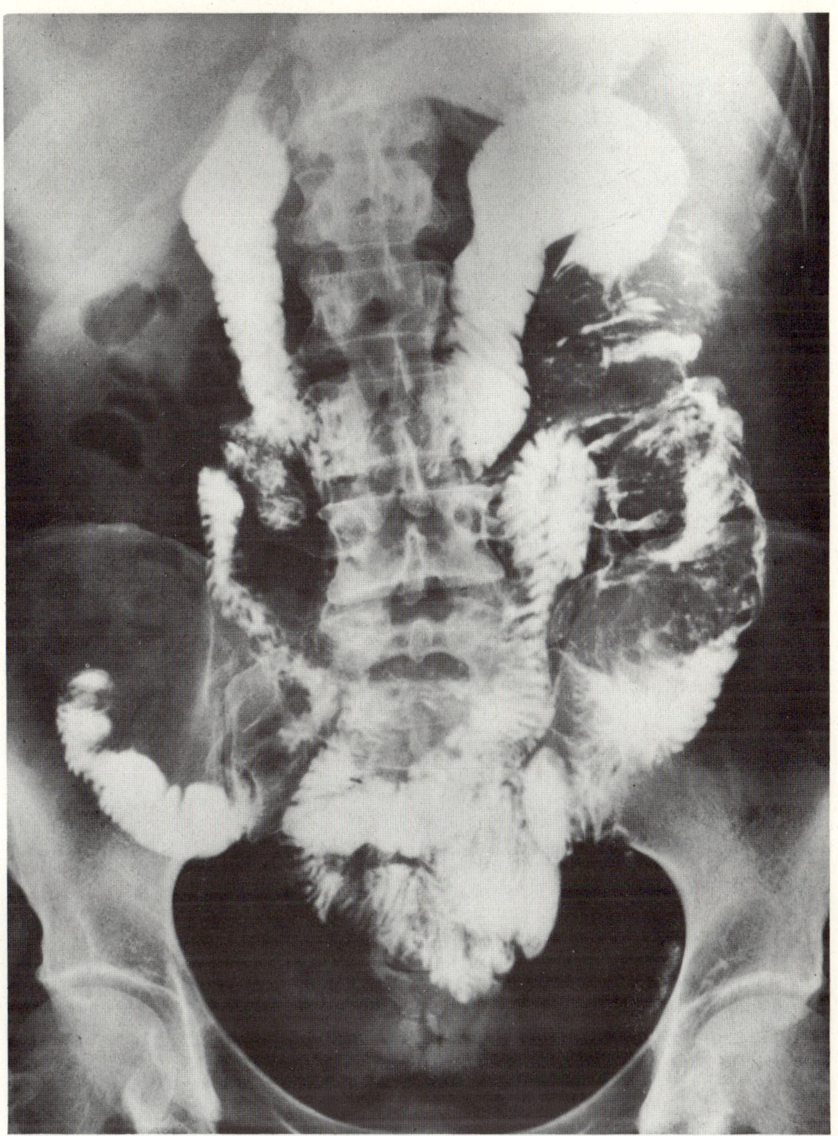

the hands of a surgeon experienced in the procedure. In the longer term, however, there appears to be an increased incidence of septicaemic deaths in treated splenectomized patients (Desser and Ultmann 1972; Hancock *et al.* 1976). The spleen is a major source of IgM and immune paresis involving IgM is a contributory factor in the genesis of septicaemia. We have shown that serum immunoglobulins, and particularly IgM levels, fall early in chemotherapy treated splenectomised patients (Hancock *et al.* 1977); at 5-years remission, progressive falls in serum immunoglobulins are seen in patients with Hodgkin's disease as a whole, but low values of IgG and IgM are particularly a feature of those having had splenectomy and chemotherapy (Hancock *et al.* 1982). The clinical relevance of these findings remains to be determined.

It is because of the possibility of such complications that the combination of peritoneoscopy with liver and spleen biopsy together with percutaneous liver biopsy has been

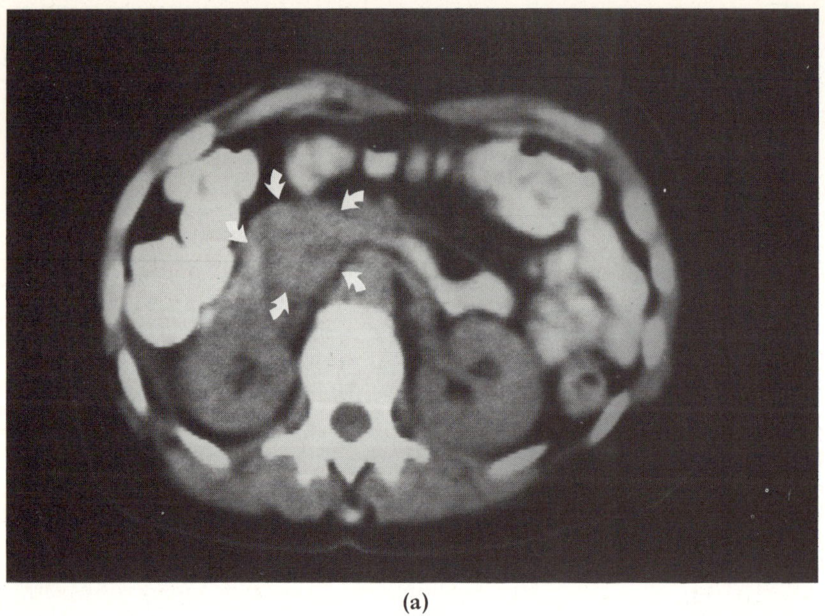

(a)

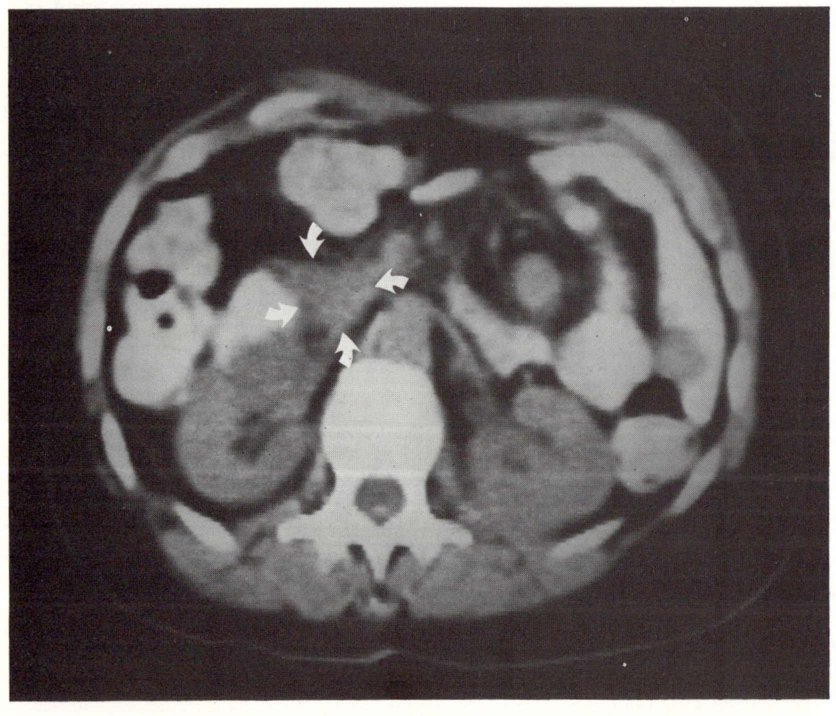

(b)

Fig. 13.20. (a, b) CT scan showing mass of enlarged lymph nodes medial and anterior to the upper pole of the right kidney before (a) and after (b) treatment.

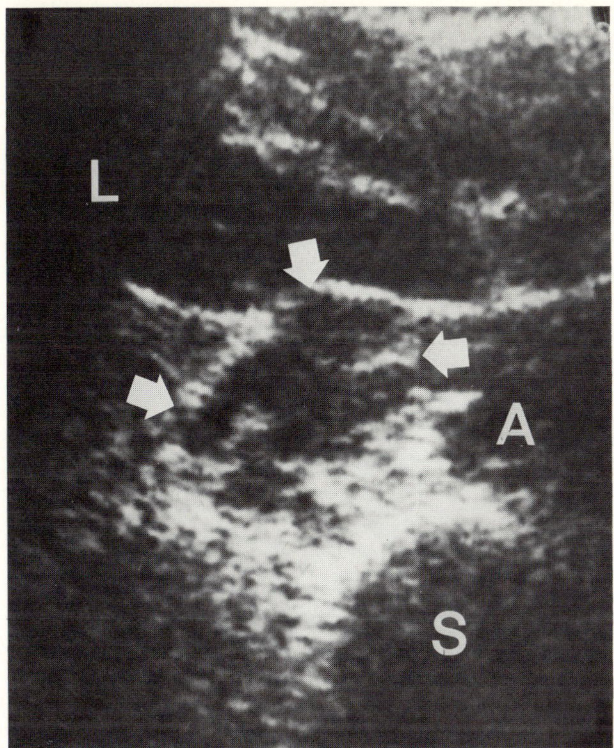

Fig. 13.21. Ultra-sound examination, transverse section at the level of the porta hepatis, showing a large mass of enlarged lymph nodes (arrowed). (L-liver, A-Aorta, S-spine.)

suggested. These procedures which have low complication rates in experienced hands may obviate the need for some patients to undergo exploratory laparotomy and could be

Table 13.1 Simplified general plan for pathological staging and treatment of Hodgkin's disease

Clinical stage	Pathological stage (laparotomy)	Treatment
IAIIA (female) ——————————→		Irradiation
IAIIA (male) ——→ IA A ———→		(local or prophylactic)
IBIIB ——————————————————→		Cyclical chemotherapy
IIIA	————————————————→	Cyclical chemotherapy
	IIIA$_{s-}$ ————————→	Total nodal irradiation
	IIIA$_{s+}$ ————————→	Cyclical chemotherapy
IIIB IVA IVB ——————————→		Cyclical chemotherapy

applied in both Hodgkin's disease and non-Hodgkin's lymphoma.

Some authorities include diagnostic laparotomy and splenectomy in the investigation of all their patients with Hodgkin's disease. Others select those patients at highest risk from abdominal involvement. If patients are to be selected it would seem that females with clinical Stage IA or IIA disease are at less risk from non-salvageable abdominal disease. Those with Stage IIIB or IV disease are obviously candidates for cytotoxic chemotherapy. Patients from these categories could therefore be spared laparotomy and splenectomy. Our own current selection policies are summarised in Table 13.1.

TREATMENT

The treatment of Hodgkin's disease, after accurate staging, now follows fairly well-established lines. For localised asymptomatic disease (Stages I, IIA) radiotherapy is usually employed; for patients with disseminated, symptomatic disease (stages IIIB, IVA and B) combination cytotoxic chemotherapy is appropriate. For stages IB, IIB and IIIA there is still considerable debate—some authorities give radiotherapy with or without chemotherapy, others give chemotherapy alone. Table 13.1 shows a simplified middle-of-the-road scheme of planned therapy (based on a selective laparotomy policy) used in Sheffield in accordance with current British National Lymphoma Investigation criteria.

Radiotherapy

The radiosensitivity of lymphomas was recognised at the turn of the century but the discriminant use of radiotherapy was not started until the 1930s when Gilbert (1939) formulated his ideas on the radiotherapeutic treatment of Hodgkin's disease. Peters (1950) later showed the importance of irradiating adjacent areas prophylactically to improve survival, and the concept of cure in a disease previously considered inexorably fatal was established by Easson and Russell (1963). Recent studies, with the evolution of histological classifications and staging criteria, have lead to considerable progress in the planned therapy of Hodgkin's disease, though the situation with non-Hodgkin's lymphoma is not yet as clear.

RADIOTHERAPY IN HODGKIN'S DISEASE

The important concepts of radiotherapy in Hodgkin's disease

traditionally involve the use of large planned fields and tumoricidal doses administered by megavoltage techniques (Fig. 13.22).

The tumoricidal dose in the standard treatment fields varies from 3500 rads in $3\frac{1}{2}$ weeks to 4500 in 4 weeks, administered by a linear accelerator or ^{60}Cobalt teletherapy apparatus. The importance of planning, marking and simulation, with check films on the treatment apparatus cannot be over-emphasized.

The *mantle* technique (opposed anterior and posterior fields) encompasses mediastinal, hilar and bilateral supraclavicular, cervical and axillary lymph nodes (Fig. 13.22a). The lungs, heart and spinal cord (the latter after 2000 rads) may be shielded with lead, or with certain low melting point alloys which are lighter and easier to work with than lead. With upper cervical lymph node involvement, the Waldeyer's ring may also be irradiated by opposed lateral fields. With large intrathoracic lymph node masses the field can be progressively modified as node regression occurs.

The *inverted Y* technique (opposed anterior and posterior fields) takes in femoral, inguinal, iliac and para-aortic nodes to almost the lower extremity of the mantle field (Fig. 13.22b). A splenic pedicle field is often incorporated and the rectum and bladder may be shielded. In young female patient the ovaries can be brought into a retro-uterine mid-line position at the time of laparotomy and splenectomy (oophoroplexy) and can thus be shielded with preservation of menstrual function. In the young male the gonads can also be shielded.

More extensive abdominal disease treatable by radiotherapy may require abdominal bath techniques (Fig. 13.22c) or appropriately modified 'spade', hepatic or pelvic fields.

Total nodal irradiation involves mantle followed after 4–6 weeks by a carefully matched inverted Y field.

Therapy selection in most patients for these standard techniques is usually straightforward though it has recently been suggested that accurately staged localised disease, i.e. PS IA IIA, may require no more than local high dose irradiation (Jelliffe 1979). Patients in the IB IIB and IIIA categories sometimes pose problems and full course chemotherapy alone may be appropriate for these groups. However, many authorities still give radiotherapy with or without intensive chemotherapy (Kaplan and Rosenberg 1975; review Kaplan 1980).

Patients with I_E or II_E staging require local radical irradiation to the extralymphatic lesion, and this is often incorporated in a mantle or inverted Y field.

In patients with IIB_E and III_E disease total nodal irradia-

tion can be followed by 6 courses of cyclical chemotherapy, or cyclical chemotherapy alone used.

The increased risk of second malignancy particularly with combined radiotherapy and chemotherapy (Valagussa *et al.* 1980) regimes must be kept in mind.

In some cases the planned treatment of Hodgkin's disease must be interrupted. For example massive intrathoracic lymphadenopathy may require mantle radiotherapy (2000 rads in two weeks) to reduce the lymph node mass interrupted by a 2-week break in which other investigations including laparotomy can be performed; the radiotherapy is then resumed with a reduced mediastinal aperture. Bulky mediastinal disease is also sometimes managed by using chemotherapy in the first instance to shrink the lesion, thus allowing smaller and less damaging radiotherapy fields.

With exceptionally large or slowly regressing tumour a local 'boost' of radiotherapy to 5000 rads in 5 weeks may be appropriate.

Most patients tolerate the radiotherapeutic regimes discussed above very well. Soreness of skin and mucous membranes may occur, also nausea, vomiting and diarrhoea, particularly with abdominal fields. Falls in blood count rarely interrupt therapy even in those patients having large areas irradiated. Symptomatic treatment (antiemetics, antidiarrhoeal agents, blood transfusion, good hydration) is generally adequate for such temporary disturbances. Loss of hair over the occipital region is possible with mantle irradiation and it is sensible to order the patient a wig sooner rather than later in treatment. With inverted Y fields the gonads, even if shielded, may receive up to 500 rads and the possibility of sterility or mutagenesis must be considered and the patient accordingly advised.

One natural consequence of radiotherapy is fibrosis, but this is usually only troublesome in the lungs where some degree of radiation pneumonitis is inevitable. In some patients the chest radiograph shows apical and paramediastinal fibrosis which may be difficult to differentiate from lymphadenopathy. Impairment of respiratory function with mantle irradiation is rarely severe.

Hypothyroidism and L'Hermittes sign (parasthesiae in the limbs particularly on neck flexion as a result of spinal cord irradiation) may occur in occasional patients.

RADIOTHERAPY IN NON-HODGKIN'S LYMPHOMAS

In non-Hodgkin's lymphoma lymphatic disease is often not contiguous and there is a higher incidence of extralymphatic involvement. The disease is therefore often more widespread

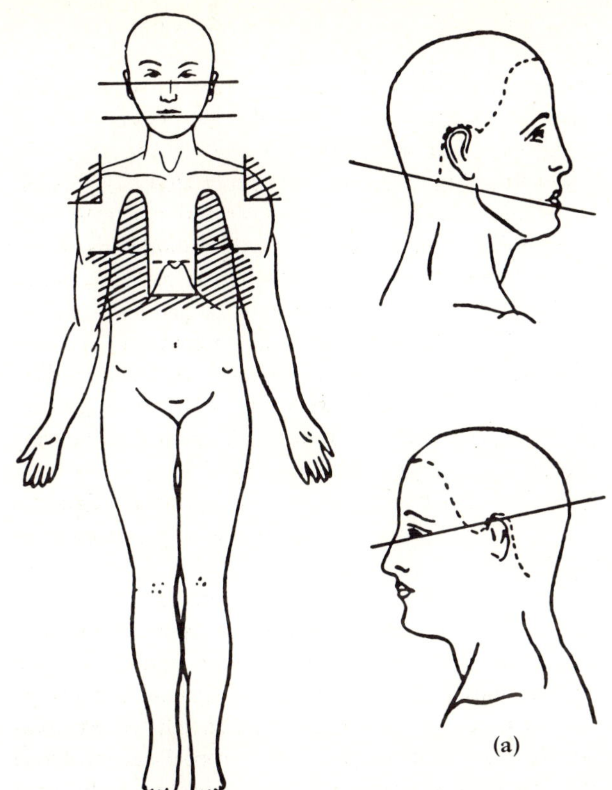

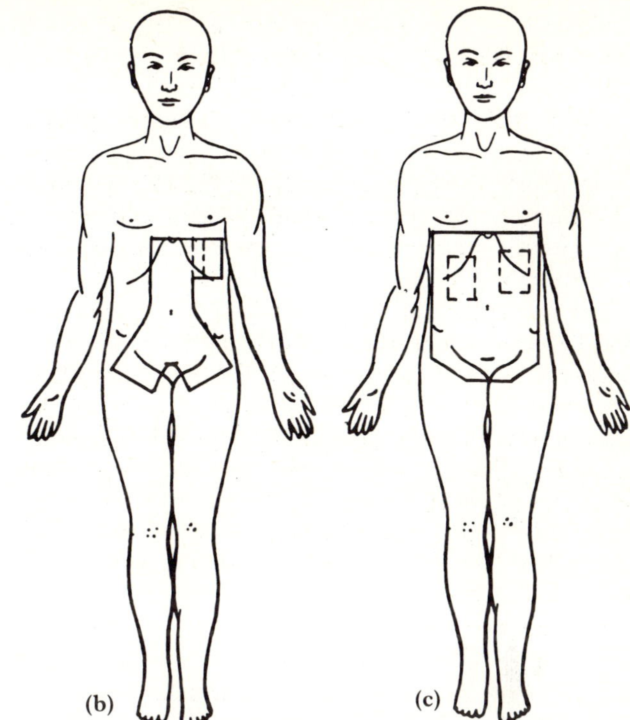

limits. **(b)** Inverted Y with splenic pedicle/spleen fields. **(c)** Abdominal bath (kidneys shielded at 2000 rads).

Fig. 13.22. Digrammatic illustrations of 'standard' radiotherapy fields as used in Sheffield. **(a)** Mantle with low/high upper field

than is clinically suspected, making planned prophylactic irradiation difficult. However, radical irradiation appears to be curative in many Stage I and I$_E$ non-Hodgkin's lymphomas. The treatment field in such cases includes the primary site with an overlap of normal tissue usually including adjacent or regional lymph node areas. Lymphomas of unfavourable histological type, particularly of head, neck and bone, are more radioresistant and may require higher doses of irradiation, e.g. 4500–6000 rads over 4–6 weeks. Lymphatic and gut tumours are more radiosensitive and may only require 3500–4000 rads over 3–4 weeks. With stage II (regional) disease, survival with local radiotherapy is not as good (Prosnitz *et al.* 1969) and systemic therapy may have to be employed. Bulky abdominal disease also carries a poor prognosis and is probably best treated with intensive chemotherapy. The prognosis with non-Hodgkin's lymphoma varies considerably according to histological type. Indeed treatment of favourable histology type lymphomas may be expectant and symptomatic particularly in older patients,

small intermittent doses of local radiotherapy being adequate. At the other end of the scale the unfavourable histological type lesions may be aggressive and rapidly fatal, whatever the therapy.

The concept of whole body irradiation, e.g. 15 rads twice weekly to 150 rads, has now regained some popularity (Hellman *et al.* 1975) in the treatment of certain low grade non-Hodgkin's lymphomas. Toxicity of this procedure is limited to the haemopoietic system.

Chemotherapy

After Billroth's attempts to treat Hodgkin's disease with arsenic in the mid-nineteenth century, little progress was made until after the second World War, when nitrogen mustard (a derivative of 'nerve gas') was used with considerable success. Since that time new agents have been developed and the importance of combining cytotoxic drugs has been realised. By use of combinations incorporating drugs each individually effective in lymphoma it is possible to increase the response rate with lower doses of drugs of non-cumulative toxicities and possibly synergistic action. Single drug resistance is avoided and by use of timed cyclical therapy it is possible to attain maximum tumour cell kill with rest periods in which normal cells (particularly in the bone marrow) can recover.

In Hodgkin's disease cyclical chemotherapy is of proven efficacy and recent advances in non-Hodgkin's lymphoma therapy have shown hearteningly improved survival in this group of conditions.

The established regimes in Hodgkin's disease are MOPP (DeVita *et al.* 1970), MVPP (Nicholson *et al.* 1970) and ABVD (Bonadonna *et al.* 1975). Most authorities give a minimum of six intensive courses of quadruple chemotherapy at 4–6 week intervals; maintenance treatment does not appear to improve disease-free survival. Less toxic regimes of ChlVPP (LOPP) and OPEC have recently proved promising (McElwain *et al.* 1977; McElwain 1982) but the most exciting development has been the use of alternating cycles of MOPP and ABVD with excellent results (Bonadonna *et al.* 1982).

Single agent chemotherapy, e.g. chlorambucil or cyclophosphamide $\pm$ prednisolone, may be appropriate for certain favourable histology non-Hodgkin's lymphomas (particularly in the older age group) but in patients with poor prognosis histology, particularly where the disease is generalised, combination chemotherapy offers the best chance of cure.

Drug regimes modified from those used in Hodgkin's disease may be effective in non-Hodgkin's lymphoma (DeVita *et al.* 1975) but the most popular regime has been COP (Hoogstraten *et al.* 1969) and its improved later modifications (CHOP, COAP, COPAd, BACOP, M-BACOD, COMLA etc.) (Table 13.2) (review Glick 1981)

The use of sequential non-cross-resistant chemotherapy regimens is also being assessed in advanced non-Hodgkin's lymphoma.

Most of the drug regimes mentioned are well-tolerated by a majority of patients. The intravenous injection of certain agents (particularly nitrogen mustard) may cause nausea and vomiting but this can be ameliorated by an effective anti-emetic drug. Superficial thrombophlebitis may also occur after intravenous injection of some drugs; this can be minimised by giving the drug into a free flowing intravenous infusion of saline.

Many patients suffer alopecia (perhaps requiring a wig), skin rashes and mucositis but these are seldom incapacitating. Bone marrow and immune depression occur, and the patient is therefore prone to infections, which should be treated promptly.

Table 13.2 Cyclical combination regimes used in lymphoma

Regimes	Drugs
MOPP	Mustine (nitrogen mustard)
	Oncovin (vincristine)
	Procarbazine
	Prednisolone (or prednisone)
MVPP	Mustine
	Velbe (vinblastine)
	Procarbazine
	Prednisolone
ABVD	Adriamycin (doxorubicin)
	Bleomycin
	Velbe
	DTIC (dacarbazine)
ABCP	Adriamycin
	Bleomycin
	CCNU (lomustine)
	Prednisolone
LOPP (ChlVPP)	Leukeran (chlorambucil)
	Oncovin or Velbe
	Procarbazine
	Prednisolone
OPEC	Oncovin
	Prednisolone
	Etoposide
	Chlorambucil
COP	Cyclophosphamide
	Oncovin
	Prednisolone
COAP	Cyclophosphamide
	Oncovin
	Ara C (cytosine arabinoside)
	Prednisolone
CHOP	Cyclophosphamide
(COPAd)	Hydroxydaunorubicin (Adriamycin)
	Oncovin
	Prednisolone
BACOP	Bleomycin
	Adriamycin
	Cyclophosphamide
	Oncovin
	Prednisolone
M-BACOD	Methotrexate (high dose) +leucovorin
	Bleomycin
	Adriamycin
	Cyclophosphamide
	Vincristine
	Dexamethasone
COM(L)A	Cyclophosphamide
	Vincristine
	Methotrexate (+leucovorin)
	Ara C (cytosine arabinoside)

Certain drugs have specific toxicities. Vincristine therapy is associated with a high incidence of neurotoxicity (including peripheral and autonomic neuropathy and cranial nerve palsies). Adriamycin is associated with cardiotoxicity and bleomycin with pulmonary fibrosis.

The effects of long term steroid therapy are well-recognized, e.g. Cushingoid appearance, osteoporosis, growth retardation, but the use of intermittent regimes appears to lessen these effects, though a careful watch must be kept for avascular necrosis of the femoral head (Hancock *et al.* 1978) and suppression of the hypothalamo-pituitary-adrenal axis (Naysmith *et al.* 1976).

Special cases

There is no evidence to date that either the administration of the contraceptive pill or pregnancy influence the prognosis in lymphoma. If a patient presents early in pregnancy with accurately staged localised disease above the diaphragm, irradiation can be safely given and further staging and treatment, if needed, carried out after delivery. Abdominal and more extensive disease occurring in the first and second trimesters of pregnancy will usually require therapeutic termination followed by the necessary radical treatment. Presentations in the third trimester can usually await prematurely induced delivery of the baby followed immediately by staging and treatment.

It is well established that pregnancy can occur after successful treatment of lymphoma. Radiotherapy to areas above the diaphragm does not affect reproductive prospects. The unprotected ovaries are ablated after full dosage radical abdominal treatment, e.g. inverted Y or abdominal bath techniques; even with repositioning and shielding they receive some irradiation. The testes may also receive irradiation in the above techniques resulting in possible mutagenesis or temporary or permanent subfertility.

Chemotherapy undoubtedly depresses testicular and ovarian function; the effects are greater in males, however, and for selected patients sperm preservation, prior to treatment, should be considered (Chapman *et al.* 1979) though many patients are oligospermic prior to treatment.

When pregnancy occurs after radiotherapy it is likely to proceed normally (Holmes and Holmes 1978); however, after chemotherapy and particularly combined modality treatments there may be an increased risk of spontaneous abortion and of foetal abnormality.

In children Hodgkin's disease is usually managed and treated in similar way to the adult disease with equally good results. More recently chemotherapy in conjunction with lower dose radiotherapy has been successfully employed in all stages in an effort to reduce the potentially adverse effects of splenectomy and radical irradiation (Jenkin and Berry 1980). Non-Hodgkin's lymphomas in childhood are generally highly malignant tumours diffusely involving the lymph nodes and rapidly spreading to bone marrow, blood and central nervous system. Truly local disease is uncommon and many authorities therefore regard chemotherapy with or without adjuvant radiotherapy as the mainstay of therapy (Malpas 1976; Murphy 1978). Regimes similar to those used in acute lymphoblastic leukaemia with central nervous system prophylaxis have been employed and improvements in survival are now becoming evident.

In patients with Hodgkin's disease over the age of 65 years, or with complicating disease, laparotomy should be avoided and conservative management may be necessary. If the disease is truly localised (IA IIA), according to clinical judgement, local or extended field irradiation is appropriate; all other patients may be better treated with less toxic regimes of combination chemotherapy, e.g. 6 cycles of LOPP, with care and appropriately reduced dosages (Aisenberg 1978).

Treatment of patients in relapse

The treatment of patients with malignant lymphoma who relapse after treatment is often difficult; their physical state may be poor and they may have little bone marrow reserve (particularly if they have had previous chemotherapy). If, in Hodgkin's disease, the patient is suffering a first relapse further investigations (including lymphogram and perhaps laparotomy) may be warranted to allow accurate assessment of disease involvement.

Patients relapsing in previously untreated lymph node regions, but without disease in treated areas, may be treated by further planned high dose radiotherapy, perhaps supplemented by 6 cycles of chemotherapy. Those with local recurrence within a treated area may tolerate further low dose radiotherapy, e.g. 2000 rads in 2 weeks, but this should be followed by 6 cycles of chemotherapy. Those with extranodal or multiple site recurrence who have had previous radiotherapy should have chemotherapy. Relapse after single agent chemotherapy should be followed by cautious cyclical quadruple chemotherapy, whilst relapse during or soon after MOPP chemotherapy will require another drug combination, e.g. ABVD. We have found that ABCP (see Table 13.2) gives complete initial remission in about 40% of such patients. Patients with recurrent disease many months or years after MOPP or MVPP may respond again to the same regime, but a careful watch must be kept on the peripheral blood counts. Treatment of patients in second and subsequent relapses is very difficult; radiotherapy or further chemotherapy may be possible.

In non-Hodgkin's lymphoma of favourable histological type local recurrence may be treated with local radiotherapy. In those patients previously treated with radiotherapy and relapsing with disseminated disease chemotherapy, e.g. chlorambucil or COP, is required. Treatment of patients relapsing after chemotherapy is again difficult particularly with unfavourable histology types though different drug regimes (incorporating for example bleomycin, methotrexate, nitrosoureas, etoposide or vindesine) may have limited success.

With interferon, partial and temporary responses may be obtained; similar to those seen with conventional treatments. Bone marrow transplantation, of immense potential in acute leukaemia, and the use of monoclonal anti-idiotype antibodies are, as yet, of unproven status in the management of lymphoma.

Neurological complications may occur during the apparently successful cytotoxic chemotherapy of malignant lymphoma. It is important to exclude vincristine neurotoxicity and, in the immunosuppressed patient, unusual central nervous system infections, e.g. *Cryptococcosis neoformans*. Recurrence of lymphoma may occur in neurological tissue since the drugs normally used in combination regimes do not penetrate the blood–brain barrier well. For acutely developing spinal cord syndromes, laminectomy and decompression may prevent complete loss of function. In most cases surgery should be followed by localised irradiation whilst cytotoxic chemotherapy, including intrathecal administration, continues.

PROGNOSIS

The prognosis in malignant lymphoma is discussed fully in Chapters 4, 5 and 6. Suffice to say that with localised Hodgkin's disease, treated by radiotherapy in specialised centres, at least 80% 5-year disease-free survival is now the rule and with disseminated disease, treated by chemotherapy, similarly improved disease free survival (over 60%) is possible. Many of these patients will be 'cured'.

With non-Hodgkin's lymphoma of unfavourable histology type the picture is not so encouraging. With localised disease 50%, and generalised disease 30%, 5-year disease-free survivals are seen, though recent research advances in this group may soon improve these figures considerably.

REFERENCES

AISENBERG A.C. (1978) Current concepts in cancer. The staging and treatment of Hodgkin's disease. *New Eng. J. Med.* **299**, 1228–32.

BLACKLEDGE G., BEST J.J.K., CROWTHER D. & ISHERWOOD I. (1980) Computed tomography (CT) in the staging of patients with Hodgkin's disease: a report on 136 patients. *Clin. Radiol.* **31**, 143–7.

BONADONNA G., SANTORO A., BONFANTE V. & VALAGUSSA P. (1982) Cyclic delivery of MOPP and ABVD combination in Stage IV Hodgkin's disease: rationale, background studies and recent results. *Cancer Treat. Rep.* **66**, 881–7.

BONADONNA G., ZUCALI R., MONFARDINI S., DE LENA M. & USLENGHI C. (1975) Combination chemotherapy of Hodgkin's disease with adriamycin, bleomycin, vinblastine and imidazole carboxamide versus MOPP. *Cancer* **36**, 252–9.

CARBONE P.P., KAPLAN H.S., MUSSHOFF N., SMITHERS D.W. & TUBIANA M. (1971) Report of the Committee on Hodgkin's Disease Staging Classification. *Cancer Res.* **31**, 1860–1.

CHAPMAN R.M., SUTCLIFFE S.B., REES L.H., EDWARD C.R.W. & MALPAS J.S. (1979) Cyclical combination chemotherapy and gonadal function. *Lancet* **i**, 285–9.

DEVITA V.T., CANELLOS G.P., CHABNER B., SCHEIN P., HUBBARD S.P. & YOUNG R.C. (1975) Advanced diffuse histiocytic lymphoma, a potentially curable disease. *Lancet* **1**, 248–50.

DEVITA V.T., SERPICK A.A. & CARBONE P.P. (1970) Combination chemotherapy in the treatment of advanced Hodgkin's disease. *Ann. Intern. Med.* **73**, 881–95.

DESSER R.K. & ULTMANN J.E. (1972) Risk of severe infection in patients with Hodgkin's disease or lymphoma after diagnostic laparotomy and splenectomy. *Ann. Intern. Med.* **77**, 143–6.

DICK F., BLOOMFIELD C.D. & BRUNNING R.D. (1974) Incidence cytology and histopathology of non-Hodgkin's lymphomas in the bone marrow. *Cancer* **33**, 1382–98.

EASSON E.C. & RUSSELL M.H. (1963) The cure of Hodgkin's disease. *Brit. Med. J.* **1**, 1704–7.

GILBERT R. (1939) Radiotherapy in Hodgkin's disease (malignant granulomatosis). Anatomic and clinical foundations; governing principles; results. *Am. J. Roent.* **41**, 198–241.

GLICK J.H. (1981) Chemotherapy for non-Hodgkin's lymphoma. In *Lymphoma*, vol. 1, pp. 388–446 (ed. Bennett J.M.). Martinus Nijhoff, The Hague.

HAN T., STUTZMAN L. & ROGUE A.L. (1971) Bone marrow biopsy in Hodgkin's disease and other neoplastic diseases. *J.A.M.A.* **217**, 1239–41.

HANCOCK B.W., BRUCE L., DUNSMORE I.R., WARD A.M. & RICHMOND J. (1977) Follow-up studies on the immune status of patients with Hodgkin's disease after splenectomy and treatment, in relapse and remission. *Br. J. Cancer* **36**, 347–54.

Hancock B.W., Bruce L., May K. & Richmond J. (1979) Ferritin a sensitising substance in the leucocyte migration inhibition test in patients with malignant lymphoma. *Br. J. Haem.* **43**, 223–33.

Hancock B.W., Bruce L., Milford Ward A. & Richmond J. (1976) Changes in immune status in patients undergoing splenectomy for the staging of Hodgkin's disease. *Brit. Med. J.* **1**, 313–15.

Hancock B.W., Bruce L., Whitham M.D., Dunsmore I.R., Ward A.M. & Richmond J. (1982) Immunity in Hodgkin's disease status after 5 years remission. *Brit. J. Cancer* **46**, 593–600.

Hancock B.W., May K., Bruce L., Dunsmore I.R., Clarke A. & Ward A.M. (1980) Haematological and immunological markers in malignant lymphoma. *Tumour Diagnostik* **3**, 140–4.

Hancock B.W., Ross B. & Huck P. (1978) A vascular necrosis of the femoral head in patients receiving intermittent cytotoxic and corticosteroid therapy for Hodgkin's disease. *Post. Grad. J. Med.* **54**, 545–6.

Hellman S., Rosenthal D.S., Moloney W.C. & Chaffey J.T. (1975) The treatment of non-Hodgkin's lymphoma. *Cancer* **36**, 804–8.

Holmes G.E. & Holmes F.F. (1978) Pregnancy outcome of patients treated for Hodgkin's disease. *Cancer* **41**, 1317–22.

Hoogstraten B., Owens A.H., Lenhard R.E., Glidewell O.J., Leone L.A., Olson K.B., Harley J.B., Townsend S.R., Miller S.P. & Spurr C.L. (1969) Combination chemotherapy in lymphosarcoma and reticulum cell sarcoma. *Blood* **33**, 370–8.

Jelliffe A.M. (1979) Hodgkin's disease: the pendulum swings. *Clin. Radiol.* **30**, 121–37.

Jenkin R.D.T. & Berry M.P. (1980) Hodgkin's disease in children. *Semin. Oncol.* **7**, 202–11.

Jones S.E., Rosenberg S.A. & Kaplan H.S. (1972) Non-Hodgkin's lymphomas I. Bone marrow involvement. *Cancer* **29**, 954–60.

Kadin M.E., Glatstein E. & Dorfman R.F. (1971) Clinopathologic studies of 117 untreated patients subjected to laparotomy for the staging of Hodgkin's disease. *Cancer* **27**, 1277–94.

Kaplan H.S. (1980) *Hodgkin's Disease* (2nd edn.) Harvard University Press, Cambridge, Mass.

Kaplan H.S. & Rosenberg S.A. (1975) The management of Hodgkin's disease. *Cancer* **36**, 796–803.

Malpas J.S. (1976) The effect of treatment on lymphomas and childhood solid tumours. *J. Roy. Coll. Physicians* **10**, 183–93.

McCready V.R. (1973) Isotope scanning. In Smithers D.W. (ed.), Hodgkin's disease, Chapter 19, pp. 179–189. Churchill Livingstone, Edinburgh.

McElwain T.J. (1982) Clinical experience of VP16 in the treatment of malignant lymphomas. In *Vepesid, its Place in the Treatment of Malignant Diseases* (Eds Ringborg U. & Davies H.C.). Professional Postgraduate Services.

McElwain T.J., Toy J. & Smith E. (1977) A combination of chlorambucil, vinblastine, procarbazine and prednisolone for the treatment of Hodgkin's disease. *Brit. J. Cancer* **36**, 276–80.

McKenna R.W., Bloomfield C.D. & Brunning R.D. (1975) Nodular lymphoma; bone marrow and blood manifestations. *Cancer* **36**, 428–40.

Murphy S.B. (1978) Current concepts in cancer. Childhood non-Hodgkin's lymphoma. *New Eng. J. Med.* **299**, 1446–8.

Naysmith A., Hancock B.W., Cullen D.R. & Richmond J. (1976) Pituitary function in patients receiving intermittent cytotoxic and corticosteroid therapy for malignant lymphoma. *Lancet* **1**, 715–17.

Nicholson W.M., Beard M.E.J., Crowther D., Stansfield A.G., Vartan C.T., Malpas J.S., Fairley G.H. & Bodley Scott R. (1970) Combination chemotherapy in generalised Hodgkin's disease. *Brit. Med. J.* **3**, 7–10.

Peters M.V. (1950) A study of survivals in Hodgkin's disease treated radiologically. *Am. J. Roent.* **63**, 299–311.

Prosnitz L.R., Hellman S., Von Essen C.F. & Kligerman M.M. (1969) The clinical course of Hodgkin's disease and other malignant lymphomas treated with radical radiation therapy. *Am. J. Roent.* **105**, 618–28.

Rosenberg S.A. (1966) Report of the Committee on the staging of Hodgkin's disease. *Cancer Res.* **26**, 1310.

Rosenberg S.A. (1971) A critique of the value of laparotomy and splenectomy in the evaluation of patients with Hodgkin's disease. *Cancer Res.* **31**, 1737–40.

Sheagren J.N., Block J.B. & Wolff S.M. (1967) Reticuloendothelial system phagocytic function in patients with Hodgkin's disease. *J. Clin. Invest.* **46**, 855–62.

Valagussa P., Santoro A., Kenda R., Fossati Bellani F., Franchi F., Banfi A., Rilke F. & Bonadonna G. (1980) Second malignancies in Hodgkin's disease: a complication of certain forms of treatment. *Brit. Med. J.* **280**, 216–19.

Viamonte M. (1971) Current status of lymphography. *Cancer Res.* **31**, 1731–2.

Webb D.I., Ubogy G. & Silver R.T. (1970) Importance of bone marrow biopsy in the clinical staging of Hodgkin's disease. *Cancer* **26**, 313–17.

L'envoi

A book like a ballade should have an ending—and the ending of lymphoreticular disease lies with the future. Perhaps others scratching despairingly in the field of lymphoreticular biology may derive the same wry amusement as I from the following poem by Gael Turnbull which might have been written about doing research.

THE SCRATCHING SOUND

The scratching sound, in case you ask, comes from my finger nails
    working at a small crevice which I've discovered in the plaster,

beyond which, you don't have to tell me, there are probably bricks
    and even concrete,

and certainly most of my time is taken up with routine or even
    compulsory activities, which is just as well since my finger nails
    would never stand up to it for long at a time,

and admittedly there is an element of deliberate eccentricity since the
    scratching has a bizarre effect upon many of my companions,
    which does help to pass the time—

none-the-less, this particular crevice is far from exhausted; and,
    finally, I can see no other way out.

GAEL TURNBULL

Reprinted by permission from
Gael Turnbull, 'Six Fancies', in
A Trampoline, Cape Goliard Press,
London.

Index